Clinical Cases in Dentistry

Clinical Cases in Dentistry

Editor: Cody Howard

AMERICAN
MEDICAL PUBLISHERS
www.americanmedicalpublishers.com

AMERICAN
MEDICAL PUBLISHERS
www.americanmedicalpublishers.com

Cataloging-in-Publication Data

Clinical cases in dentistry / edited by Cody Howard.
p. cm.
Includes bibliographical references and index.
ISBN 979-8-88740-628-2
1. Dentistry. 2. Oral medicine. 3. Teeth. I. Howard, Cody.
RK51 .E95 2023
617 .6--dc23

American Medical Publishers,
41 Flatbush Avenue,
1st Floor, New York,
NY 11217, USA

ISBN 979-8-88740-628-2 (Hardback)

Contents

Preface

The purpose of the book is to provide a glimpse into the dynamics and to present opinions and studies of some of the scientists engaged in the development of new ideas in the field from very different standpoints. This book will prove useful to students and researchers owing to its high content quality.

The specialized field of healthcare which is focused on diagnosing, preventing, and treating various diseases and conditions that affect the oral cavity is known as dentistry. It plays a crucial role in the maintenance of oral health and treatment of dental issues to ensure overall well-being. There are several common diseases and conditions treated in dentistry such as tooth decay, gum disease and oral cancer. Tooth decay is a medical condition caused by the accumulation of plaque and bacteria on the teeth, leading to cavities and tooth loss if left untreated. Gum disease, such as gingivitis and periodontitis, affects the gums and supporting structures of the teeth, leading to inflammation, bleeding, and ultimately tooth loss. Other dental problems which are dealt with under this field are bad breath, dental abscesses, tooth sensitivity, malocclusion, and temporomandibular joint disorder. This book unravels the recent studies in the field of dentistry. It will help new researchers by foregrounding their knowledge in this branch of medicine.

At the end, I would like to appreciate all the efforts made by the authors in completing their chapters professionally. I express my deepest gratitude to all of them for contributing to this book by sharing their valuable works. A special thanks to my family and friends for their constant support in this journey.

Editor

1

Mandibular Body Reconstruction Utilizing a Three-Dimensional Custom-Made Porous Titanium Plate: A Four-Year Follow-Up Clinical Report

Carlos-Martín Ardila[1] **Yuritza Hernández-Arenas**[2] **and Efraín Álvarez-Martínez**[1]

[1]*Titular Professor University of Antioquia, Medellín, Colombia*
[2]*University of Antioquia, Medellín, Colombia*

Correspondence should be addressed to Carlos-Martín Ardila; martin.ardila@udea.edu.co

Academic Editor: Wen Lin Chai

A clinical case of a 42-year-old woman patient, who had a mandibular reconstruction utilizing a three-dimensional (3D) custom-made porous titanium plate dental restoration, is presented. She showed a recurrence of a unicystic ameloblastoma involving the left hemimandible. The patient declined to be managed by a bone-free flap. A mandibular resection in the healthy areas was provided, followed by reconstruction utilizing a 3D custom-made porous titanium plate dental restoration with a hybrid dental prosthesis. The 3D rehabilitation was created considering slim tomodensitometric sections. The cutting guides and custom-created 3D plate were fabricated employing medical software via computer-aided design and fabricating with locations planned for healing abutments. The patient was contented with the rehabilitation, and the condition continued stable at the four-year follow-up.

1. Introduction

Bone free flaps are the standard treatment approach for the reconstruction of significant mandibular defects; thus, the main bone sources include the scapula and iliac crest [1]. The recommended technique for mandibular reconstruction is the pedicled flap plus a titanium megaplate [2]. Although this method offers the filling tissue required and specific support, distinct limitations have been described: the establishment of a new surgical place, megaplate exposure or fractures, complications with the articulation, and several esthetic consequences [3–5]. Recently, three-dimensional (3D) custom-made porous titanium plates have been used for mandibular reconstructions, which offer an alternative in those cases of free flap contraindications or refusal by the patient; however, only very short-term follow-ups have been reported. This case report presents a mandibular reconstruction including a custom-made porous titanium plate with a hybrid dental prosthesis followed for 4 years.

2. Case Report

A 42-year-old woman showed a recurrence of a unicystic ameloblastoma involving the left hemimandible (Figures 1(a)–1(c)). She was intervened twice, with an interval of six years. The two operations included a curettage of the neoplasm cavity down to the apparently healthy bone tissue. She declined to be managed by a free flap. Thus, a mandibular resection in the healthy areas was chosen and provided, followed by reconstruction utilizing a 3D custom-made porous titanium plate with a hybrid dental prosthesis. Preoperative and postoperative radiographs are shown in Figure 2. Written consent of the patient according to ethical principles was signed.

The 3D rehabilitation was created considering slim tomodensitometric sections (Figures 3(a)–3(e)). The cutting guides and custom-created 3D plate were fabricated employing medical software via computer-aided design and fabricating (CAD-CAM) with locations planned for healing abutments, followed by the implant sustained prosthesis

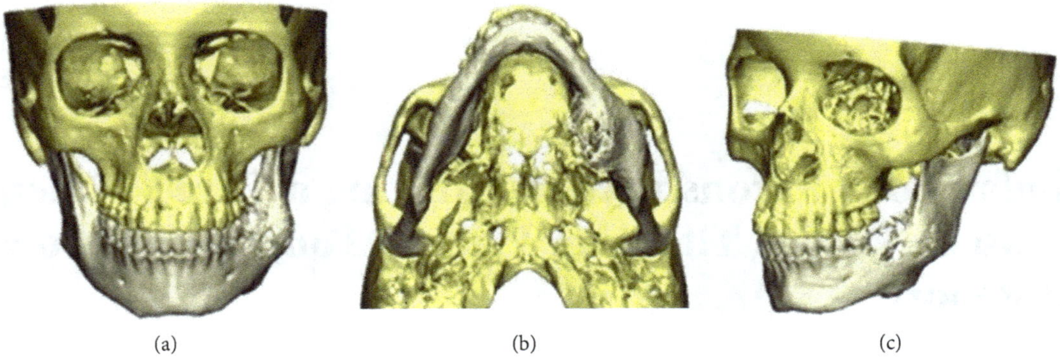

FIGURE 1: 3D reconstruction showing ameloblastoma. (a) Frontal view. (b) Sagittal view. (c) Axial view.

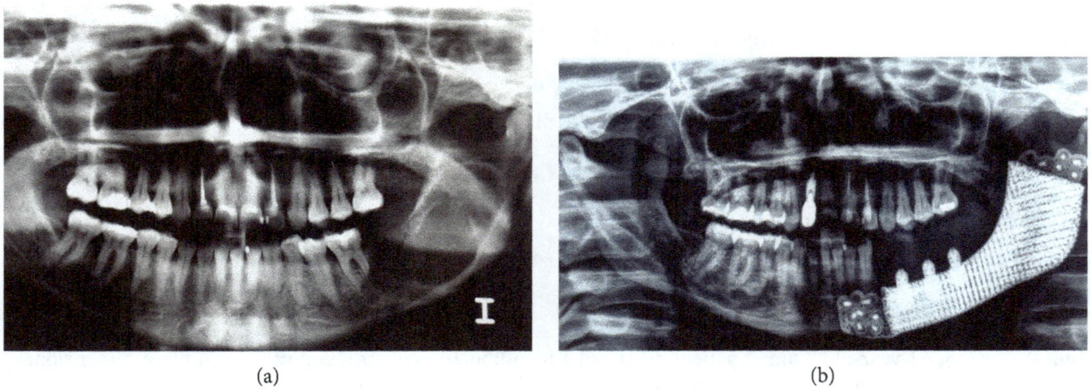

FIGURE 2: Preoperative (a) and postoperative (b) radiographs.

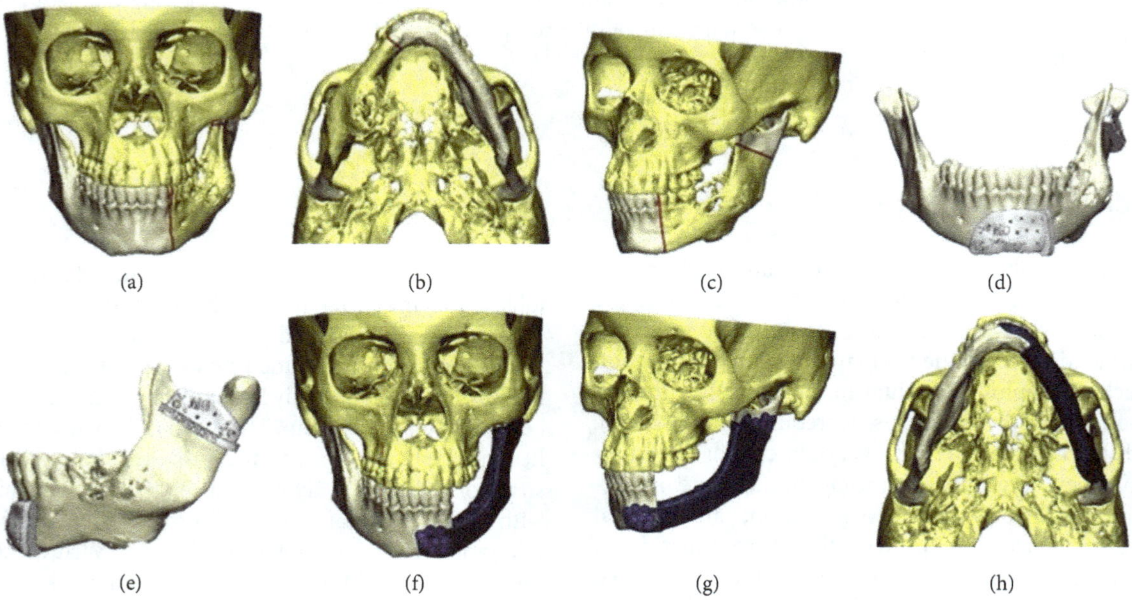

FIGURE 3: (a–e) Three-dimensional simulation cutting guides. (f–h) Simulation of the custom implant in porous titanium.

(Figures 3(f)–3(h)). The titanium plate was designed to allow the placement of dental implants (4.1 mm × 10 mm) at the same time. The designed titanium plate (thickness of 12 mm) was printed with medial grade powder (constituted of porous grade 2 titanium).

The surgery was completed under general anesthesia and nasotracheal intubation. The surgical method was intraoral and preauricular (Figures 4(a) and 4(b)). The cutting guides were fixed considering the formerly described markers at the level of the left mandibular condyle and the symphyseal area.

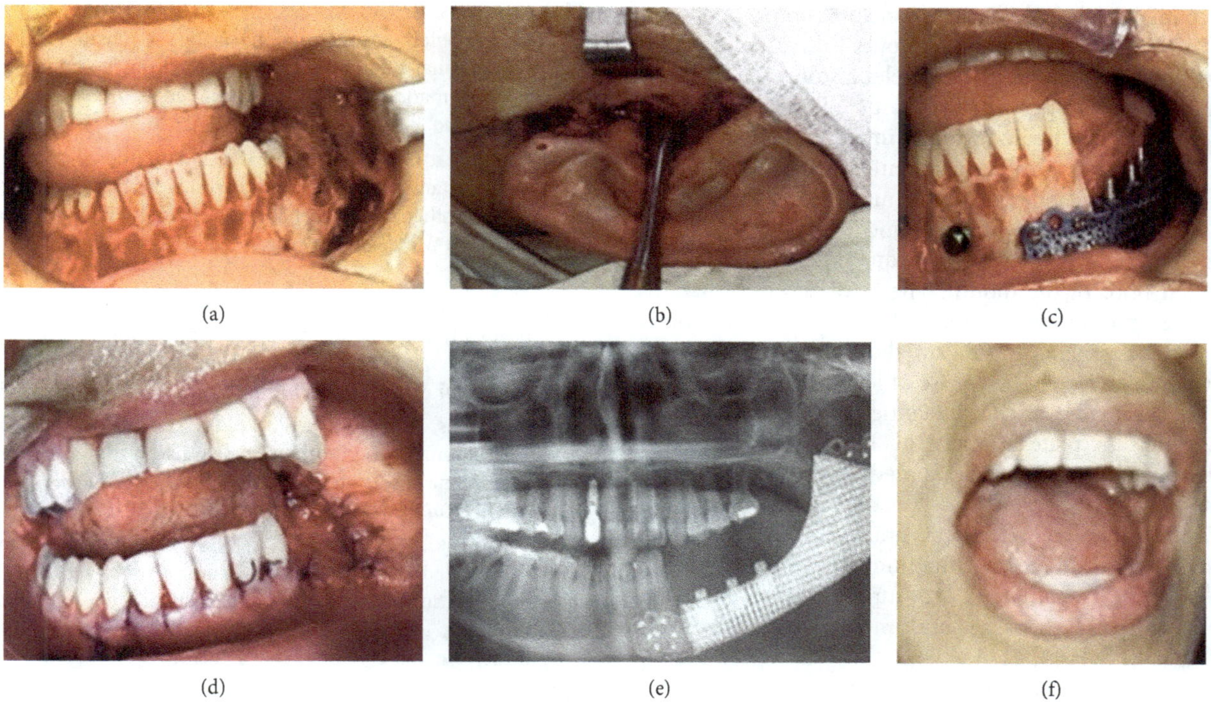

Figure 4: Surgical procedure. (a) Intraoral approach. (b) Preauricular approach. (c) Plate in position. (d) immediate postoperative. (e) Radiograph view at four years postoperative. (f) Intraoral view at four years postoperative.

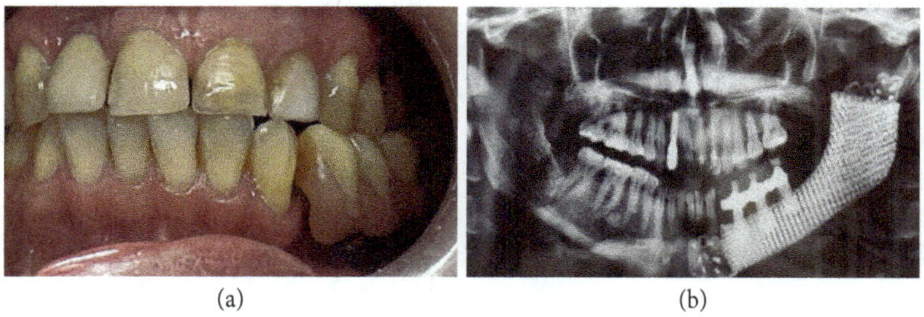

Figure 5: Intraoral view and radiograph after prosthesis.

The plate was subsequently retained in position using screws for fixation (Figure 4(c)).

Three healing abutments were connected to the porous titanium plate substituting the mandible (Figure 4(c)). The hybrid dental prosthesis was made and attached to the porous titanium plate after two months following the operation. Moreover, miniconical abutments were used to support hybrid prostheses. A metal framework was created for the mandibular hybrid prosthesis, and the definitive prosthesis was completed by means of standard procedures.

The patient was given postoperative cleaning guidelines and educated about regular maintenance and possible difficulties associated to the prosthesis. The patient was recalled after 2 days to examine satisfaction and was followed-up further at regular 3-month intervals a year. At all recall intervals, the prostheses were removed, and soft tissue condition was perceived. The patient was satisfied with the rehabilitation, and the condition continued stable at the four-year of follow-up (Figures 4(d) and 4(f)). Intraoral view and radiograph after prosthesis are shown in Figure 5.

3. Discussion

The current case presents a mandibular body reconstruction utilizing 3D custom-made porous titanium plate with a hybrid dental prosthesis. The 3D scheme permits respect for the anatomy, and the intervention is considerably shortened than other approaches with the application of the cutting guides. Additionally, this design warrants an impeccable rearrangement of the inferior border and, subsequently, the competence to rebuild a quality mandibular form in contrast with traditional mega-plates [3]. Moreover, the porous titanium permits its tissue ingrowth from the adjacent tissues allowing improved integration [6]. Interestingly, its mechanical strength was equated to cortical bone [7, 8].

To our knowledge, only a few publications have presented 3D custom-made porous titanium plates for mandibular reconstructions; additionally, follow-ups of more than 2 year have not been reported. Qassemyar et al. [3] described two cases demanding reconstruction of the mandibular body, but for whom a bone-free flap was contraindicated.

Those patients had a history of ameloblastoma and squamous cell carcinoma. Touré and Gouet [5] treated a patient with a massive recurrence of ameloblastoma of the right hemimandible. The period of patient's follow-up was up to 18 months and was treated with an implant-supported prosthesis. Rachmiel et al. [9] documented a case of a patient with a large deficiency in the ramus. One-year follow-up revealed an appropriate function and form. Lee et al. [10] showed a case with a history of squamous cell carcinoma on the left floor of the mouth. There was no postoperative difficulty in the follow-up phase of 14 months. In contrast to the present case that was followed during four years, those cases were followed in the course of less than one and a half years; however, one of the difficulties of 3D custom-made porous titanium plates is that the long-term tolerance is not recognized, but it can be assumed that the tolerance will undoubtedly not be inferior to that of traditional plates [3, 11]. Even though the alloplastic graft utilized in this case was 3D CAD/CAM porous titanium, these mechanics do not remove the probability of exposure; therefore, it is essential to assess patient's tissues and, most importantly, evade the symphysis area [3, 11, 12].

The present case, together with the cases previously described by Qassemyar et al. [3] and Touré and Gouet [5], has used dental implants. The different advantages presented by this kind of 3D custom-made porous titanium plates for complete reconstructions together with dental implants are relevant [3, 5, 13, 14]. A meticulous oral-dental follow-up is crucial for the stability of these procedures [5, 13, 15].

The 3D custom-made porous titanium plates for bone reconstructions are simple, rapid, and predictable. Moreover, dental rehabilitation does not demand an osseointegration stage.

Consent

The patient signed the informed consent related to hospital care and for academic purposes.

Acknowledgments

The authors acknowledge their employment relationship with the Universidad de Antioquia.

References

[1] A. Takushima, K. Harii, H. Asato, T. Nakatsuka, and Y. Kimata, "Mandibular reconstruction using microvascular free flaps: a statistical analysis of 178 cases," *Plastic and Reconstructive Surgery*, vol. 108, no. 6, pp. 1555–1563, 2001.

[2] Y. Shnayder, D. Lin, S. C. Desai, B. Nussenbaum, J. P. Sand, and M. K. Wax, "Reconstruction of the lateral mandibular defect," *JAMA Facial Plastic Surgery*, vol. 17, no. 5, pp. 367–373, 2015.

[3] Q. Qassemyar, N. Assouly, S. Temam, and F. Kolb, "Use of a three-dimensional custom-made porous titanium prosthesis for mandibular body reconstruction," *International Journal of Oral and Maxillofacial Surgery*, vol. 46, no. 10, pp. 1248–1251, 2017.

[4] Y. Y. Jo, S. G. Kim, M. K. Kim, S. H. Shin, J. Ahn, and H. Seok, "Mandibular reconstruction using a customized three-dimensional titanium implant applied on the lingual surface of the mandible," *The Journal of Craniofacial Surgery*, vol. 29, no. 2, pp. 415–419, 2018.

[5] G. Touré and E. Gouet, "Use of a 3-dimensional custom-made porous titanium prosthesis for mandibular body reconstruction with prosthetic dental rehabilitation and lipofilling," *Journal of Oral and Maxillofacial Surgery*, vol. 77, no. 6, pp. 1305–1313, 2019.

[6] J. Matena, S. Petersen, M. Gieseke et al., "SLM produced porous titanium implant improvements for enhanced vascularization and osteoblast seeding," *International Journal of Molecular Sciences*, vol. 16, no. 12, pp. 7478–7492, 2015.

[7] A. Barbas, A. S. Bonnet, P. Lipinski, R. Pesci, and G. Dubois, "Development and mechanical characterization of porous titanium bone substitutes," *Journal of the Mechanical Behavior of Biomedical Materials*, vol. 9, pp. 34–44, 2012.

[8] P. Lipinski, A. Barbas, and A. S. Bonnet, "Fatigue behavior of thin-walled grade 2 titanium samples processed by selective laser melting. Application to life prediction of porous titanium implants," *Journal of the Mechanical Behavior of Biomedical Materials*, vol. 28, pp. 274–290, 2013.

[9] A. Rachmiel, D. Shilo, O. Blanc, and O. Emodi, "Reconstruction of complex mandibular defects using integrated dental custom-made titanium implants," *The British Journal of Oral & Maxillofacial Surgery*, vol. 55, no. 4, pp. 425–427, 2017.

[10] Y. W. Lee, H. J. You, J. A. Jung, and D. W. Kim, "Mandibular reconstruction using customized three-dimensional titanium implant," *Archives of Craniofacial Surgery*, vol. 19, no. 2, pp. 152–156, 2018.

[11] J. H. Oh, "Recent advances in the reconstruction of cranio-maxillofacial defects using computer-aided design/computer-aided manufacturing," *Maxillofacial Plastic and Reconstructive Surgery*, vol. 40, no. 1, p. 2, 2018.

[12] G. S. Zheng, Y. X. Su, G. Q. Liao et al., "Mandible reconstruction assisted by preoperative virtual surgical simulation," *Oral Surgery, Oral Medicine, Oral Pathology, Oral Radiology*, vol. 113, no. 5, pp. 604–611, 2012.

[13] A. Cohen, A. Laviv, P. Berman, R. Nashef, and J. Abu-Tair, "Mandibular reconstruction using stereolithographic 3-dimensional printing modeling technology," *Oral Surgery, Oral Medicine, Oral Pathology, Oral Radiology, and Endodontics*, vol. 108, no. 5, pp. 661–666, 2009.

[14] R. Kontio, "Update on mandibular reconstruction: computer-aided design, imaging, stem cells and future applications," *Current Opinion in Otolaryngology & Head and Neck Surgery*, vol. 22, no. 4, pp. 307–315, 2014.

[15] C. Linz, H. Collmann, A. Kübler, H. Böhm, and T. Schweitzer, "Patient-specific biodegradable implant in pediatric craniofacial surgery," *Journal of Cranio-Maxillo-Facial Surgery*, vol. 45, no. 8, p. 1111, 2017.

2

A Case of Synovial Chondromatosis of Temporomandibular Joint with Numerous Loose Bodies

Yumiko Matsusue,[1,2] Kazuhiko Yamamoto,[1] Nobuhiro Yamakawa,[1] Ikumi Yamamoto,[1] Shinpei Matsuda,[3] Hitoshi Yoshimura,[3] Tetsuji Kawakami,[1,2] and Tadaaki Kirita[1]

[1]*Department of Oral and Maxillofacial Surgery, Nara Medical University, Japan*
[2]*Department of Oral and Maxillofacial Surgery, Takita Hospital, Japan*
[3]*Department of Dentistry and Oral Surgery, Unit of Sensory and Locomotor Medicine, Division of Medicine, Faculty of Medical Science, University of Fukui, Japan*

Correspondence should be addressed to Yumiko Matsusue; yumikoch@naramed-u.ac.jp

Academic Editor: Rui Amaral Mendes

Here, we report a case of synovial chondromatosis of the temporomandibular joint (TMJ) with numerous loose bodies. A 56-year-old woman was examined in the oral surgery department for trismus and pain in the left TMJ when opening the mouth. Imaging indicated TMJ synovial chondromatosis, and the patient was referred to our department for further examination. Her facial features were symmetrical, and no occlusal abnormalities were found. The maximum mouth opening was 30 mm, and movement of the left mandibular condyle was restricted and accompanied by pain and joint sounds. Panoramic radiography showed deformation of the left mandibular condyle and radiopaque lesions surrounding it. Computed tomography showed numerous small granules around the left mandibular condyle, some of which were calcified. Magnetic resonance imaging showed anterior disc displacement without reduction in the left TMJ and hypointense lesions on T2-weighted images. Bone scintigraphy showed an accumulation in the area of the left TMJ. Based on the diagnosis of the left TMJ synovial chondromatosis, the lesions were removed, and plastic surgery on the mandibular condyle was performed under general anesthesia. We removed 386 white loose bodies. Histopathologically, the loose bodies were consistent with synovial chondromatosis lesions. The postoperative course was uneventful, with no recurrence or TMJ dysfunction approximately 5 years after the surgery, indicating that open surgery is the best course of intervention in such cases.

1. Introduction

Synovial chondromatosis is a benign disease in which synovial cells create cartilaginous metaplasia in synovial tissue, resulting in loose cartilage bodies in the joint cavity. The most common sites include the knee, elbow, and hip. Synovial chondromatosis of the temporomandibular joint (TMJ) was first described by Von Haller in 1764 [1]. Synovial chondromatosis is not frequently encountered in the TMJ, but reports of such cases have increased along with recent advances in diagnostic imaging, including magnetic resonance imaging (MRI). Here, we report a case of TMJ synovial chondromatosis with numerous loose bodies to draw attention to this rare condition and suggest a suitable course of action for its treatment. We also review the related literature of reported TMJ synovial chondromatosis cases.

2. Case Presentation

A 56-year-old woman presented to our department with a chief complaint of pain in her left TMJ in December 2014. Around November 2012, the patient had noticed pain in her left TMJ when widely opening her mouth, but the symptoms disappeared, and she did not address the matter. Around July 2014, the symptoms recurred, and she began experiencing trismus. She visited the dental and oral surgery department at a hospital for examination. Both computed tomography (CT) and MRI indicated synovial chondromatosis of the TMJ, and she was referred to our department for treatment.

Clinical examination found that she had a fairly healthy physique and no signs of nutritional deficiency. There was no visible facial deformation, and the maximum mouth opening was 30 mm. Movement of the left mandibular condyle was poor, and there was pain as well as joint sounds when widely opening the mouth but no occlusal abnormality (Figure 1).

Panoramic radiography showed that the left mandibular condyle was flattened, with a radiopaque image near the superior joint cavity (Figure 2). The TMJ radiograph also showed deformation in the left mandibular fossa. With mouth opening, both mandibular condyles were able to move to near the lowest point of the articular eminence. CT showed that the left mandibular condyle was flattened, and small and granular nodules were observed in the joint capsule of the left TMJ, some of which were calcified (Figure 3).

T1-weighted MRI of the left TMJ showed deformity of the left mandibular condyle and anterior disc displacement without reduction, and T2-weighted MRI showed fine nodular areas of hypointensity in the superior joint cavity (Figures 4(a)–4(c)). Bone scintigraphy showed accumulation at an area matching the left TMJ (Figure 4(d)). Based on these findings, the final diagnosis was of left synovial chondromatosis of the TMJ.

Approximately 2 months after the initial examination, the masses were removed, and plastic surgery was performed on the mandibular condyle under general anesthesia. Incision lines were set according to the Al-Kayat–Bramley method [2]. The skin incisions were made, detaching up to the temporal fascia. An incision was made in the superficial temporal fascia, then in between the superficial and deep layers to the zygomatic arch, where the periosteum was incised to expose the joint capsule. The joint capsule was punctured, and approximately 2 mL of slightly viscous synovial fluid was collected. Incising the joint capsule revealed numerous white loose bodies around the mandibular condyle and in the superior joint cavity. The loose bodies were not adherent to the surrounding tissue and were carefully removed.

Although the articular disc was preserved, the mandibular condyle was deformed. Therefore, plastic surgery of the mandibular condyle was performed using an ultrasonic cutting instrument (Piezosurgery®, Mectron Medical Technology, Carasco, Italy). A closed drain was placed in the wound, and the incision was sutured to complete the operation (Figure 5).

At the time of writing, it has been more than 5 years since the surgery. There have been no signs of local recurrence or trismus. Image findings have also not indicated any recurrence (Figures 6 and 7).

The loose bodies removed were 2 to 5 mm in diameter, white, bone-like, hard, and numbered 386 in total (Figure 8).

Histopathologically, there was proliferation of cartilage tissue with chondrocytes forming round or irregular small masses surrounded by fibrous tissue, along with fibrosis and ossification. There were no signs of malignancy, which is consistent with synovial chondromatosis (Figure 9).

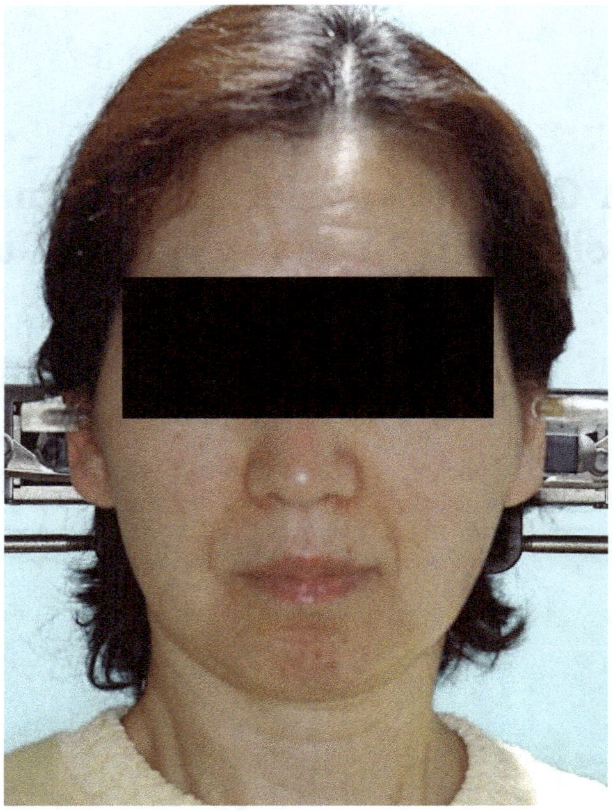

FIGURE 1: Facial photograph from the first examination. There is no visible facial deformation.

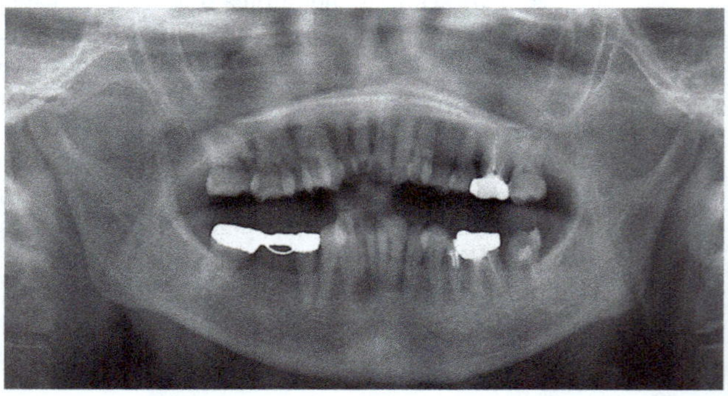

FIGURE 2: Panoramic radiograph from the first examination. The left mandibular condyle is flattened, and radiopaque images are seen near the superior joint cavity.

3. Discussion

In this report, we presented the case of a patient with TMJ synovial chondromatosis with numerous loose bodies who was successfully treated with surgery and has remained symptom free 5 years after the operation. Synovial chondromatosis of the temporomandibular joint presents with clinical symptoms similar to TMJ disorder, including trismus, restricted movement of the TMJ, pain, and noise [3, 4]. Thus, patients are sometimes treated for TMJ disorder for an extended period rather than receiving proper treatment [5]. Imaging is essential for diagnosing this disease, but

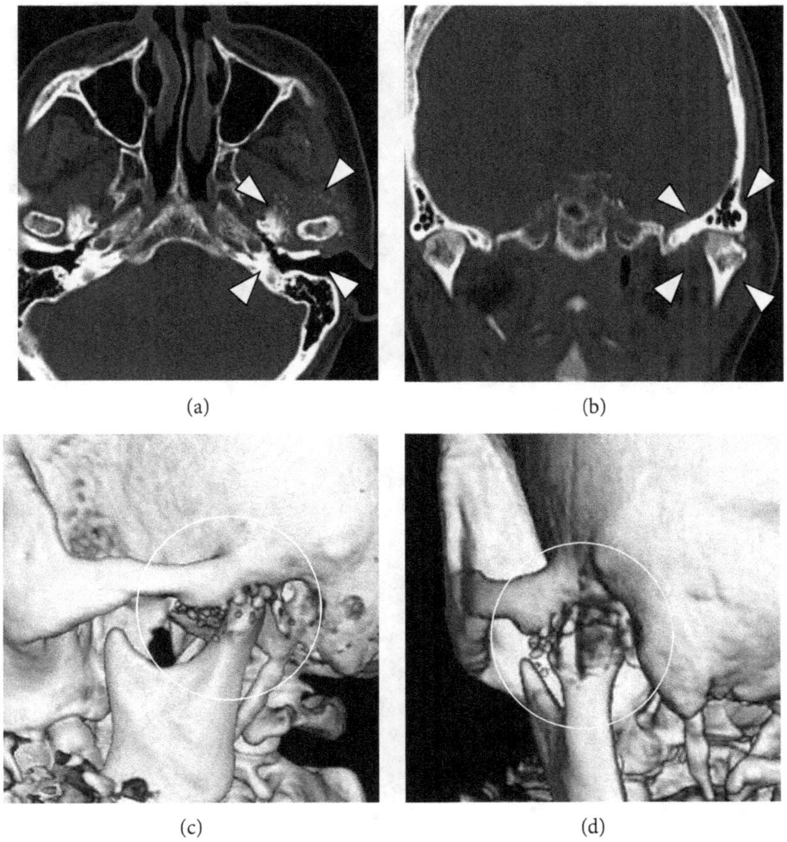

FIGURE 3: CT images from first examination: (a) axial image, (b) coronal image, and (c, d) 3D image. Deformation of the left mandibular condyle is seen, with many small, granular nodules in the area of the left TMJ, some of which are calcified.

simple radiography often does not show any changes. CT depicts joint and soft tissue swelling, multiple calcifications in a joint, or hardening and resorption of joint surfaces, but lesions may not be depicted in the absence of obvious calcification or bone changes. MRI shows enlargement of the joint cavity, synovial fluid retention, and a swollen joint capsule with multiple hypointense masses in T2-weighted images [6–8]. Diagnosis is relatively easy in cases with numerous calcifications, such as the present one, but when these are not visible, diagnosis can be complicated. Therefore, both CT and MRI should be used to ensure a comprehensive diagnosis incorporating all clinical findings [9–11]. This condition must be differentiated from other possible diagnoses such as TMJ internal derangement, tuberculous arthritis, osteochondrosis ossificans, osteochondral fracture, and pseudogout [12]. If accompanied by intracranial progression [13], conditions such as meningioma, schwannoma, chondrosarcoma, lymphoma, and cholesteatoma should be considered [4].

Milgram [14, 15] classified synovial chondromatosis of the knee, elbow, and hip into three stages and considered it a self-limited disease that progresses from stages 1 to 3 in this order. In stage 3, synovectomy is not necessary if the loose bodies are removed, and even in stage 2, synovectomy is not always required. Gerard et al. [16] classified the disease into four stages of histopathological changes in synovial activity. They recommend expansion surgery in the early stages and reduction surgery in the late stages of synovial chondromatosis. Our case presented as stage 3 according to Milgram's classification and stage 2 according to Gerard's classification. By carefully removing as many of the numerous loose bodies as possible and performing plastic surgery of the mandibular condyle, we minimized postoperative dysfunction, indicating that this intervention was appropriate.

We located 202 case reports of TMJ synovial chondromatosis, including the present one, published from 2009 to 2019 [7, 11, 17–58] (Table 1). The cases covered a wide age range from 15 to 86 years and included 144 women and 58 men. The clinical symptoms were swelling in 60 cases, pain in 104 cases, trismus in 97 cases, and joint sounds in 67 cases. All patients were examined at a medical institution for these symptoms. Approximately 90% of patients had open surgeries, but approximately 10% had arthroscopic surgeries. In addition to removing the lesions, resection arthroplasty was performed in 14 cases, mandibular plastic surgery or resection in 8 cases, discectomy in 11 cases, and synovectomy in 12 cases. Conservative surgery was selected if the surrounding tissue was normal. Loose bodies were found in most cases, but ours was the only one where more than 300 loose bodies were removed.

The therapy for TMJ synovial chondromatosis is principally surgical intervention, as the number of loose bodies increases or the symptoms worsen [59]. If the loose bodies are confined to the superior joint space, arthroscopic surgery can be selected, although some studies have reported recurrence after arthroscopic surgery [60]. If the goal is definite

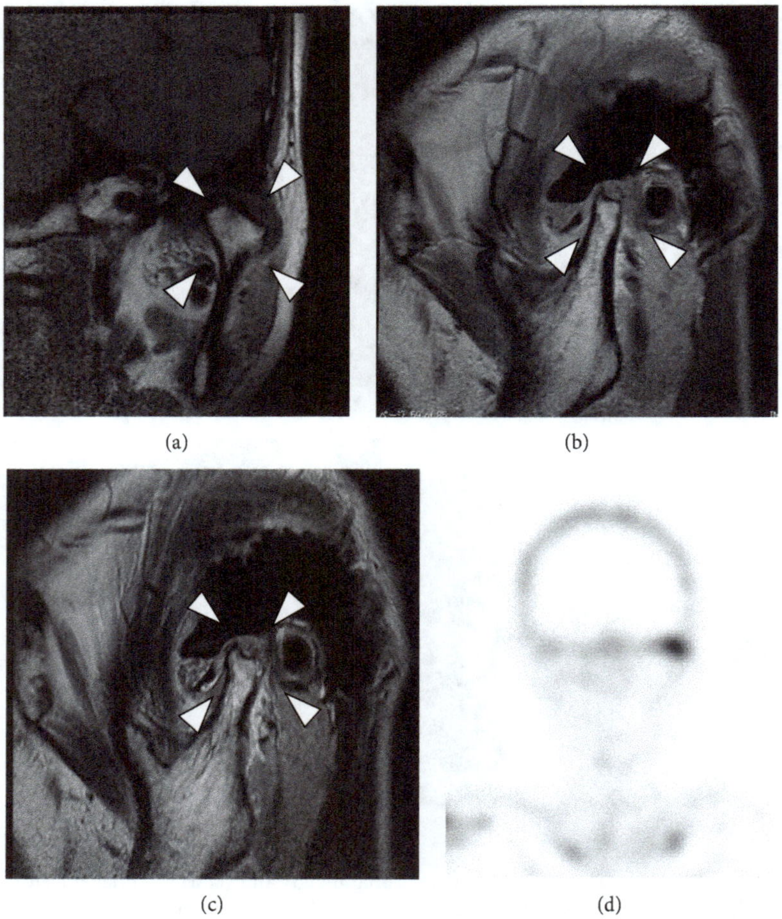

Figure 4: MR image and bone scintigraphy from the first examination. (a, b) T1-weighted image; (c) T2-weighted image. In the left TMJ, T1-weighted images show deformity of the left mandibular condyle and anterior disc displacement without reduction, and T2-weighted images show areas of small, nodular hypointensity around the left mandibular condyle. (d) Bone scintigraphy. An accumulation is seen in the area of the left TMJ.

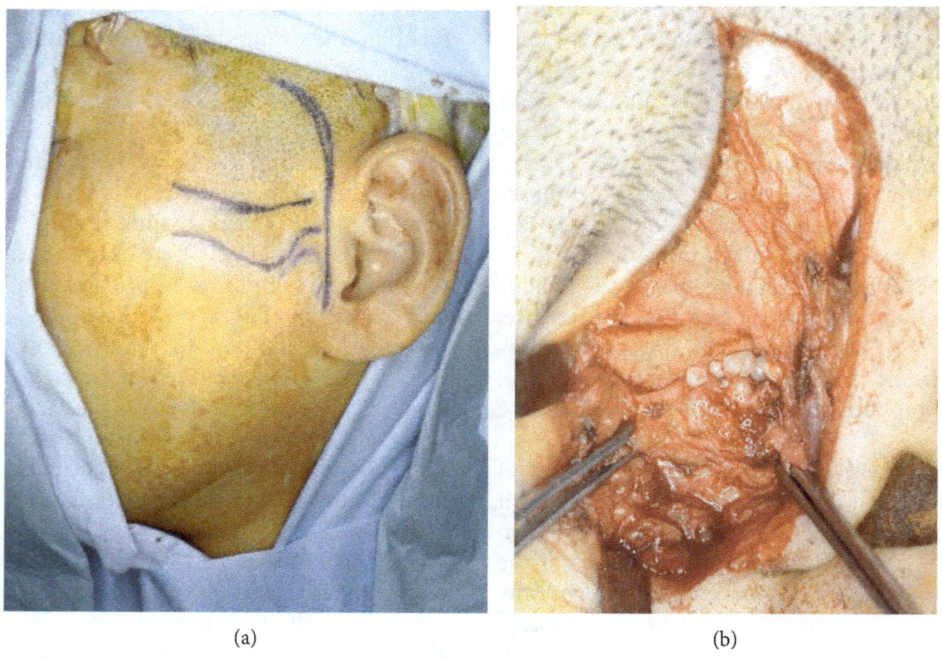

Figure 5: Intraoperative findings: (a) skin incision line (arrowhead); (b) numerous white loose bodies exposed after incision of the joint capsule.

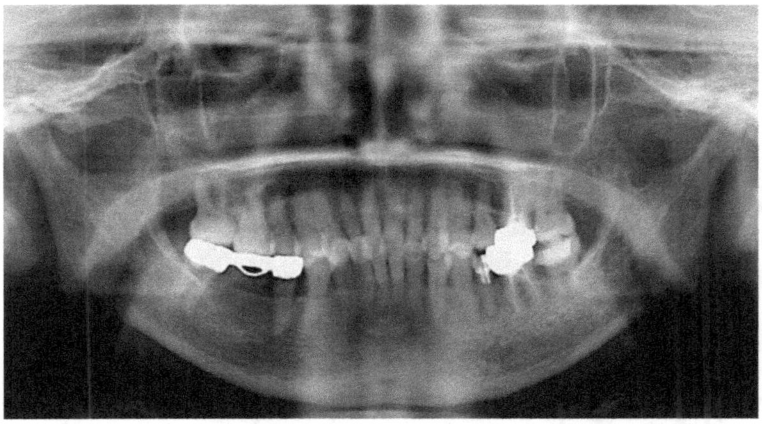

FIGURE 6: Panoramic radiograph approximately 2 years after the surgery. There are no findings suggesting recurrence.

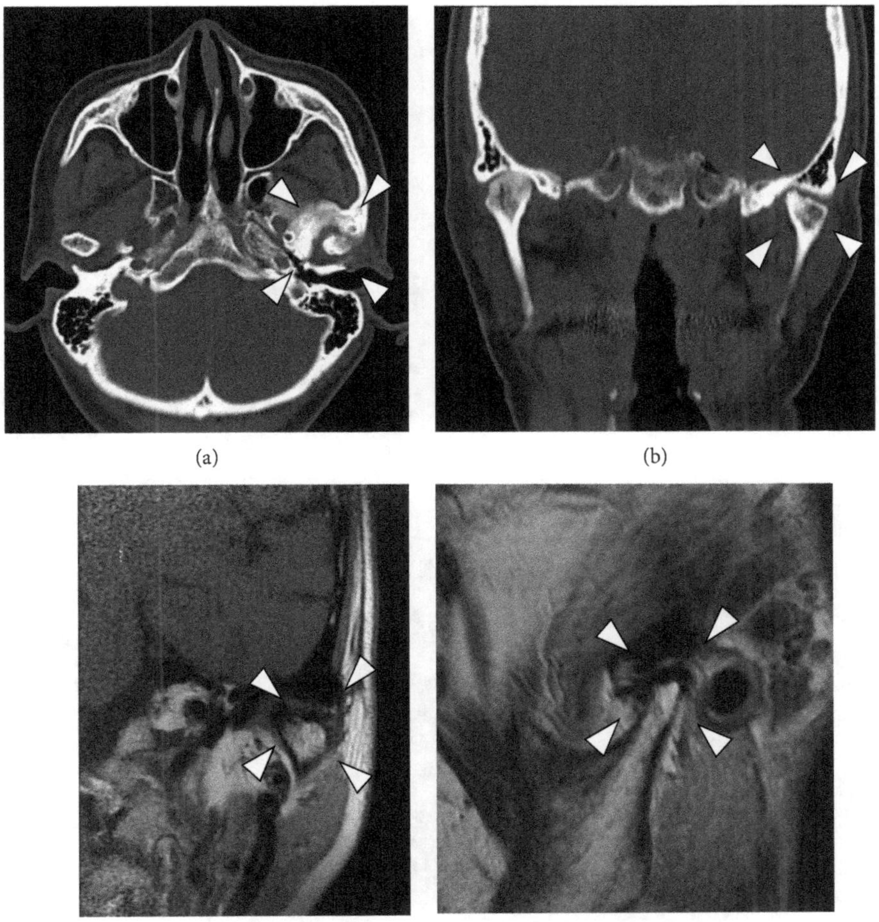

(a) (b) (c) (d)

FIGURE 7: CT and MR images approximately 2 years after the surgery: (a, b) CT images—(a) axial image and (b) coronal image; (c, d) MR images, T1-weighted image. None of the images suggest recurrence.

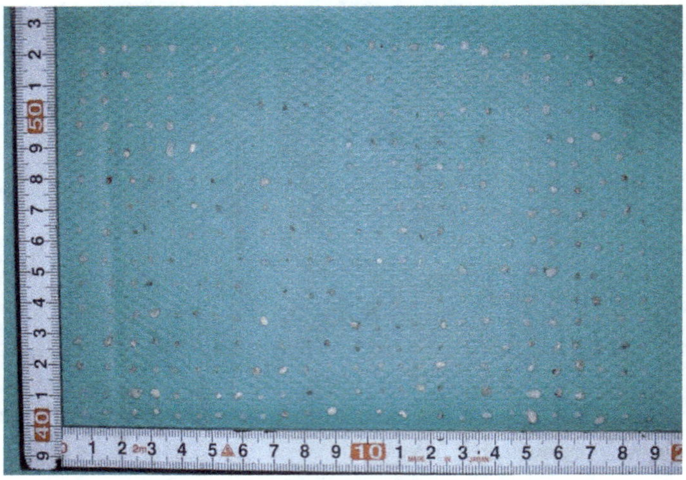

FIGURE 8: Extracted specimens. A total of 386 white, bone-like, hard, loose bodies of 2–5 mm in diameter were removed.

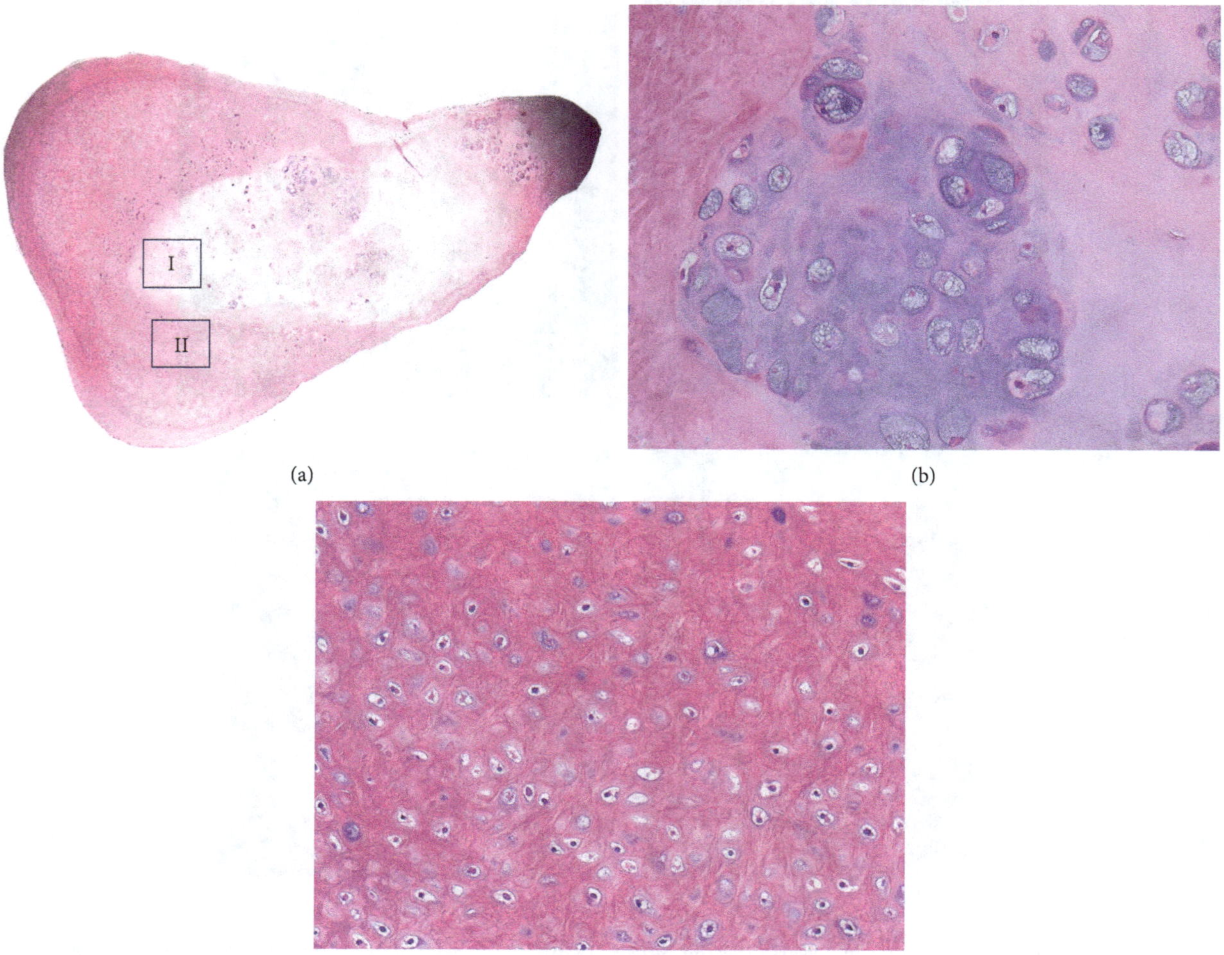

(a) (b) (c)

FIGURE 9: Histopathological findings: (a) hematoxylin-eosin staining ×1.25, low magnification; (b) hematoxylin-eosin staining ×200, high magnification of AI; (c) hematoxylin-eosin staining ×200, high magnification of AII. Cartilage tissue with growth of chondrocytes forming round or irregular small masses surrounded by fibrous tissue. Fibrosis and ossification are observed in some areas.

Table 1: Summary of data from the studies included in the review, 2009 through 2019.

No.	First author	Year	No. of cases	Age	Sex	Site	Clinical manifestations				Imaging			Loose bodies		Treatments (other than synovial chondrectomy)				Remarks
							Swelling	Pain	LJO	Crepitation	CT	MRI	CBCT	No.	Size (mm)	Arthrotomy	Condylectomy	Discectomy	Synovectomy	Such as arthroscopy
1	Peng [17]	2009	1	58	F	R	+	+	+	—	+	—	—	—	—	—	—	+	+	
2	Cai [18]	2009	1	21	F	L	—	+	+(28 mm)	+	—	+	—	7	5 × 8	—	—	—	—	Only arthroscopy
3	Balasundaram [19]	2009	1	82	M	L	+	—	+(35 mm)	—	—	—	+	—	—	NL	NL	NL	NL	
4	Zha [20]	2009	1	44	M	L	+	+	+	+	+	+	—	90-95	NL	—	—	—	+	
5	Sato [21]	2010	1	74	F	L	+	+	+(35 mm)	—	+	+	—	180	1-5	—	—	—	—	Arthroscopy
6	Goizueta-Adame [22]	2010	1	15	F	L	—	+	+(29 mm)	—	+	+	—	—	—	+	—	—	—	Osteotomy of the zygomatic arch
7	Goizueta-Adame [22]	2010	1	74	F	L	—	+	+(14 mm)	—	+	+	—	—	—	+	—	—	—	
8	Boffano [23]	2010	1	55	F	R	+	+	—	+	+	—	—	<6	<5	—	—	—	+	
9	Pimenta e Souza [24]	2010	1	28	M	R	+	—	—	+	+	—	—	10	NL	NL	NL	NL	NL	
10	Guarda-Nardini [25]	2010	1	53	F	R	+	+	+(20 mm)	—	X-P only	—	—	2	10-25	NL	NL	NL	NL	
11	Cai [26]	2010	1	48	F	L	—	+	—	+	—	+	—	3	16 × 9	—	—	—	—	Only arthroscopy
12	González-Pérez [27]	2010	1	50	M	L	+	+	+(20 mm)	+	+	+	—	35	2-10	—	+	—	—	
13	Shah [28]	2011	1	25	F	L	—	+	—	—	+	—	—	43	<1.5 × 2.5	—	—	+	+	
14	Mori [29]	2011	1	52	F	L	—	+	-(48 mm)	+	+	—	—	N	VS	—	—	—	—	
15	Lim [30]	2011	1	49	M	R	+	+	+(27 mm)	+	+	—	—	N	VS	—	—	—	—	
16	Chen [31]	2011	1	50	M	L	+	+	+(28 mm)	—	—	—	+	N	VS	+	—	—	—	Arthroscopy
17	Guijarro-Martínez [32]	2011	1	38	F	B	+	—	-(40 mm)	—	—	+	—	N	NL	—	—	—	—	
18	Matsumura [33]	2012	1	46	M	R	—	—	+(24 mm)	+	+	+	—	+	NL	—	+	—	+	Aspiration biopsy
19	Matsumoto [34]	2013	1	34	F	R	—	—	-(42 mm)	+	+	+	+	N	NL	—	—	—	—	Assisted with arthroscopy
20	Coleman [35]	2013	1	63	F	L	+	—	—	—	+	+	—	—	—	—	+	—	—	Aspiration biopsy
21	Valentini [36]	2013	1	60	F	L	+	+	—	—	+	+	—	—	—	—	—	—	—	
22	Sink [37]	2014	1	82	M	L	—	—	-(40 mm)	—	—	+	—	—	—	—	—	—	—	Aspiration biopsy
23	Pau [38]	2014	1	70	M	R	+	+	+	—	+	+	—	—	—	—	+	—	—	Reconstruction of the cranial base
24	Cascone [39]	2914	1	30	M	L	—	+	—	—	—	+	—	11	20-30	—	—	—	+	
25	Pinto [40]	2015	1	54	F	L	+	+	+(20 mm)	—	+	+	—	11	<10	—	—	—	—	
26	Ivask [41]	2015	1	45	F	L	—	+	+(38 mm)	+	+	—	—	N	3-10	+	—	—	—	Arthroscopy
27	Sozzi [42]	2015	1	68	F	R	+	+	+(20 mm)	+	+	+	—	N	VS	—	—	—	—	

Table 1: Continued.

No.	First author	Year	No. of cases	Age	Sex	Site	Clinical manifestations				Imaging			Loose bodies		Treatments (other than synovial chondrectomy)				Remarks
							Swelling	Pain	LJO	Crepitation	CT	MRI	CBCT	No.	Size (mm)	Arthrotomy	Condylectomy	Discectomy	Synovectomy	Such as arthroscopy
28	Yoshitake [43]	2016	1	72	M	R	+	+	+(30 mm)	—	+	+	—	—	—	—	—	—	—	
29	Selvi [44]	2016	1	45	F	R	+	+	+(24 mm)	—	—	+	—	N	NL	+	—	+	—	Arthroscopy, arthroplasty, eminectomy
30	McCaffery [45]	2017	1	34	M	R	+	—	—	—	+	+	—	—	—	—	+	—	—	Osteotomy of the zygomatic arch
31	Khanna [46]	2017	1	43	M	L	+	+	+	—	+	—	—	—	—	—	—	—	—	
32	Khanna [46]	2017	1	35	M	R	+	+	+	—	+	+	—	+	NL	—	—	—	—	Osteotomy of the zygomatic arch
33	Kim [47]	2017	1	26	F	R	—	+	—	—	+	+	—	+	2	—	—	—	—	
34	Kim [47]	2017	1	31	F	L	—	+	-(45 mm)	—	+	+	—	+	7-10	—	—	—	—	
35	Kim [48]	2018	1	50	M	L	+	+	—	—	+	+	—	120	Small	—	—	—	—	
36	Holtmann [49]	2018	1	63	F	R	+	+	—	—	+	+	—	25	14 × 6 VS	—	—	—	—	
37	Matsuda [50]	2019	1	73	F	L	+	+	—	—	+	+	—	44	VS	—	—	—	—	*1
38	Tang [51]	2019	1	60	F	R	—	+	—	—	+	—	—	—	—	—	—	—	—	
39	Tang [51]	2019	1	38	F	R	+	—	+(25 mm)	—	+	—	+	+	NL	—	—	—	—	
40	Tang [51]	2019	1	30	F	L	+	+	+(28 mm)	—	+	—	+	+	NL	—	—	—	—	
41	Meng [52]	2010	20	44.0 (32-67)	8/12	12/7/1	13	17	14	5	15	13	—	40 > N	VS	8	2	9	—	Arthroscopy: 1
42	Wang [11]	2012	22	45.3 (17-64)	7/15	12/10/0	NL	NL	NL	NL	—	22	—	NL	NL	NL	NL	NL	NL	
43	Cai [53]	2016	33	43.0 (21-62)	7/26	18/15/0	3	20	16/30.5 mm(15-55 mm)	18	4	33	—	N	0.5-16	—	—	—	—	Only arthroscopy: 32 Assisted with arthroscopy: 1
44	Liu [7]	2016	10	47.2 (31-67)	2/8	2/8/0	7	7	7	5	1	—	9	6 * 2	NL	—	—	—	—	
45	Bai [54]	2017	36	48.11 (29-65)	11/25	14/22/0	NL	NL	22	9	36	36	—	4 * 2	NL	—	—	—	—	Assisted with arthroscopy: 36
46	Brabyn [55]	2018	6	42.0 (33-57)	0/6	0/6/0	2	2	32.3 mm (20-46 mm)	4	5	5	—	6 * 2	0.5-3.0	—	—	—	—	
47	Maffia [56]	2019	6	48.6 (30-61)	2/4	2/4/0	5	6	5	3	6	6	—	NL	NL	—	—	—	6	
48	Lee [57]	2019	16	32.68 (19-49)	2/14	7/9/0	—	10	4	8	2	15	—	40-100	0.5-6.5	—	—	—	—	Only arthroscopy: 16

Table 1: Continued.

No.	First author	Year	No. of cases	Age	Sex	Site	Clinical manifestations				Imaging			Loose bodies		Treatments (other than synovial chondrectomy)				Remarks
							Swelling	Pain	LJO	Crepitation	CT	MRI	CBCT	No.	Size (mm)	Arthrotomy	Condylectomy	Discectomy	Synovectomy	Such as arthroscopy
49	Benslama [58]	2019	12	50.5 (43-86)	4/8	3/9/0	4	10	6	2	2	6	—	2-30	VS	—	—	—	—	Assisted with arthroscopy: 1
50	Present case	2020	1	56	F	L	—	+	+(30 mm)	+	+	+	—	386	2-5	+	+	—	—	

cure, we believe that open surgical resection is the best option.

Synovial chondromatosis is characterized by multiple chondrodysplasia or osteochondrodysplasia and free body formation in a joint due to synovial metaplasia, but its underlying pathological mechanism remains unclear. Possible triggers are trauma and continuous irritation to the synovial membrane [61]. Trauma is considered to lead to the production of cartilage from secondary synovial changes, while continuous stimulation may trigger cartilage formation from synovial cell metaplasia due to internal joint damage. However, our patient had no history of trauma. We believe that anterior disc displacement allows rich connective tissue growth in the posterior synovium, which is chronically stimulated by the mandibular condyle. Although the molecular mechanism of this disease is not understood, immunohistochemical studies of loose bodies from synovial chondromatosis have found expression of fibroblast growth factor-2 and fibroblast growth factor receptor-1 in chondrocytes, suggesting their involvement in the pathology [62, 63]. In a study of synovial tissue from TMJ synovitis, interleukin-1β and tumor necrosis factor α were expressed in both the synovial cell layer and the vascular wall [64, 65]. These reports indicate that the onset of this disease is influenced by a mechanism involving inflammatory cytokines and other substances produced by the synovial membrane or microvascular disorders that regulate the growth and activity of synovial cells against a background of genetic or environmental factors [66, 67]. However, in addition to the above factors, various cytokines, growth factors, pain-producing substances, and other substances involved in inflammation and cell proliferation are known to be expressed in the synovial fluid and synovial cells of the TMJ [65, 68]. Clarifying the locations and effects of these substances could help provide diagnostic indicators for the diagnosis of this type of synovial chondritis and its pathological progression.

The prognosis of this disease is relatively good, and recurrence is uncommon. However, because of reports of malignant transformation to chondrosarcoma in other joints [6, 69, 70], we plan to continue to follow-up this patient.

In conclusion, we reported a rare case of TMJ synovial chondromatosis with 386 loose bodies, which were removed using open surgery. There has been no recurrence in the 5-year follow-up period, indicating that open surgery is the best course of intervention in such cases.

References

[1] A. Von Haller, *Elementa physiologiae corporus humani*, Sumptibus Societatis Typographicae; Bernae, 1765.

[2] A. Al-Kayat and P. Bramley, "A modified pre-auricular approach to the temporomandibular joint and malar arch," *Journal of Oral Surgery*, vol. 17, no. 2, pp. 91–103, 1979.

[3] K. Forssell, R. P. Happonen, and H. Forssell, "Synovial chondromatosis of the temporomandibular joint: report of a case and review of the literature," *International Journal of Oral and Maxillofacial Surgery*, vol. 17, no. 4, pp. 237–241, 1988.

[4] O. Lieger, J. Zix, E. J. Stauffer-Brauch, and T. Iizuka, "Synovial chondromatosis of the temporomandibular joint with cranial extension: a case report and literature review," *Journal of Oral and Maxillofacial Surgery*, vol. 65, no. 10, pp. 2073–2080, 2007.

[5] F. R. Carls, A. von Hochstetter, W. Engelke, and H. F. Sailer, "Loose bodies in the temporomandibular joint: the advantages of arthroscopy," *Journal of Cranio-Maxillo-Facial Surgery*, vol. 23, no. 4, pp. 215–221, 1995.

[6] L. Ardekian, W. Faquin, M. J. Troulis, L. B. Kaban, and M. August, "Synovial chondromatosis of the temporomandibular joint: report and analysis of eleven cases," *Journal of Oral and Maxillofacial Surgery*, vol. 63, no. 7, pp. 941–947, 2005.

[7] X. Liu, Z. Huang, W. Zhu, P. Liang, and Q. Tao, "Clinical and imaging findings of temporomandibular joint synovial chondromatosis: an analysis of 10 cases and literature review," *Journal of Oral and Maxillofacial Surgery*, vol. 74, no. 11, pp. 2159–2168, 2016.

[8] A. M. Noyek, R. C. Holgate, S. M. Fireman, P. Rosen, and K. P. Pritzker, "The radiologic findings in synovial chondromatosis (chondrometaplasia) of the temporomandibular joint," *The Journal of Otolaryngology. Supplement*, vol. 3, pp. 45–48, 1977.

[9] E. Balliu, V. Medina, J. Vilanova et al., "Synovial chondromatosis of the temporomandibular joint: CT and MRI findings," *Dento Maxillo Facial Radiology*, vol. 36, no. 1, pp. 55–58, 2007.

[10] S. Ginaldi, "Computed tomography feature of synovial osteochondromatosis," *Skeletal Radiology*, vol. 5, no. 4, pp. 219–222, 1980.

[11] P. Wang, Z. Tian, J. Yang, and Q. Yu, "Synovial chondromatosis of the temporomandibular joint: MRI findings with pathological comparison," *Dento Maxillo Facial Radiology*, vol. 41, no. 2, pp. 110–116, 2012.

[12] D. P. Von Arx, M. T. Simpson, and P. Batman, "Synovial chondromatosis of the temporomandibular joint," *The British Journal of Oral & Maxillofacial Surgery*, vol. 26, no. 4, pp. 297–305, 1988.

[13] Q. Yu, J. Yang, P. Wang, H. Shi, and J. Luo, "CT features of synovial chondromatosis in the temporomandibular joint," *Oral Surgery, Oral Medicine, Oral Pathology, Oral Radiology, and Endodontics*, vol. 97, no. 4, pp. 524–528, 2004.

[14] J. W. Milgram, "Synovial osteochondromatosis: a histopathological study of thirty cases," *The Journal of Bone and Joint Surgery. American Volume*, vol. 59, no. 6, pp. 792–801, 1977.

[15] J. W. Milgram, "The classification of loose bodies in human joints," *Clinical Orthopaedics and Related Research*, vol. 124, pp. 282–291, 1977.

[16] Y. Gerard, A. Shall, and M. Ameil, "Synovial osteochondromatosis. Therapeutic indications based on a histological classification," *Chirurgie; memoires de l'Academie de chirurgie*, vol. 119, no. 4, pp. 190–195, 1993.

[17] L. W. Peng, D. M. Yan, Y. G. Wang, and Y. D. Li, "Synovial chondromatosis of the temporomandibular joint: a case report with bilateral occurrence," *Journal of Oral and Maxillofacial Surgery*, vol. 67, no. 4, pp. 893–895, 2009.

[18] X. Y. Cai, C. Yang, M. J. Chen, and B. Yun, "Simultaneous pigmented villonodular synovitis and synovial chondromatosis of the temporomandibular joint: case report," *International Journal of Oral and Maxillofacial Surgery*, vol. 38, no. 11, pp. 1215–1218, 2009.

[19] A. Balasundaram, J. R. Geist, S. C. Gordon, and G. D. Klasser, "Radiographic diagnosis of synovial chondromatosis of the temporomandibular joint: a case report," *Journal of the Canadian Dental Association*, vol. 75, no. 10, pp. 711–714, 2009.

[20] W. Zha, Y. F. Zhao, Y. Liu, and L. Jiang, "A case of synovial chondromatosis of the temporomandibular joint secondary

to preauricular trauma," *International Journal of Oral and Maxillofacial Surgery*, vol. 38, no. 11, pp. 1212–1215, 2009.

[21] J. Sato, K. I. Notani, J. Goto, M. Shindoh, and Y. Kitagawa, "Synovial chondromatosis of the temporomandibular joint accompanied by loose bodies in both the superior and inferior joint compartments: case report," *International Journal of Oral and Maxillofacial Surgery*, vol. 39, no. 1, pp. 86–88, 2010.

[22] C. C. Goizueta-Adame and R. González-García, "Synovial chondromatosis of the temporomandibular joint: report of 2 patients whose joints were reconstructed with costochondral graft and alloplastic prosthesis," *The British Journal of Oral & Maxillofacial Surgery*, vol. 48, no. 5, pp. 374–377, 2010.

[23] P. Boffano, S. Viterbo, and G. F. Bosco, "Diagnosis and surgical management of synovial chondromatosis of the temporomandibular joint," *The Journal of Craniofacial Surgery*, vol. 21, no. 1, pp. 157–159, 2010.

[24] D. P. Souza, C. C. Loureiro, P. F. Falchet, L. F. Leandro, and R. Raitz, "Synovial chondromatosis of the temporomandibular joint: an asymptomatic case report and literature review," *Cranio*, vol. 28, no. 1, pp. 67–71, 2010.

[25] L. Guarda-Nardini, F. Piccotti, G. Ferronato, and D. Manfredini, "Synovial chondromatosis of the temporomandibular joint: a case description with systematic literature review," *International Journal of Oral and Maxillofacial Surgery*, vol. 39, no. 8, pp. 745–755, 2010.

[26] X. Y. Cai, C. Yang, M. J. Chen, B. Jiang, and B. L. Wang, "Arthroscopically guided removal of large solitary synovial chondromatosis from the temporomandibular joint," *International Journal of Oral and Maxillofacial Surgery*, vol. 39, no. 12, pp. 1236–1239, 2010.

[27] L. M. González-Pérez, J. Congregado-Córdoba, and M. V. Salinas-Martín, "Temporomandibular joint synovial chondromatosis with a traumatic etiology," *International Journal of Oral and Maxillofacial Surgery*, vol. 40, no. 3, pp. 330–334, 2011.

[28] S. B. Shah, S. Ramanojam, P. K. Gadre, and K. S. Gadre, "Synovial chondromatosis of temporomandibular joint: journey through 25 decades and a case report," *Journal of Oral and Maxillofacial Surgery*, vol. 69, no. 11, pp. 2795–2814, 2011.

[29] Y. Mori, K. Kakudo, M. Gotoh et al., "A case of synovial chondromatosis of the temporomandibular joint followed for 17 years," *Oral Surgery, Oral Medicine, Oral Pathology, Oral Radiology, and Endodontics*, vol. 112, no. 1, pp. e35–e39, 2011.

[30] S. W. Lim, S. J. Jeon, S. S. Choi, and K. H. Choi, "Synovial chondromatosis in the temporomandibular joint: a case with typical imaging features and pathological findings," *The British Journal of Radiology*, vol. 84, no. 1007, pp. e213–e216, 2011.

[31] M. J. Chen, C. Yang, X. H. Zhang, and Y. T. Qiu, "Synovial chondromatosis originally arising in the lower compartment of temporomandibular joint: a case report and literature review," *Journal of Cranio-Maxillo-Facial Surgery*, vol. 39, no. 6, pp. 459–462, 2011.

[32] R. Guijarro-Martínez, M. Puche Torres, M. Marqués Mateo et al., "Bilateral synovial chondromatosis of the temporomandibular joint," *Journal of Cranio-Maxillo-Facial Surgery*, vol. 39, no. 4, pp. 261–265, 2011.

[33] Y. Matsumura, J. Nomura, K. Nakanishi, S. Yanase, H. Kato, and T. Tagawa, "Synovial chondromatosis of the temporomandibular joint with calcium pyrophosphate dihydrate crystal deposition disease (pseudogout)," *Dento Maxillo Facial Radiology*, vol. 41, no. 8, pp. 703–707, 2012.

[34] K. Matsumoto, T. Sato, S. Iwanari et al., "The use of arthrography in the diagnosis of temporomandibular joint synovial chondromatosis," *Dento Maxillo Facial Radiology*, vol. 42, no. 1, p. 15388284, 2013.

[35] H. Coleman, E. Chandraratnam, G. Morgan, L. Gomes, and F. Bonar, "Synovial chondrosarcoma arising in synovial chondromatosis of the temporomandibular joint," *Head and Neck Pathology*, vol. 7, no. 3, pp. 304–309, 2013.

[36] V. Valentini, P. Arangio, S. Egidi et al., "Diagnosis and treatment of synovial chondromatosis of the TMJ: a clinical case," *Ann Stomatol*, vol. 4, no. 3-4, pp. 269–272, 2013.

[37] J. Sink, B. Bell, and H. Mesa, "Synovial chondromatosis of the temporomandibular joint: clinical, cytologic, histologic, radiologic, therapeutic aspects, and differential diagnosis of an uncommon lesion," *Oral Surgery, Oral Medicine, Oral Pathology, Oral Radiology*, vol. 117, no. 3, pp. e269–e274, 2014.

[38] M. Pau, Á. Bicsák, K. E. Reinbacher, M. Feichtinger, and H. Kärcher, "Surgical treatment of synovial chondromatosis of the temporomandibular joint with erosion of the skull base: a case report and review of the literature," *International Journal of Oral and Maxillofacial Surgery*, vol. 43, no. 5, pp. 600–605, 2014.

[39] P. Cascone, P. Gennaro, G. Gabriele et al., "Temporomandibular synovial chondromatosis with numerous nodules," *The Journal of Craniofacial Surgery*, vol. 25, no. 3, pp. 1114-1115, 2014.

[40] A. A. Pinto, R. Ferreira e Costa, S. F. de Sousa, M. R. P. Chagas, M. A. V. do Carmo, and J. C. T. de Lacerda, "Synovial chondromatosis of the temporomandibular joint successfully treated by surgery," *Head and Neck Pathology*, vol. 9, no. 4, pp. 525–529, 2015.

[41] O. Ivask, E. Leibur, and Ü. Voog-Oras, "Synovial chondromatosis in the temporomandibular joint: case report with review of the literature," *Stomatologija*, vol. 17, no. 3, pp. 97–101, 2015.

[42] D. Sozzi, G. Bocchialini, G. Novelli, M. G. Valente, F. Moltrasio, and A. Bozzetti, "A rare case of synovial chondromatosis of the inferior TMJ compartment. Diagnosis and treatment aspect," *Annali di stomatologia*, vol. 6, no. 3-4, pp. 91–95, 2015.

[43] H. Yoshitake, K. Kayamori, R. Nakamura, S. Wake, and K. Harada, "Pseudotumor in the temporomandibular joint: a case report," *International Journal of Surgery Case Reports*, vol. 15, pp. 5–9, 2015.

[44] F. Selvi, J. Messina, W. C. Faquin, and D. A. Keith, "Relapsing polychondritis concomitant with synovial chondromatosis of the temporomandibular joint," *Journal of Oral and Maxillofacial Surgery*, vol. 74, no. 11, pp. 2207–2215, 2016.

[45] C. McCaffery, M. Dodd, F. Bekiroglu, and E. Twohig, "Synovial chondromatosis of the temporomandibular joint with extension into the middle cranial fossa and internal carotid canal," *International Journal of Oral and Maxillofacial Surgery*, vol. 46, no. 7, pp. 867–870, 2017.

[46] J. N. Khanna and R. Ramaswami, "Synovial chondromatosis of the temporomandibular joint with intracranial extension–report of two cases," *International Journal of Oral and Maxillofacial Surgery*, vol. 46, no. 12, pp. 1579–1583, 2017.

[47] D. H. Kim, E. H. Lee, E. S. Cho et al., "Temporomandibular joint synovial chondromatosis extending to the temporal bone: a report of two cases," *Journal of the Korean Association of Oral and Maxillofacial Surgeons*, vol. 43, no. 5, pp. 336–342, 2017.

[48] H. S. Kim, W. Lee, J. W. Choi, W. J. Han, and E. K. Kim, "Temporomandibular joint synovial chondromatosis accompanying

temporal bone proliferation: a case report," *Imaging Sci Dent*, vol. 48, no. 2, pp. 147–152, 2018.

[49] H. Holtmann, T. Böttinger, N. R. Kübler et al., "Intra- and extracapsular synovial chondromatosis of the temporomandibular joint: rare case and review of the literature," *SAGE open medical case reports*, vol. 6, 2018.

[50] S. Matsuda, H. Yoshimura, and K. Sano, "Application of a real-time 3-dimensional navigation system for treatment of synovial chondromatosis of the temporomandibular joint: a case report," *Medicine (Baltimore)*, vol. 98, no. 18, article e15382, 2019.

[51] B. Tang, K. Wang, H. Wang, and G. Zheng, "Radiological features of synovial chondromatosis affecting the temporomandibular joint: report of three cases," *Oral Radiology*, vol. 35, no. 2, pp. 198–204, 2019.

[52] J. Meng, C. Guo, B. Yi, Y. Zhao, H. Luo, and X. Ma, "Clinical and radiologic findings of synovial chondromatosis affecting the temporomandibular joint," *Oral Surgery, Oral Medicine, Oral Pathology, Oral Radiology, and Endodontics*, vol. 109, no. 3, pp. 441–448, 2010.

[53] X. Y. Cai, C. Yang, M. J. Chen et al., "Arthroscopic management for synovial chondromatosis of the temporomandibular joint: a retrospective review of 33 cases," *Journal of Oral and Maxillofacial Surgery*, vol. 70, no. 9, pp. 2106–2113, 2012.

[54] G. Bai, C. Yang, Y. Qiu, and M. Chen, "Open surgery assisted with arthroscopy to treat synovial chondromatosis of the temporomandibular joint," *International Journal of Oral and Maxillofacial Surgery*, vol. 46, no. 2, pp. 208–213, 2017.

[55] P. J. Brabyn, A. Capote, M. F. Muñoz-Guerra, I. Zylberberg, F. J. Rodríguez-Campo, and L. Naval-Gías, "Arthroscopic management of synovial chondromatosis of the temporomandibular joint. Case series and systematic review," *J Maxillofac Oral Surg*, vol. 17, no. 4, pp. 401–409, 2018.

[56] F. Maffia, V. Vellone, C. De Quarto, M. Runci Anastasi, and P. Cascone, "Synovial chondromatosis of the temporomandibular joint with glenoid fossa erosion: disk preservation for spontaneous anatomical recovery," *Journal of Cranio-Maxillo-Facial Surgery*, vol. 47, no. 12, pp. 1898–1902, 2019.

[57] L. M. Lee, Y. M. Zhu, D. D. Zhang, Y. Q. Deng, and Y. Gu, "Synovial chondromatosis of the temporomandibular joint: a clinical and arthroscopic study of 16 cases," *Journal of Cranio-Maxillo-Facial Surgery*, vol. 47, no. 4, pp. 607–610, 2019.

[58] L. Benslama, T. Schouman, S. Toure, J. Chardain, and P. Goudot, "Synovial chondromatosis of the temporomandibular joint: report and analysis of 12 cases," *J Stomatol Oral Maxillofac Surg*, vol. 120, no. 5, pp. 476–479, 2019.

[59] J. Ishii, K. Kino, J. Kobayashi, and T. Amagasa, "Synovial chondromatosis of the temporomandibular joint: long-term postoperative follow-up of the residual calcification," *Journal of Medical and Dental Sciences*, vol. 50, no. 1, pp. 133–137, 2003.

[60] Z. X. Han, M. J. Chen, C. Yang, and M. J. Dong, "Recurrent synovial chondromatosis of the temporomandibular joint: report of two cases," *The British Journal of Oral & Maxillofacial Surgery*, vol. 55, no. 9, pp. 965–967, 2017.

[61] A. Deboise and Y. Roche, "Synovial chondromatosis of the temporomandibular joint possibly secondary to trauma: a case report," *International Journal of Oral and Maxillofacial Surgery*, vol. 20, no. 2, pp. 90–92, 1991.

[62] Y. Li, L. A. El Mozen, H. Cai et al., "Transforming growth factor beta 3 involved in the pathogenesis of synovial chondromatosis of temporomandibular joint," *Scientific Reports*, vol. 5, no. 1, 2015.

[63] J. Sato, N. Segami, T. Suzuki, Y. Yoshitake, and K. Nishikawa, "The expression of fibroblast growth factor-2 and fibroblast growth factor receptor-1 in chondrocytes in synovial chondromatosis of the temporomandibular joint. Report of two cases," *International Journal of Oral and Maxillofacial Surgery*, vol. 31, no. 5, pp. 532–536, 2002.

[64] T. Ikebe, E. Nakayama, M. Shinohara, H. Takeuchi, and Y. Takenoshita, "Synovial chondromatosis of the temporomandibular joint: the effect of interleukin-1 on loose-body-derived cells," *Oral Surgery, Oral Medicine, Oral Pathology, Oral Radiology, and Endodontics*, vol. 85, no. 5, pp. 526–531, 1998.

[65] T. Suzuki, N. Segami, M. Nishimura, H. Hattori, and T. Nojima, "Analysis of 70Kd heat shock protein expression in patients with internal derangement of the temporomandibular joint," *International Journal of Oral and Maxillofacial Surgery*, vol. 29, no. 4, pp. 301–304, 2000.

[66] P. Anract, M. Katabi, M. Forest, J. Benoit, J. Witvoët, and B. Tomeno, "Synovial chondromatosis and chondrosarcoma. A study of the relationship between these two diseases," *Revue de Chirurgie Orthopédique et Réparatrice de l'Appareil Moteur*, vol. 82, no. 3, pp. 216–224, 1996.

[67] J. Morales-Ducret, E. Wayner, M. J. Elices, J. M. Alvaro-Gracia, N. J. Zvaifler, and G. S. Firestein, "Alpha 4/beta 1 integrin (VLA-4) ligands in arthritis. Vascular cell adhesion molecule-1 expression in synovium and on fibroblast-like synoviocytes," *Journal of Immunology*, vol. 149, pp. 1424–1431, 1992.

[68] S. Fujita, H. Yoshida, I. Tojyo, T. Wada, K. Murakami, and T. Iizuka, "Synovial chondromatosis of the temporomandibular joint: clinical and immunohistopathological considerations," *The British Journal of Oral & Maxillofacial Surgery*, vol. 42, no. 3, pp. 259-260, 2004.

[69] S. Kenan, I. F. Abdelwahab, M. J. Klein, and M. M. Lewis, "Case report 817: synovial chondrosarcoma secondary to synovial chondromatosis," *Skeletal Radiology*, vol. 22, no. 8, pp. 623–626, 1993.

[70] D. I. Campbell, R. K. De Silva, H. De Silva, S. H. Sinon, and A. M. Rich, "Temporomandibular joint synovial chondromatosis with intracranial extension: a review and observations of patient observed for 4 years," *Journal of Oral and Maxillofacial Surgery*, vol. 69, no. 8, pp. 2247–2252, 2011.

3

Nasopalatine Duct Cyst with Impacted Inverted Mesiodens: A Rare Case Report and Literature Review

Shamimul Hasan,[1] **Deepika Bablani Popli**,[2] **Syed Ansar Ahmad**,[3] **Keya Sircar**,[2] **Shahnaz Mansoori**,[1] **and Kirti Dua**[4]

[1]*Department of Oral Medicine and Radiology, Faculty of Dentistry, Jamia Millia Islamia, New Delhi, India*
[2]*Department of Oral Pathology, Faculty of Dentistry, Jamia Millia Islamia, New Delhi, India*
[3]*Department of Oral and Maxillofacial Surgery, Faculty of Dentistry, Jamia Millia Islamia, New Delhi, India*
[4]*Faculty of Dentistry, Jamia Millia Islamia, New Delhi, India*

Correspondence should be addressed to Shamimul Hasan; shasan1@jmi.ac.in

Academic Editor: Sreekanth Kumar Mallineni

Nasopalatine duct cyst (NPDC) is a non-odontogenic, developmental epithelial cyst that accounts for 1% of maxillary cysts. It often arises due to the spontaneous proliferation of the epithelial tissue remnants, although trauma, bacterial infection, and mucous retention may also trigger the proliferation. Owing to its slow-growing, asymptomatic nature, the cyst is often discovered as an accidental finding during routine clinical and radiographic examinations. However, the majority of cases present as a tiny, asymptomatic swelling just posterior to the palatine papillae. Radiographically, it appears as a well-defined oval or round radiolucency in the maxillary anterior teeth region and should be differentially diagnosed with inflammatory periapical lesions and a wide incisive foramen. A pulp vitality test is essential to rule out lesions of endodontic origin. Microscopically, NPDCs display a mixed pattern of the epithelial lining and exhibit neurovascular bundles (small to medium-sized nerves, arteries, and veins), and minor salivary glands in the cystic connective tissue, a distinctive feature facilitating a confirmatory diagnosis. Enucleation and marsupialization remain the treatment of choice. NPDC associated with impacted mesiodens is an extremely uncommon entity. A comprehensive literature search carried out on the PubMed and Google Scholar search engines revealed only three cases of NPDC with impacted mesiodens to date. The purpose of this study is to report an extremely rare case of NPDC associated with an impacted inverted mesiodens in a 19-year-old male patient who presented with an asymptomatic swelling in the maxillary anterior teeth region. To the best of our knowledge, this is only the fourth reported case of NPDC with impacted mesiodens.

1. Introduction

Supernumerary teeth refer to an extra tooth as compared to normal dentition, with a reported prevalence rate of 0.3–0.8% and 0.5–3.8% in the primary and permanent dentitions, respectively [1].

The precise etiopathogenesis of supernumerary teeth is still debatable, although trauma, drugs, infections, radiation, genetic, environmental, and hormonal factors may serve as potential triggers that might have an impact on tooth development. Phylogenetic reversion (Atavism) theory, dental lamina hyperactivity theory, and dichotomy theory are the different recommended theories in etiopathogenesis [2, 3]. Various syndromic conditions (cleidocranial dysplasia, Gardner's syndrome, cleft lip and palate, oral-facial-digital syndrome, and chondroectodermal dysplasia) may also be associated with supernumerary teeth [4].

Studies have demonstrated that panoramic radiographs are inaccurate in the identification of supernumerary teeth due to a narrow image layer in the maxillary anterior region and spinal superimposition [5, 6]. About 50% of supernumerary teeth might go undetected on the panoramic radiographs; hence, a higher level of dental training and more accurate diagnostic aids are imperative for detecting the precise location of supernumerary teeth and their relation with the contiguous vital structures [6].

Localization of supernumerary teeth is cardinal to ascertain the surgical technique and also to avert the potential iatrogenic injury to the adjacent anatomic structures during the surgical procedure [7]. Published literature has demonstrated that various radiographic techniques, including the horizontal tube shift technique (HTST) and vertical tube shift technique (VTST), have been employed to locate supernumerary teeth [8, 9]. However, there is no scientific affirmation to validate the relative accuracy of HTST and VTST for the exact localization of supernumerary teeth. Mallineni et al. analyzed the relative accuracy of these two techniques and affirmed that the VTST is more precise in the localization of unerupted supernumerary teeth in the maxillary anterior region [7]. Recently, artificial intelligence models using deep learning (DL) algorithms with convolutional neural networks have been developed for the detection of mesiodens on panoramic radiographs. A study by Kuwada et al. focused on the automated detection of mesiodens in permanent dentition using DL algorithms [10]. However, a study by Ha et al. focused on the automated detection of mesiodens on panoramic radiographs for primary, mixed, and permanent dentition groups [11].

Supernumerary teeth may be associated with an array of complications, such as delay/failure of permanent teeth eruption, rotation/displacement/impaction/crowding and dilacerations of adjacent permanent teeth, and mid-line diastema. Resorption of the adjacent tooth roots, dentigerous cyst, and ameloblastoma development has also been reported with supernumerary teeth [3, 12]. Dentigerous cysts in association with supernumerary teeth account for 5–6% of all dentigerous cysts, of which about 90% have accompanying mesiodens [2].

Nasopalatine duct cyst (NPDC) is a development, non-odontogenic, epithelial cyst that constitutes 1% of all maxillary cysts [13]. Meyer in 1914 was the first to describe it as an accessory paranasal sinus [14]. NPDC is now the favored term for the synonymous "incisive canal cyst" as it may be seen within the nasopalatine canal (NPC) or in the palatal soft tissues or at the canal opening [15].

NPDC associated with impacted mesiodens is an extremely uncommon entity. A comprehensive literature search carried out on the Google Scholar and PubMed search engines revealed only three case reports of NPDC with impacted mesiodens [16–18]. The purpose of this study is to report an extremely rare case of NPDC associated with an impacted inverted mesiodens in a 19-year-old male patient who presented with asymptomatic swelling in the maxillary anterior teeth region. To the best of our knowledge, this is only the fourth reported case of NPDC with impacted mesiodens.

2. Case Description

A 19-year-old male patient presented with a slow-progressing, painless swelling in the maxillary anterior teeth region for the last 4 months. The initially smaller swelling has gradually increased with time to reach the present size. The past medical and family anamnesis was non-contributory, with no history of preceding trauma. The patient consulted a private practitioner one month back, who prescribed him antibiotics and analgesics for 7 days (tablet Augmentin 625 mg twice daily and tablet Ketorol DT 10 mg twice daily). However, the swelling persisted, and the patient visited our outpatient department. On physical examination, a diffuse swelling roughly 5cm × 5cm in size, involving the left mid-facial region, was seen. The swelling extended up to 2 cm below the left infra-orbital margin to about 2 cm inferior to the lower aspect of the upper lip with a slight elevation of the upper lip and anteroposteriorly extended from the right nasal alae to about 3 cm anterior to the left tragus of the ear. A slight superior deviation of the left nasal alae with left nasolabial fold obliteration was also noticeable. Palpatory findings elicited a non-tender, firm-hard consistency swelling with no increase in the surface temperature [Figures 1(a) and 1(b)]. On intraoral examination, a solitary, well-demarcated, 5cm × 4cm sized swelling in the maxillary anterior vestibule region with labial cortex expansion was appreciated. The swelling extended from the distal margin of tooth #12 to the mesial aspect of tooth #14 anteroposteriorly. Superiorly, the swelling obliterated the labial mucobuccal fold and inferiorly extended up to the gingival teeth margins. Palpatory features were suggestive of a non-tender swelling, with peripheral firm consistency and central fluctuations [Figure 1(c)]. The dentition showed normal tooth count and color with no clinically carious or missing teeth.

The maxillary anterior teeth elicited a positive response (representing a vital pulp tissue) with pulp vitality tests. Fine-needle aspiration yielded a brownish-yellow, blood-tinged cystic aspirate [Figure 2(a)]. An intraoral periapical radiograph (IOPAR) revealed a well-demarcated, heart-shaped unilocular radiolucency, peripherally encircled with a thin corticated border, and an impacted inverted mesiodens in the anterior maxillary region. The radiolucent lesion extended mesiodistally from the distal aspect of tooth #11 to the mesial margin of tooth #23 and inferiorly up to the root apices of the maxillary incisors. Root resorption of teeth #21 and #22 with distal flaring of the roots of teeth #11 and #21 was also noticed [Figure 2(b)]. Orthopantomogram (OPG) showed a well-circumscribed, ovoid, unilocular radiolucent lesion with peripheral corticated borders in the maxillary anterior region. The radiolucency extended from the mesial aspect of tooth #12 to the distal margin of tooth #25 and encircled the pericoronal aspect of the impacted inverted mesiodens. The floor of the left maxillary sinus was slightly pushed superiorly, and a slight distal displacement of the roots of teeth 11 and 21 with root resorption of teeth #21, #22, #24, and #25 was also apparent [Figure 2(c)].

Cone-beam computed tomography (CBCT) was advised to ascertain the extent of the lesion and three-dimensional (3D) location of the mesiodens and their relation with the adjacent vital structures. However, the patient denied the radiographic investigation due to financial constraints; thus, the exact localization of the mesiodens and its relationship with the lesion and adjacent structures could not be ascertained. Hence, in the absence of a CBCT scan, it is likely that

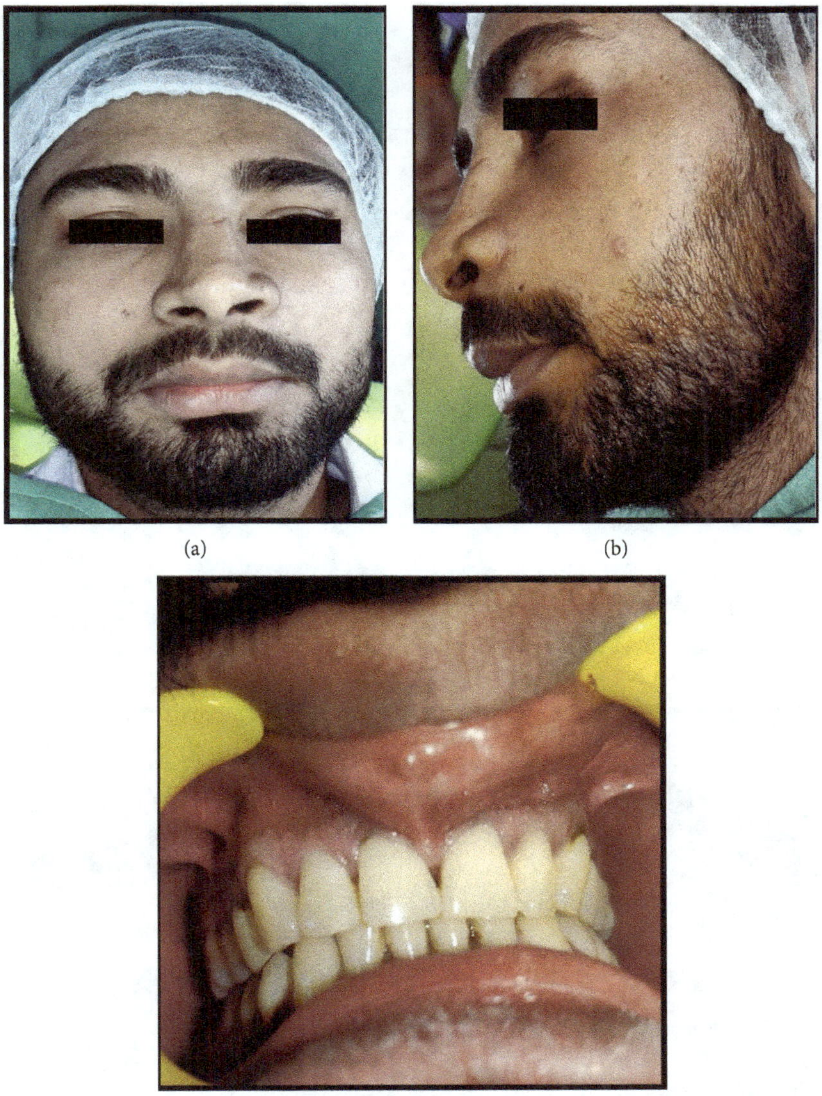

(a) (b) (c)

FIGURE 1: (a) and (b) Extraoral swelling on the left mid-facial region. (c) Intraoral swelling in the maxillary anterior region.

the patient had a cystic lesion and also a mesiodens without a relationship between them.

Considering the patient's age, location, and radiographic features, radicular cyst, dentigerous cyst, and adenomatoid odontogenic tumor were considered in the differential diagnosis.

Surgical enucleation of the lesion was considered (after an unremarkable hematological evaluation and obtaining written patient consent). A crevicular incision from the right maxillary canine to the left second molar was made, and the flap was reflected. Eight milliliters of blood-tinged, straw-colored fluid was aspirated from the cystic cavity, and impacted mesiodens was seen between the two maxillary central incisors. The impacted mesiodens was attached to the bone and not adherent to the cystic lining. Carnoy's solution was used to completely remove the cystic lining. Iodoform gauze was inserted in the cavity, and one end of the gauze was taken out from below the alae of the nose. Sutures were placed, and the enucleated specimen was sent for histopathologic evaluation [Figures 3(a), 3(b), and 3(c)].

The submitted hemotoxylin and eosin (H&E) sections (100×) showed a cystic epithelial lining with a fibrous connective tissue wall. The epithelial lining displayed a combination of epithelial varieties with the dominant type being ciliated pseudostratified columnar epithelium with goblet cells. Non-keratinized stratified squamous epithelium and primitive flat epithelium resembling reduced enamel epithelium were also present in places. Few areas show prominent juxta-epithelial hyalinization. The cystic wall revealed numerous mucous acini, muscular arteries, small veins, and nerves. Inflammatory cells along with cholesterol clefts and giant cells were also noted in some sections. These microscopic features were suggestive of a NPDC [Figures 4(a) and 4(b)].

There was uneventful postoperative healing, and no recurrences were noted during the 3-month-periodic follow-up.

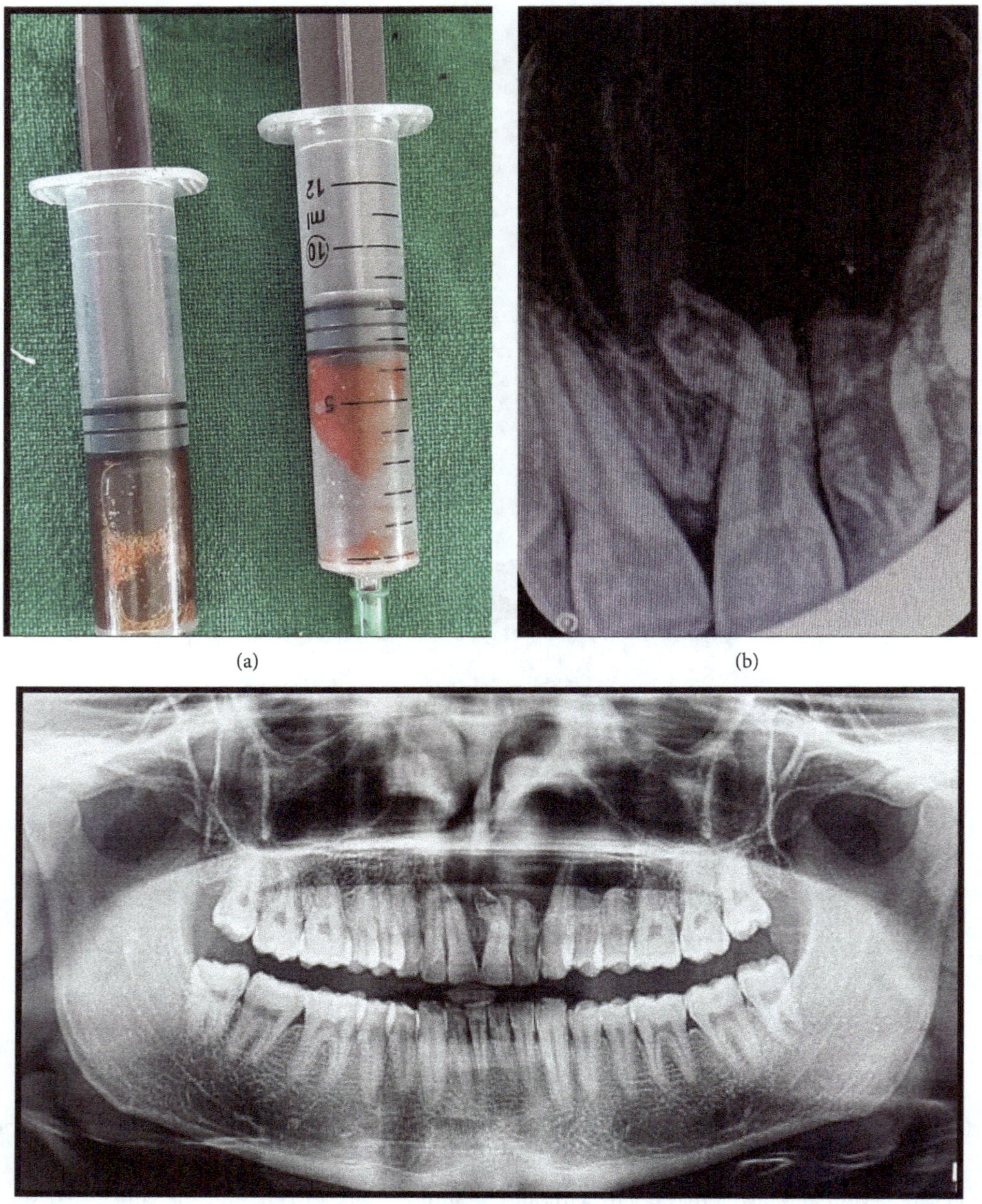

(a) (b) (c)

Figure 2: (a) Fine-needle aspiration revealed yellow-brown, blood-tinged cystic aspirate. (b) and (c) IOPAR and OPG demonstrate a well-defined unilocular radiolucency with an impacted inverted mesiodens in the maxillary anterior region.

3. Discussion

Mesiodens occurring in the maxillary anterior tooth region is the commonest reported supernumerary teeth, with a prevalence of 0.15–1.9%. [19]. They describe a common developmental deformity in mixed dentition [20]. Based on their appearance, mesiodens can be classified as rudimentary mesiodens and supplementary mesiodens in permanent and deciduous dentition, respectively. They are termed conical, tuberculate, or molariform based on their morphology [21].

Generally, mesiodens has no evident manifestations and only present as an increase in the tooth number [22]. However, mesiodens can give rise to numerous complications related to both the adjacent teeth and other vital structures. The likely dental complications with mesiodens include crowding with delayed permanent incisors eruption, midline diastema, rotation/displacement of the permanent incisors, caries, periodontitis, occlusal discrepancies, root resorption/abnormal root formation of the adjacent teeth, and infection. Mesiodens may also exert an impact on the neighboring vital anatomical structures, causing NPC /nasal floor perforation or the development of cysts [19].

Mesiodens is usually identified as incidental findings on routine radiographic investigations or in cases where the tooth fails to erupt normally [19]. Published literature has appraised various techniques for the localization of

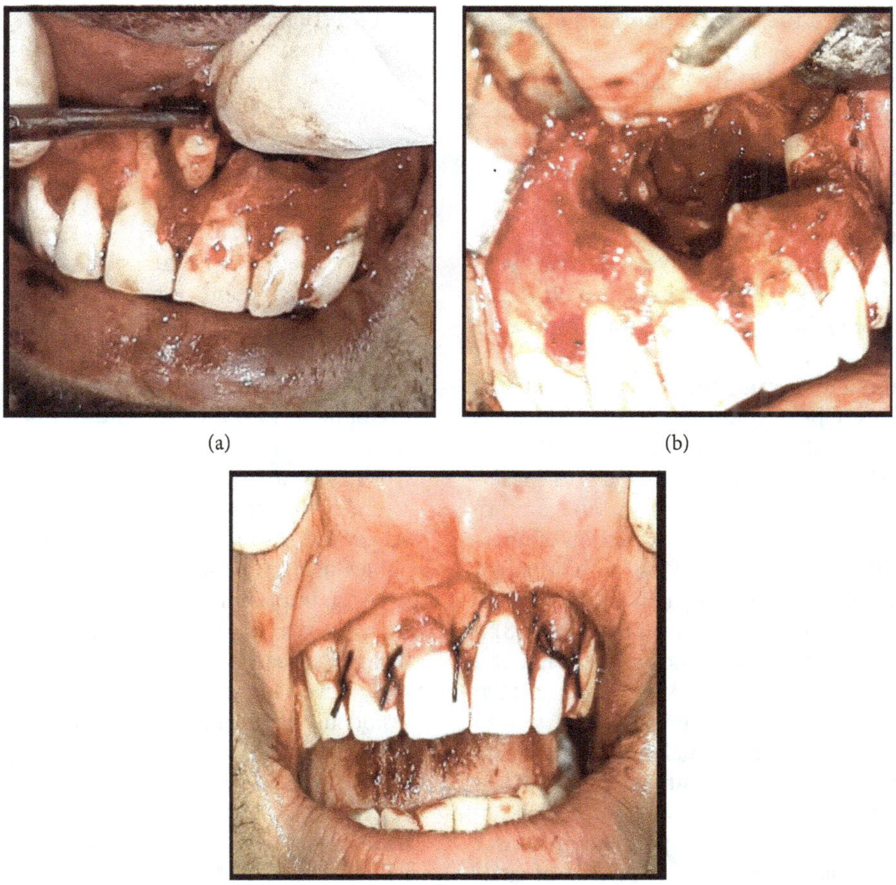

(a) (b) (c)

Figure 3: (a)–(c) The surgical enucleation of the lesion.

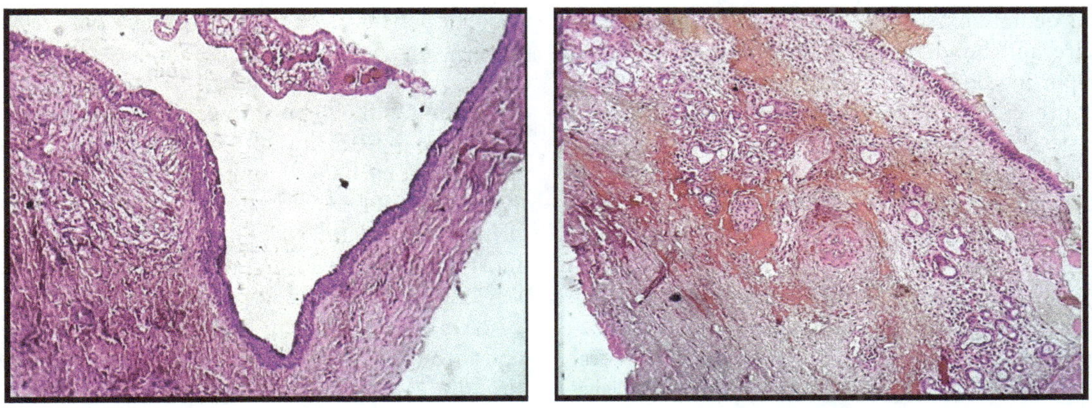

(a) (b)

Figure 4: (a) and (b) Epithelial lining showing a combination of pseudostratified ciliated columnar and nonkeratinized stratified squamous epithelium varieties, with mucous glands and neurovascular bundles in the cystic wall (H&E stain, 100×).

mesiodens. Conventional radiographic techniques, such as periapical radiographs, maxillary occlusal, and panoramic radiographs, have been employed for mesiodens diagnosis, localization, and management in the past. However, due to the imprecise localization of the mesiodens, they fail to fulfill the requirements of mesiodens extraction under the defined treatment protocol [23, 24]. The anterior maxillary and mandibular regions frequently pose a diagnostic challenge due to a narrow focal trough, vertebral superimposition, and the air space between the palate and the tongue, thus questioning the precise localization of the mesiodens with panoramic radiographs [11]. Although, the same lingual opposite buccal (SLOB) radiographic technique has demonstrated some diagnostic utility, however, the loss of image clarity, magnification, and superimposition limits the use of plain two-dimensional (2D) radiographs. Hence, it is imperative to delineate the 3D location of the mesiodens for a precise diagnosis and treatment plan [25, 26]. CBCT can ascertain not only the 3D location, shape, and axial inclination of mesiodens but also their relationship with adjacent vital structures. Over the years, CBCT has become an indispensable preoperative radiographic investigation for mesiodens localization and management [27].

In the present case, only 2D imaging (IOPAR and panoramic radiography) was carried out and revealed a well-defined unilocular radiolucency with impacted inverted mesiodens. However, 3D imaging (CBCT) was imperative in this case to ascertain the precise extent of the lesion and 3D location of the mesiodens, and their relation with the adjacent vital structures. CBCT could not be carried out as the patient was not willing due to financial constraints.

A surgical extraction is the primary treatment of mesiodens, and repositioning it in the dental arch may be another treatment option. However, the timing of extraction of unerupted mesiodens is still debatable [23]. Most authors advocate early intervention and surgical extraction of the unerupted mesiodentes as soon as they are identified [28].

Hence, an impacted mesiodens should be extracted at a young age when it appears to cause injury to the adjacent tissues. The optimal age for mesiodens extraction has been documented to be 6–7 years, after which more complications may be anticipated [29]. Other authors propose that extraction of the impacted mesiodens should be delayed until the root formation of the adjacent permanent incisor tooth is completed. This may avert the potential loss of vitality or root resorption of the adjacent permanent teeth. Moreover, early surgical intervention in a young patient necessitates the treatment under general anesthesia, which be associated with potential complications and might create psychological dental anxiety in the child [30]. In addition, early exposure and bonding of the impacted incisor may result in supporting bone loss and formation of scar tissue, thus further preventing the tooth eruption [31]. However, extraction is not always the mainstay of treatment for supernumerary teeth. Unerupted mesiodentes that do not appear to cause potential damage to the adjoining dentition and structures are routinely monitored without undergoing extraction [23, 24, 28].

The NPC, also referred to as the incisive canal or anterior palatine canal, is generally seen in the midline, just posterior to the maxillary central incisors. The anterior oral opening and the nasal opening of NPC are known as incisive foramen (IF) and Stenson's foramina, respectively [32]. NPC connects the oral and nasal cavities by linking the IF and the nasal foramen [33].

The content of the NPC comprises a neurovascular bundle (formed by the nasopalatine nerve, the terminal branches of the nasopalatine artery, and the veins) encircled by the connective tissue, fat, and seromucous glands [34]. Another anatomical structure called the nasopalatine duct may occasionally be seen within the NPC. The nasopalatine duct generally exhibits gradual degeneration; hence, it is now regarded as a vestigial structure in humans, embryologically and phylogenetically [35].

The etiopathogenesis of these cysts is still ambiguous, although some researchers have suggested that NPDCs arise from the spontaneous proliferation of the epithelial tissue remnants [13, 35–38]. Trauma (ill-fitting dentures/orthodontic appliances, previous endodontic treatment, or implant placement), bacterial infection, or mucous retention may also act as triggering factors for the proliferation of the epithelial tissue remnants [13, 37, 38]. As these cysts occur in incisive canals of the human fetus, spontaneous cystic degeneration of epithelial remnants is also proposed [13, 37].

However, in our case, there was no history of trauma, and the clinical evaluation did not exhibit periodontal pockets in the maxillary anterior teeth region. Hence, cystic development in our case could not be attributed to any factor other than spontaneous proliferation.

NPDCs associated with impacted mesiodens are an extremely uncommon entity. A detailed literature search was carried out on the Google Scholar and PubMed search engines using the following keywords: NPDC, supernumerary teeth, impacted teeth, and mesiodens. Case reports published in the English language up to August 2022 were extensively searched. This comprehensive literature search finally revealed only three cases of NPDC with impacted mesiodens, as summarized in Table 1 [16–18].

NPDC is one of the many gnathic pathologies but is distinctive in that it is site-specific (seen in only the midline of the maxillary anterior region) [36, 39]. NPDCs generally exhibit an age predilection (frequently seen in the age range of 40–60 years), although it may affect any age group [36, 37, 39–41]. However, age should not be a criterion to rule out its occurrence in the younger age group, as a case of NPDC has been documented in a 7-year-old child [35, 42]. NPDCs usually exhibit a male predilection (M : F 3 : 1) [43, 44].

Our patient was a 19-year-old male who reported a slow-progressing, painless swelling in the maxillary anterior teeth region for the past 4 months.

Owing to their slow-growing asymptomatic nature (40% of cases), they are usually observed as incidental findings during regular clinical and radiographic investigations [13, 17, 37, 38, 40, 43, 44]. A tiny asymptomatic swelling just behind the palatine papilla is the presenting symptom in most cases; however, a few cases may present a midline swelling on the labial aspect of the alveolar ridge. Larger cysts may cause severe destruction and exhibit "through and through" fluctuation between the palatal and labial cortex [17, 36, 37]. The size of the swelling is usually <2 cm in diameter. However, larger and more aggressive lesions up to 52 mm may cause complete perforation of the labial and palatal cortex [13, 45]. The superficial cyst usually presents as a fluctuant swelling with a bluish hue, in contrast to the deeper cysts covered by masticatory mucosa, unless ulcerated. Few cases of nasopalatine nerve impingement may cause numbness and tingling sensations [13, 17, 36, 37]. Depending on the discharge, the patient may experience either a salty taste (in cases of mucoid discharge) or a foul taste (in cases of purulent discharge). A cyst with mesiodens and tooth displacement as seen in the present case is a rarity [17, 36, 37].

Table 1: Reported NPDC cases with impacted mesiodens.

S.no.	Author(s)	Age (years)/sex	Clinical findings	Radiographic features	Treatment plan
1.	Gopal et al. [16]	18/M	Swelling and recurrent pus discharge in teeth #12–#22	Impacted inverted mesiodens within a well-circumscribed unilocular radiolucency	Surgical enucleation and removal of the mesiodens
2.	Tariq Salamm et al. [17]	55/F	Pain and swelling in teeth #12–#21	Impacted supernumerary tooth within a heart-shaped radiolucency	Surgical enucleation and removal of the mesiodens
3.	Bereket and Kaynar [18]	27/M	Swelling in the anterior palatal region of teeth #15–#25	Horizontally located supernumerary tooth within a lytic lesion in the anterior maxilla	Cystic decompression followed by surgical enucleation

Radiographically, NPDC generally exhibits a well-circumscribed, unilocular midline radiolucency, with an oval/round shape [35–37, 40, 43]. However, a few cases may present as a heart-shaped lesion, either due to notching by the nasal septum or superimposition of the nasal spine on the radiolucent area [36, 37, 43]. Divergence of the central incisor roots is a frequent radiographic feature of NPDCs, although root resorption is an infrequent occurrence. Superior displacement of the nasal floor has also been reported [46]. Computed tomography not only renders superior delineation of the lesion and the contiguous anatomical structures but also facilitates the best surgical treatment strategy [17, 36, 37, 44].

Radiographic appearance in our case was in sync with the previously published literature. Radiographically, a well-circumscribed unilocular radiolucent lesion with corticated borders, encompassing an impacted inverted mesiodens, was seen in the maxillary anterior region. Root resorption of the involved teeth, with a distal displacement of central incisor roots and superior displacement of the floor of the left maxillary sinus, was also noticed.

CBCT could not be performed as the patient was not willing due to financial constraints.

Microscopically, NPDCs display mixed patterns of epithelial linings. Ciliated columnar epithelium and squamous epithelium predominate the nasal floor and the oral cavity region, respectively, and the intermediate region is lined by the cuboidal epithelium [36, 37, 45]. NPDC is the only cyst in the oral and maxillofacial regions that exhibit neurovascular bundles (small to medium-sized nerves, arteries, and veins) and minor salivary glands in the cystic connective tissue. This distinctive histopathological feature facilitates a confirmatory diagnosis [41].

Our case demonstrated a combination of epithelial varieties, with the ciliated pseudostratified columnar epithelium in predominance. Numerous mucous acini, muscular arteries, small veins, nerves, and inflammatory cells were also appreciated microscopically.

Inflammatory lesions, such as periapical cysts and granulomas [37, 40, 41, 44, 46], wide IF [9, 36, 37, 41, 44–46], odontogenic keratocyst [40], nasolabial cyst [40, 47], and adenomatoid odontogenic tumor [48], may be given a place in the differential diagnosis of NPDCs. The radiographic appearance of a periapical cyst/granuloma with a maxillary central incisor tooth often simulates that of an asymmetric NPDC. However, a periapical cyst usually involves the periapical region of non-vital teeth with a discontinuity of the lamina dura. NPDCs typically appear as well-delineated, round/ovoid/pear/heart-shaped radiolucencies in between the roots of a vital maxillary central incisor with a continuous lamina dura. In addition, a shift in the horizontal angulation alters the position of an NPDC, whereas the periapical cyst sustains its location around the maxillary central incisors periapex [17, 37, 44, 46]. In such situations, the pulp vitality test is essential to rule out lesions of endodontic origin [17, 18, 37, 40, 43].

A positive pulp vitality test with the associated teeth was seen in the present case, thus negating any periapical inflammatory lesion.

NPDCs may be clinically differentiated from a widened IF by aspiration of the lesion. An ill-defined radiolucency with a diameter of 0.6–0.8 cm in the maxillary central incisor region is often considered a wide IF. On the other hand, NPDCS usually appear as well-circumscribed, spherical radiolucent lesions, often with the superior cystic margin at a higher position than that of an IF [36, 37, 44].

Odontogenic keratocysts often exhibit an aggressive growth pattern and appear as ostelytic lesions with defined borders in the inter radicular/periapical areas of maxillary anterior teeth. However, they are mostly seen as multilocular radiolucent lesions in the mandibular posterior teeth [40]. Furthermore, microscopically, the cystic lumen is composed of a "cheesy" material, often with a parakeratinized epithelium lining [48].

Nasolabial cysts are soft tissue cysts and do not exhibit bone involvement, hence not apparent on the radiographic examination. In addition, the nasolabial cysts most commonly occur in the nasolabial sulcus, lateral to the midline [40, 47].

Adenomatoid odontogenic tumors most commonly occur in the maxillary anterior teeth region of young females. The radiolucency extends apically beyond the cementoenamel junction. In addition, these lesions display a mixed radiolucent-radiopaque radiographic pattern [48].

Enucleation, marsupialization, and decompression are the frequently employed treatment regimens. NPDCs are generally managed with enucleation, although marsupialization is recommended for large aggressive cystic lesions [18]. Cystic aspiration is generally performed before surgical enucleation. Surgical enucleation has a favorable prognosis and low recurrence rates. [35]. Malignant transformation of NPDCs is an extremely uncommon complication [41].

In our case, the lesion was surgically enucleated, and uneventful postoperative healing was observed. There was no recurrence during the 3-month follow-up period.

The main limitation in this case report was that a CBCT scan could not be performed due to the lack of facility and the patient's unwillingness due to financial constraints. Hence, a 3D extent of the lesion, the precise localization of the mesiodens, and its relation with the contiguous structures could not be ascertained. The 2D radiographic imaging (IOPAR and panoramic radiography) performed in this case was not sufficient to ascertain the 3D localization of the mesiodens and its relationship with the cystic lesion and adjacent vital structures.

4. Conclusion

Mesiodens seen in the maxillary anterior tooth region is the most frequently occurring supernumerary teeth. However, NPDCs in association with mesiodens are an extremely uncommon finding with only three reported cases to date. This study aims to report a case of NPDC with an impacted inverted mesiodens. Surgical enucleation was carried out and favorable healing with no recurrences was observed during the 3-month follow-up.

5. Recommendations

(i) A 3D radiographic examination, such as CBCT, is essential to delineate the exact shape, orientation, and location of the mesiodens, and also to evaluate their relationship with the contiguous vital structures.

(ii) NPDCs should also be given a place in the differential diagnosis of the radiolucent lesions in the anterior maxillary region.

(iii) Pulp vitality should be carried out to exclude the lesions of endodontic origin and ensure precise diagnosis and treatment strategy.

6. Patient Feedback

The patient experienced uneventful favorable healing after the enucleation of the cystic lesion and was completely satisfied with the treatment protocol. The patient has been carefully examined and followed up for 3 months, during maintenance visits scheduled every 4 weeks. The patient did not report any signs of recurrences and was completely asymptomatic during the follow-up period.

Consent

Written informed consent has been obtained from the patient.

Acknowledgments

Self-funded.

References

[1] A. Lao, S. Bi, H. Cheng, L. Tiehan, H. Shengbin, and Z. Shufan, "A combination of kissing molars, maxillary bilateral supernumerary teeth and macrodontia: a rare case report," *BMC Oral Health*, vol. 20, no. 1, p. 112, 2020.

[2] S. Hasan, S. A. Ahmed, and L. B. Reddy, "Dentigerous cyst in association with impacted inverted mesiodens: report of a rare case with a brief review of literature," *International Journal of Applied & Basic Medical Research*, vol. 4, no. 3, pp. 61–64, 2014.

[3] D. M. Talaat, I. Y. Hachim, M. M. Afifi, I. M. Taalat, and M. A. ElKateb, "Assessment of risk factors and molecular biomarkers in children with supernumerary teeth: a single-center study," *BMC Oral Health*, vol. 22, no. 1, p. 117, 2022.

[4] S. M. Mallinneni, "Supernumerary teeth: review of the literature with recent updates," *Conference Papes in Science*, vol. 2014, p. 6, 2014.

[5] T. P. Witcher, S. Brand, J. R. Gwilliam, and F. McDonald, "Assessment of the anterior maxilla in orthodontic patients using upper anterior occlusal radiographs and dental panoramic tomography: a comparison," *Oral Surgery, Oral Medicine, Oral Pathology, Oral Radiology, and Endodontics*, vol. 109, no. 5, pp. 765–774, 2010.

[6] R. P. Anthonappa, N. M. King, A. B. Rabie, and S. K. Mallineni, "Reliability of panoramic radiographs for identifying supernumerary teeth in children," *International Journal of Paediatric Dentistry*, vol. 22, no. 1, pp. 37–43, 2012.

[7] S. K. Mallineni, R. P. Anthonappa, and N. M. King, "Reliability of horizontal and vertical tube shift techniques in the localisation of supernumerary teeth," *European Archives of Paediatric Dentistry*, vol. 17, no. 6, pp. 455–460, 2016.

[8] C. A. Clark, "A method of ascertaining the relative position of unerupted teeth by means of film radiographs," *Proceedings of the Royal Society of Medicine*, vol. 3, no. Odontol_Sect, pp. 87–90, 1910.

[9] J. J. Keur, "Radiographic localization techniques," *Australian Dental Journal*, vol. 31, no. 2, pp. 86–90, 1986.

[10] C. Kuwada, Y. Ariji, M. Fukuda et al., "Deep learning systems for detecting and classifying the presence of impacted supernumerary teeth in the maxillary incisor region on panoramic radiographs," *Oral Surgery, Oral Medicine, Oral Pathology, Oral Radiology*, vol. 130, no. 4, pp. 464–469, 2020.

[11] E. G. Ha, K. J. Jeon, Y. H. Kim, J. Y. Kim, and S. S. Han, "Automatic detection of mesiodens on panoramic radiographs using artificial intelligence," *Scientific Reports*, vol. 11, no. 1, p. 23061, 2021.

[12] X. Ma, Y. Jiang, H. Ge et al., "Epidemiological, clinical, radiographic characterization of non-syndromic supernumerary teeth in Chinese children and adolescents," *Oral Diseases*, vol. 27, no. 4, pp. 981–992, 2021.

[13] K. S. Swanson, G. E. Kaugars, and J. C. Gunsolley, "Nasopalatine duct cyst: an analysis of 334 cases," *Journal of Oral and Maxillofacial Surgery*, vol. 49, no. 3, pp. 268–271, 1991.

[14] A. W. Meyer, "A unique supernumerary para-nasal sinus directly above superior incisors," *Journal of Anatomy and Physiology*, vol. 48, pp. 118–120, 1914.

[15] M. Shear and P. M. Speight, *Cysts of the Oral and Maxillofacial Regions*, Blackwell Munksgaard, Oxford, 4th edition, 2007.

[16] D. Gopal, A. Telang, L. A. Telang, K. Loganathan, and B. T. Reddy, "Nasopalatine duct cyst associated with a mesiodens: misdiagnosis or missed diagnosis?," *Journal of Clinical and Diagnostic Research*, vol. 9, no. 5, pp. ZD21–ZD22, 2015.

[17] A. R. Tariq Salamm, V. Parthiban, Gopinath, and R. Karpagam, "Extensive nasopalatine duct cyst causing nasolabial protrusion," *Indian Journal of Multidisciplinary Dentistry*, vol. 1, no. 5, pp. 285–288, 2011.

[18] C. Bereket and M. Kaynar, "Nasopalatine duct cyst concurrent with supernumerary tooth: a case report," *Journal of Dental Faculty of Atatürk University*, vol. 23, no. 1, pp. 98–102, 2013.

[19] M. Barham, S. Okada, M. Hisatomi et al., "Influence of mesiodens on adjacent teeth and the timing of its safe removal," *Imaging Science in Dentistry*, vol. 52, no. 1, pp. 67–74, 2022.

[20] R. P. Anthonappa, N. M. King, and A. B. Rabie, "Diagnostic tools used to predict the prevalence of supernumerary teeth: a meta-analysis," *Dento Maxillo Facial Radiology*, vol. 41, no. 6, pp. 444–449, 2012.

[21] J. Alarcón, J. Guzmán, T. S. Masuko, P. N. Caceres, and R. Fuentes, "Non-syndromic familial mesiodens: presentation of three cases," *Diagnostics*, vol. 12, no. 8, p. 1869, 2022.

[22] J. Kong, Z. Peng, T. Zhong et al., "Clinical analysis of approach selection of extraction of maxillary embedded mesiodens in children," *Disease Markers*, vol. 2022, 2022.

[23] F. Ata-Ali, J. Ata-Ali, D. Peñarrocha-Oltra, and M. Peñarrocha-Diago, "Prevalence, etiology, diagnosis, treatment and complications of supernumerary teeth," *Journal of Clinical and Experimental Dentistry*, vol. 6, no. 4, pp. e414–e418, 2014.

[24] L. D. Rajab and M. A. Hamdan, "Supernumerary teeth: review of the literature and a survey of 152 cases," *International Journal of Paediatric Dentistry*, vol. 12, no. 4, pp. 244–254, 2002.

[25] Y. Kim, T. Jeong, J. Kim, J. Shin, and S. Kim, "Effects of mesiodens on adjacent permanent teeth: a retrospective study in Korean children based on cone-beam computed tomography," *International Journal of Paediatric Dentistry*, vol. 28, no. 2, pp. 161–169, 2018.

[26] D. G. Liu, W. L. Zhang, Z. Y. Zhang, Y. T. Wu, and X. C. Ma, "Three-dimensional evaluations of supernumerary teeth using cone-beam computed tomography for 487 cases," *Oral Surgery, Oral Medicine, Oral Pathology, Oral Radiology, and Endodontics*, vol. 103, no. 3, pp. 403–411, 2007.

[27] P. L. Alberto, "Surgical exposure of impacted teeth," *Oral and Maxillofacial Surgery Clinics of North America*, vol. 32, no. 4, pp. 561–570, 2020.

[28] O. Sarne, Y. Shapira, S. Blumer et al., "Supernumerary teeth in the maxillary anterior region: the dilemma of early versus late surgical intervention," *The Journal of Clinical Pediatric Dentistry*, vol. 42, no. 1, pp. 55–61, 2018.

[29] R. S. M. Omer, R. P. Anthonappa, and N. M. King, "Determination of the optimum time for surgical removal of unerupted anterior supernumerary teeth," *Pediatric Dentistry*, vol. 32, no. 1, pp. 14–20, 2010.

[30] S. Gupta and N. Marwah, "Impacted supernumerary teeth-early or delayed intervention: decision making dilemma?," *International Journal of Clinical Pediatric Dentistry*, vol. 5, no. 3, pp. 226–230, 2012.

[31] C. Mason, N. Azam, R. D. Holt, and D. C. Rule, "A retrospective study of unerupted maxillary incisors associated with supernumerary teeth," *The British Journal of Oral & Maxillofacial Surgery*, vol. 38, no. 1, pp. 62–65, 2000.

[32] S. Harbilen and G. Magat, "Evaluation of anatomical and morphological characteristics of the nasopalatine canal in a Turkish population by cone beam computed tomography," *Folia Morphologica*, vol. 77, no. 3, pp. 527–535, 2018.

[33] A. I. Linjawi and H. Y. A. Marghalani, "Relationship between maxillary central incisors and incisive canal: a cone-beam computed tomography study," *Folia Morphologica*, vol. 81, no. 2, pp. 458–463, 2022.

[34] P. Milanovic, D. Selakovic, M. Vasiljevic et al., "Morphological characteristics of the nasopalatine canal and the relationship with the anterior maxillary bone-a cone beam computed tomography study," *Diagnostics*, vol. 11, no. 5, p. 915, 2021.

[35] S. Lake, J. Iwanaga, S. Kikuta, R. J. Oskouian, M. Loukas, and R. S. Tubbset, "The incisive canal: a comprehensive review," *Cureus*, vol. 10, no. 7, p. e3069, 2018.

[36] S. Shylaja, K. Balaji, and A. Krishna, "Nasopalatine duct cyst: report of a case with review of literature," *Indian Journal of Otolaryngology and Head & Neck Surgery*, vol. 65, no. 4, pp. 385–388, 2013.

[37] J. E. Francolí, N. A. Marqués, L. B. Aytés, and C. G. Escoda, "Nasopalatine duct cyst: report of 22 cases and review of the literature," *Medicina Oral, Patología Oral y Cirugía Bucal*, vol. 13, no. 7, pp. E438–E443, 2008.

[38] R. Vasconcelos, M. F. de Aguiar, W. Castro, V. C. de Araújo, and R. Mesquita, "Retrospective analysis of 31 cases of nasopalatine duct cyst," *Oral Diseases*, vol. 5, no. 4, pp. 325–328, 1999.

[39] N. Ely, E. C. Sheehy, and F. McDonald, "Nasopalatine duct cyst: a case report," *International Journal of Paediatric Dentistry*, vol. 11, no. 2, pp. 135–137, 2001.

[40] I. L. Cavalcante, C. C. Barros, J. L. Cunha et al., "Clinicopathologic features of nasopalatine duct cysts: a retrospective study in two Brazilian oral and maxillofacial pathology referral centers," *Medicina Oral, Patología Oral y Cirugía Bucal*, vol. 26, no. 5, pp. e676–e683, 2021.

[41] M. J. Lang, Y. P. Lee, M. J. Hwang, and C. P. Chiang, "Nasopalatine duct cyst—case report," *Journal of Dental Sciences*, vol. 16, no. 3, pp. 1047–1049, 2021.

[42] P. Scolozzi, A. Martinez, M. Richter, and T. Lombardi, "A nasopalatine duct cyst in a 7-year-old child," *Pediatric Dentistry*, vol. 30, no. 6, pp. 530–534, 2008.

[43] J. D. Gnanasekhar, S. V. Walvekar, A. M. Al-Kandari, and Y. Al-Duwairi, "Misdiagnosis and mismanagement of a nasopalatine duct cyst and its corrective therapy. A case report," *Oral Surgery, Oral Medicine, Oral Pathology, Oral Radiology, and Endodontics*, vol. 80, no. 4, pp. 465–470, 1995.

[44] M. Aparna, A. Chakravarthy, S. R. Acharya, and R. Radhakrishnan, "A clinical report demonstrating the significance of distinguishing a nasopalatine duct cyst from a radicular cyst," *BML Case Reports*, vol. 2014, p. bcr2013200329, 2014.

[45] D. Sankar, V. Muthusubramanian, J. A. Nathan, R. S. Nutalapati, Y. M. Jose, and Y. N. Kumar, "Aggressive nasopalatine duct cyst with complete destruction of palatine bone," *Journal of Pharmacy & Bioallied Sciences*, vol. 8, no. 5, pp. 185–188, 2016.

[46] S. C. White and M. J. Pharoah, "Cysts of the jaws," in *Oral Radiology: Principles and Interpretation*, S. C. White and M. J. Pharoah, Eds., pp. 11661167, Mosby-Elsevier, Maryland Heights, MO, 5th edition edition, 2019.

[47] B. T. G. Rodrigues, A. Fischer, M. J. Romañach, B. A. B. de Andrade, N. de Almeida Freire, and M. S. Israel, "Nasolabial cyst in an elderly patient: a case report," *Gerodontology*, vol. 38, no. 3, pp. 317–320, 2021.

[48] Q. Jiang, G. Z. Xu, C. Yang, C. Q. Yu, D. M. He, and Z. Y. Zhang, "Dentigerous cysts associated with impacted supernumerary teeth in the anterior maxilla," *Experimental and Therapeutic Medicine*, vol. 2, no. 5, pp. 805–809, 2011.

4

A Rare Anatomical Finding: Bilateral Accessory Mental Foramen

Zülfikar Karabıyık[1] and Mustafa Kıranatlı[2]

[1]Kütahya Health Science University, Dentistry Faculty, Department of Oral and Maxillofacial Surgery, Turkey
[2]Kütahya Health Science University, Dentistry Faculty, Department of Oral and Maxillofacial Radiology, Turkey

Correspondence should be addressed to Zülfikar Karabıyık; zulfikarkarabiyik60@gmail.com

Academic Editor: Darko Macan

Aim. Accessory mental foramen (AMF) is a not common anatomical variation. During the surgical procedures involving the mandible such as implant surgery, periapical surgery, jaw surgeries, and periapical surgery and enucleation of pathologies at the mental region, obvious attention should be given to prevent postoperative sequelae. *Case Report.* Orthopantomograph (OPG) is routinely taken to visualize the maxillofacial region at a dental clinic. OPG shows exactly upper and lower jaw and teeth but superficially reveals some pathology or anatomic variation. It misses sometimes an anatomic landmark such as AMF. As the surgery is planned to a maxillofacial region, a detailed knowledge should be known before going into surgery to not interfere with anatomic landmarks. A 52-year-old male patient was referred to Kütahya Health Science University Dental Hospital, Turkey, to rehabilitate his bilateral partial edentulous lower jaw region. Implant surgery was planned in our patient. OPG was taken to evaluate the maxillofacial region but was unremarkable. Before the implant surgery, CBCT was obtained from our patient. CBCT and a three-dimensional reconstructed model of the male patient showed bilateral accessory mental foramen (AMF). *Conclusion.* Accessory mental foramen (AMF) carries additional innervation to the chin, mandibular anterior gingiva, and mental region. Reflection and protection of the AMF during the surgery can prevent hemorrhage and neurosensory disturbance at the mental region and can improve quality of life for the patient. CBCT has higher precision but also a higher price and radiation dose. Although anatomical variations are uncommon, they can be found on digital panoramic radiographs but in limited percentage.

1. Introduction

The path and shape of the mandibular canal and mental foramen are significant milestones in surgical operations performed on the mandible such as implant placement, periapical surgeries, enucleations of pathologies, surgical correction of jaw deformities, and extraction of impacted teeth [1]. The mental foramen (MF) is placed on the anterolateral side of the mandible [2, 3]. MF is generally located in an inferior position which is between root apexes of the bicuspids. It usually opens a superior-posterior position and carries neurovascular bundle named as the mental nerve. The mental nerve branches while it was exiting from the MF. The mental nerve innervates the skin of the mental and lower lip region. A buccal mucous membrane and buccal gingiva from the lower midline to the second premolar region is also innervated by the mental nerve [4].

Any foramen in addition to MF is regarded as accessory mental foramen (AMF) [2, 5]. Accessory foramen showing a connection with the mandibular canal is defined as accessory mental foramen, and accessory foramen revealing no connection with the mandibular canal is defined as nutrient foramen [6]. AMF is generally smaller than MF [7]. It can be found in the apical region of the first molar and in the posterior or superior region of the mental foramen as in our case. Detailed knowledge regarding the possible location, incidence, shape, and size of the AMF helps clinician to perform local anesthesia correctly and adequately. Identification of AMF on radiograph prevents misdiagnosis of bone lesions [8]. Identification and protection of AMF result in operation

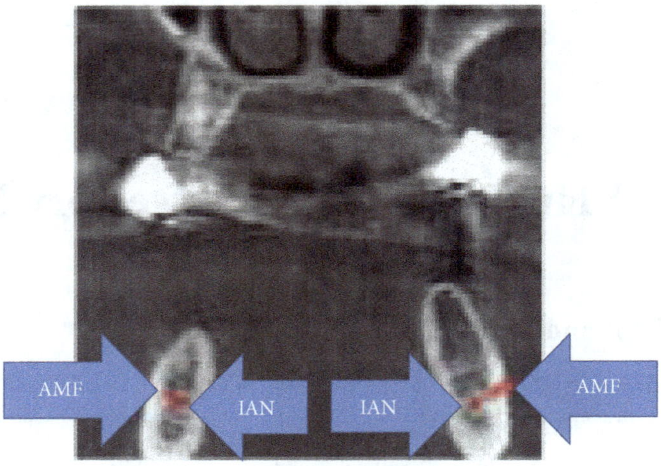

Figure 1: Right and left AMF at coronal CBCT.

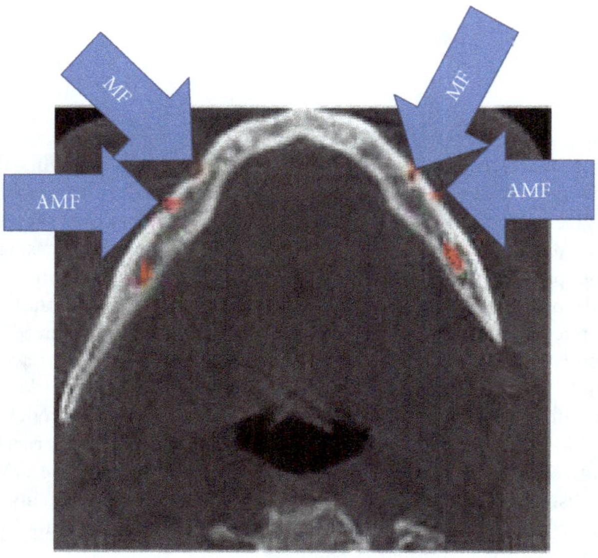

Figure 2: Right and left AMF at axial CBCT.

involving the mental region with minimal nerve injury and morbidity [9].

The present paper reports a case of AMF using CBCT.

2. A Case Report

A 52-year-old male patient came to the Department of Oral and Maxillofacial Surgery, Kütahya Health Science University Dental Hospital, Turkey, for the implant rehabilitation. His medical history was unremarkable. On the clinical examination, he was partially edentulous. On the panoramic radiograph, MF was identified. For the detailed examination, CBCT was obtained from the patient. Bilateral small round-shaped radiolucency distal to MF was seen at the axial CBCT section and a three-dimensional reconstructed model. These small foramina were connected to the inferior alveolar nerve canal (IAN) (Figure 1). It was referred to as AMF.

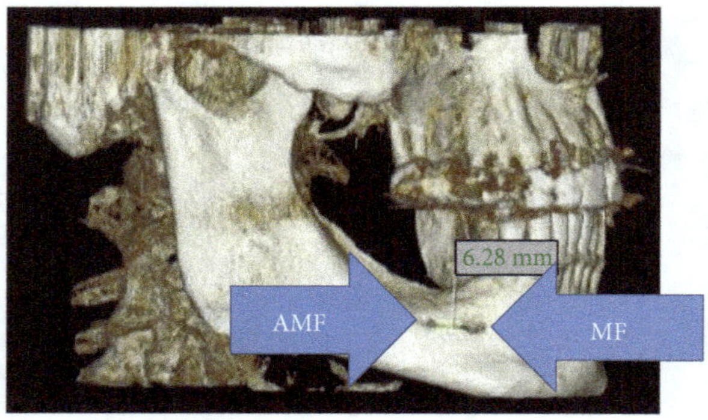

Figure 3: Right AMF at reconstructed CBCT.

3. Discussion

MF is generally only one exit on each side of the lower jaw. MF is not developed until the 12th gestational week. Balcioğlu and Kocaelli asserted that splitting of the mental nerve from the inferior alveolar nerve before the exit to mental foramen may be a reason for the formation of AMF [2]. Double mental foramina are reported in literature [10]. AMF can change from a small indistinct bar to separate foramina [11]. Sawyer et al. added that the number of AMF can change from one to three foramina [4]. In the present case, two distinct foramina distal to MF were seen at axial CBCT and 3D reconstructed model bilaterally (Figures 2–4). Prevalence of AMF ranges from 1.4 to 12% [11–14]. Studies showed no gender differences according to the incidence of AMF [2]. Paraskevas et al. studied cadavers and found that the average diameter of AMF was 1 mm [8]. In our case, the diameter of the AMF was found to be 1.65 mm at the right side and 1.52 mm at the left site (Figures 5 and 6). AMF incidence can differ in ethnic groups [15]. Its incidence does not differ in right and left sides. Paraskevas et al. found that the mean distance from MF to AMF is 5.24 mm [8]. In our case, the distance from the MF to AMF was found to be 6.28 mm at the right side and 3.97 mm at the left side. MF can be observed by periapical radiography and OPG, but it can be detected with CBCT

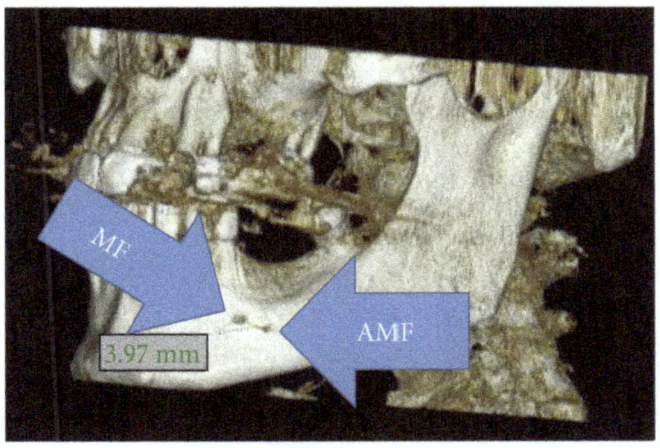

Figure 4: Left AMF at reconstructed CBCT.

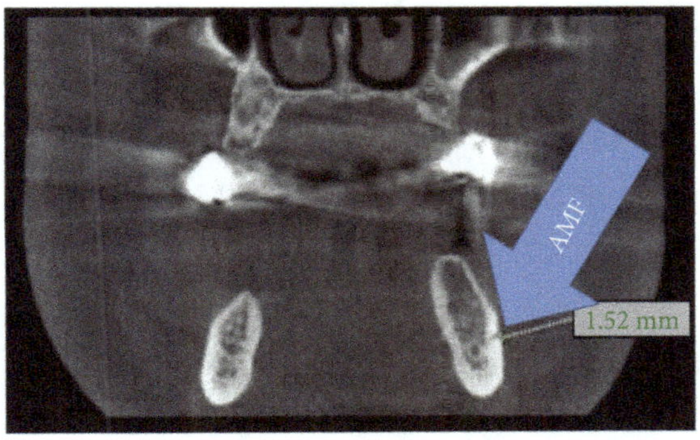

Figure 5: Left AMF at coronal CBCT.

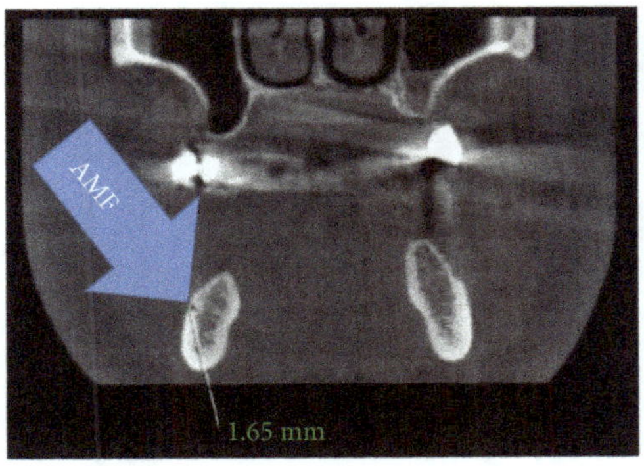

Figure 6: Right AMF at coronal CBCT.

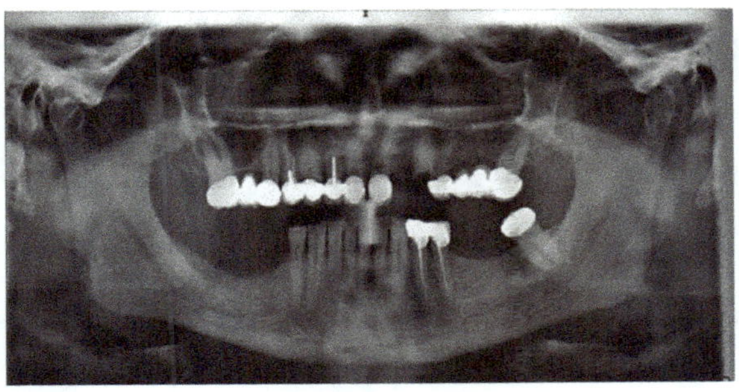

Figure 7: Patient's orthopantomograph.

without exception [2]. AMF was detected on CBCT not on orthopantomograph in our case (Figure 7).

While it can be difficult to differentiate MF from AMF on radiographs, the presence of connection between the mandibular canal and such foramina supports the case of AMF.

4. Conclusıon

Neurosensory sequelae during the surgery involving the mental region are not scarce. In order to avoid neurovascular complications during the surgery, a possibility of AMF should be kept in mind. Knowledge about anatomic variations can prevent the complications and increase the quality of life after the surgery. CBCT has higher precision but also a higher price and radiation dose. Although anatomical variations (AMF) are uncommon, they can be found on digital panoramic radiographs but in limited percentage. AMF is detected on CBCT without exception.

References

[1] M. Naitoh, K. Yoshida, K. Nakahara, K. Gotoh, and E. Ariji, "Demonstration of the accessory mental foramen using rotational panoramic radiography compared with cone-beam computed tomography," *Clinical Oral Implant Research*, vol. 22, no. 12, pp. 1415–1419, 2011.

[2] H. A. Balcioglu and H. Kocaelli, "Accessory mental foramen," *North American Journal of Medical Sciences*, vol. 1, no. 6, pp. 314-315, 2009.

[3] R. Singh, "Evaluation of position, shape, size and incidence of mental foramen and accessory mental foramen in Indian adult human skulls," *Anatomy*, vol. 5, pp. 23–29, 2011.

[4] D. R. Sawyer, L. M. Kiely, and A. M. Pyle, "The frequency of accessory mental foramina in four ethnic groups," *Archieves of Oral Biology*, vol. 43, no. 5, pp. 417–420, 1998.

[5] S. Gupta and S. J. Soni, "Study of anatomical variations and incidence of mental foramen and accessory mental foramen in dry human mandibles," *National Journal Of Medical Research*, vol. 2, pp. 28–30, 2012.

[6] Y. Sisman, H. Sahman, E. A. Sekerci, T. T. Tokmak, Y. Aksu, and E. Mavili, "Detection and characterization of the mandibular accessory buccal foramen using CT," *Dentomaxillofacial Radiology*, vol. 41, no. 7, pp. 558–563, 2012.

[7] N. S. T. Imada, R. S. P. M. L. Fernandes, B. S. Centurion, C. de Oliveira-Santos, H. M. Honório, and I. R. F. Rubira-Bullen, "Accessory mental foramina: prevalence, position and diameter assessed by cone-beam computed tomography and digital panoramic radiographs," *Clinical Oral Implants Research*, vol. 25, no. 2, pp. e94–e99, 2014.

[8] G. Paraskevas, A. Mavrodi, and K. Natsis, "Accessory mental foramen: an anatomical study on dry mandibles and review of the literature," *Mund Keifer Gesichtschirurgie*, vol. 19, no. 2, pp. 177–181, 2015.

[9] A. Voljevica, E. Talovic, and A. Hasanović, "Morphological and morphometric analysis of the shape, position, number and size of mental foramen on human mandibles," *Acta Medica Academica*, vol. 44, no. 1, pp. 31–38, 2015.

[10] N. J. Serman, "The mandibular incisive foramen," *Journal of Anatomy*, vol. 167, pp. 195–198, 1989.

[11] J. Kieser, D. Kuzmanovic, A. Payne, J. Dennison, and P. Herbison, "Patterns of emergence of the human mental nerve," *Archives of Oral Biology*, vol. 47, no. 10, pp. 743–747, 2002.

[12] C. Igarashi, K. Kobayashi, A. Yamamoto, Y. Morita, and M. Tanaka, "Double mental foramina of the mandible on computed tomography images: a case report," *Oral Radiology*, vol. 20, no. 2, pp. 68–71, 2004.

[13] L. B. Çağirankaya and H. Kansu, "An accessory mental foramen: a case report," *The Journal of Contemporary Dental Practice*, vol. 9, no. 1, pp. 98–104, 2008.

[14] H. Toh, J. Kodama, M. Yanagisako, and T. Ohmori, "Anatomical study of the Accessory mental foramen and the distribution of Its nerve," *Okajimas Folia Anatomica Japonica*, vol. 69, no. 2-3, pp. 85–88, 1992.

[15] N. S. Mamatha, N. S. Kedarnath, M. Singh, and G. Patel, "Accessory mental nerve: a case report," *Journal of Clinical and Diagnostic Research*, vol. 7, pp. 2078-2079, 2013.

5

Actinomycosis of the Lower Lip: Report of a Case

Manabu Shigeoka,[1] Daisuke Takeda,[2] and Masaya Akashi[2]

[1]*Division of Pathology, Department of Pathology, Kobe University Graduate School of Medicine, Kobe, Japan*
[2]*Division of Oral and Maxillofacial Surgery, Department of Surgery Related, Kobe University Graduate School of Medicine, Kobe, Japan*

Correspondence should be addressed to Manabu Shigeoka; shigeokamanabu@gmail.com

Academic Editor: Paolo Giacomo Arduino

Actinomycosis is usually a chronic infectious disease caused by *Actinomyces* species, which are anaerobic Gram-positive bacteria that normally colonize the human oral cavity and digestive and urogenital tracts. Although this lesion often occurs on soft tissue around the mandible, cases localized in the lip are very uncommon. We encountered a patient with actinomycosis in the lower lip. A 76-year-old woman with a 5-mm submucosal nodule of the lower lip was referred to our hospital from a dental clinic. The clinical diagnosis was a benign submucosal tumor. Total excision and histological examination were conducted. No oral antibiotic therapy was prescribed. The histological diagnosis was actinomycosis. The postoperative course was uneventful with no signs of recurrence during the 6 months after surgery.

1. Introduction

Actinomycosis is a chronic disease caused by the anaerobic Gram-positive bacterium Actinomyces, and *Actinomyces israelii* is known as the most common causative organism [1, 2]. Although cervicofacial actinomycosis is the most frequent clinical form of actinomycosis, this disease is rare nowadays due to its high sensitivity to most antibiotics and the general improvement in oral hygiene [3]. Actinomycosis of the lip is very rare; we identified only six cases in the international literature in a search of the PubMed database using the search terms "actinomycosis" and "lip" [3–8]. In this report, we present an additional case of actinomycosis of the lip and discuss the diagnostics, therapeutics, and pathogenesis.

2. Case Presentation

A 76-year-old woman with a 2-month history of a submucosal mass on her lower lip was referred to our hospital. She had not received any treatment for the lesion as she had no history of fever, pain, or trauma. An intraoral clinical examination revealed a nonmovable asymptomatic submucosal nodule ~5 mm in diameter on the right side of the lower lip (Figure 1(a)). A whitish color with a creamy tinge was visible through the mucosa. Dental panoramic radiography provided little useful information (Figure 1(b)). The patient had a history of fatty liver, cholecystolithiasis, and spinal canal stenosis.

The clinical diagnosis of a possible benign submucosal tumor was based on the clinical examination findings and the lesion's appearance. A complete excision was performed with the patient under local anesthesia to obtain the histological diagnosis. The surgeon decided not to prescribe antibiotics because the excision was not complex.

Low-power microscopy revealed the bacterial colony within a dilated salivary gland duct in a submucosal area which was covered by non-atypical squamous epithelium (Figure 2(a)). An abscess with numerous inflammatory cells was observed surrounding the bacterial colony. In the high-power view, the colony consisted of a central mass of bacteria surrounded by an eosinophilic club-like structure arranged in radiating rosette pattern with calcification and a dense infiltration of inflammatory cells including neutrophils (Figure 2(b)). The histological diagnosis was actinomycosis. At 6 months after the lesion's excision, the wound had healed well and no symptoms of recurrence were observed.

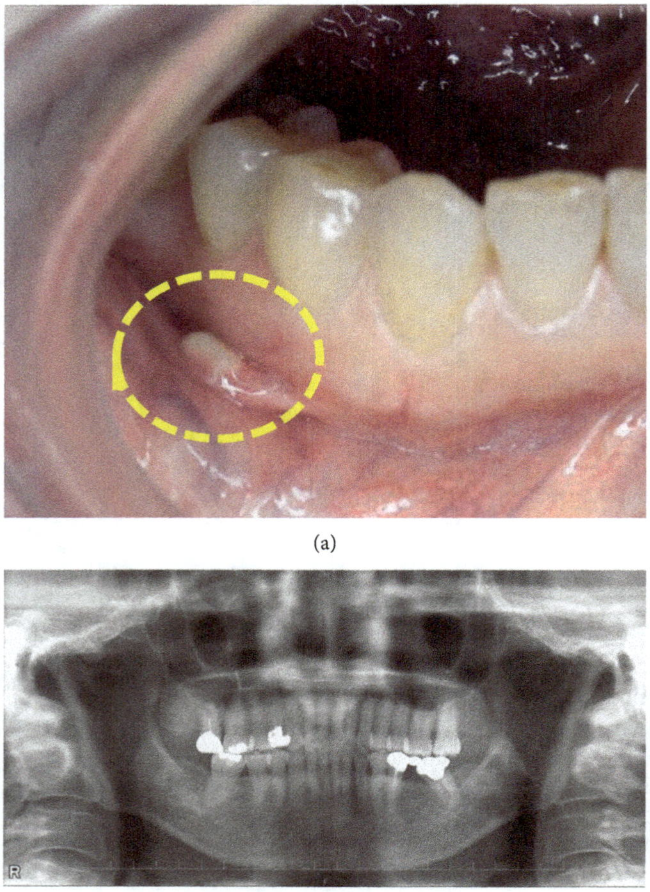

(a)

(b)

FIGURE 1: Intraoral clinical findings and imaging findings of the 76-year-old female patient. (a) A whitish-colored submucosal mass covered with normal mucosa was observed on the mucosal aspect of the right lower lip. The *dotted line* indicates the extent of the lesion. This lesion was 5 mm in max. Dia. and was clinically diagnosed as a benign tumor. (b) Dental panoramic radiography provided no significant findings that seemed to be associated with the mass.

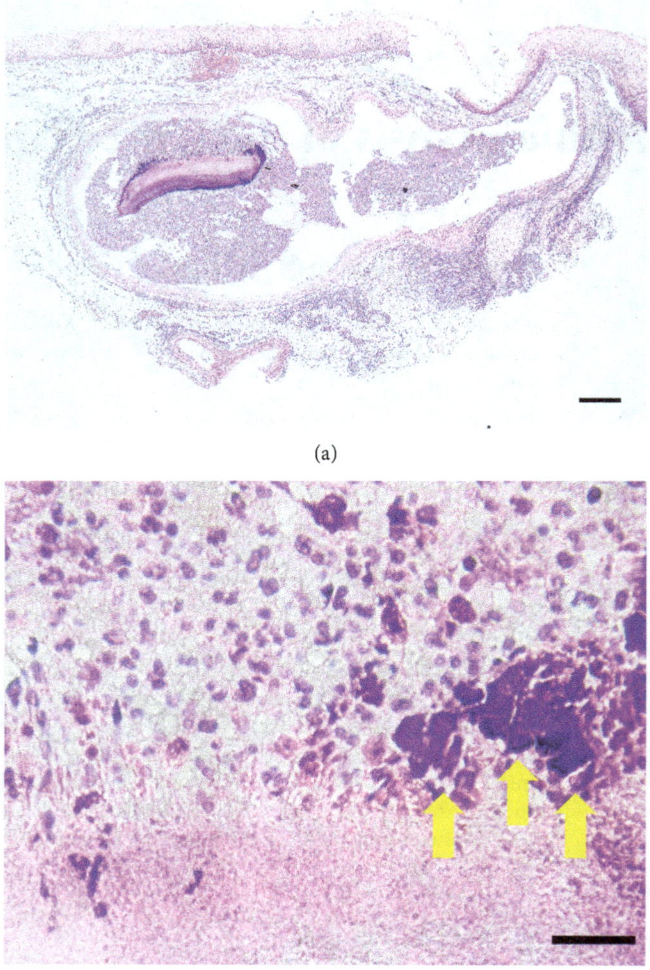

(a)

(b)

FIGURE 2: Histological findings. (a) Low-power image. The lesion consisted of an abscess formation with a basophilic bacterial colony contained within a dilated salivary gland duct. Squamous epithelium with little reactive cell atypia covering them was observed. Scale bar: 20 μm. (b) High-power image. The central bacterial colony was characterized by peripheral eosinophilic club-like structures with calcification (*arrows*) and surrounded by inflammatory cells including neutrophils. Scale bar: 200 μm.

3. Discussion

Several clinical types of actinomycosis have been described, including actinomycosis at a cervicofacial, thoracic, abdominal, or female genitalia site; ~50% of the reported cases occurred in the cervicofacial region [9, 10]. The typical presentation of cervicofacial actinomycosis is the formation of an abscess with a fistula on the skin surface or the oral mucosa and an induration of the soft tissue [2]. Although poor dental hygiene, oral mucosal trauma, and dental intervention have been considered as predisposing conditions for this disease [2], actinomycosis is rare nowadays due to its high sensitivity to most antibiotics and the general improvement in oral hygiene [3]. The majority of cervicofacial sites affected by actinomycosis are the parotids and the mandible [11]. From the anatomical viewpoint, it is speculated that the lip is unlikely to be infected with anaerobic Gram-positive bacteria. In fact, we identified only six cases of actinomycosis of lip in a search of the PubMed database [3–8]. We have presented a patient with actinomycosis of the lip treated by surgical excision and would like to stress three important points learned from this case.

First, an excisional biopsy is practical for the final diagnosis of actinomycosis involving the lip. A histological examination plus bacterial culture has been considered the gold standard for diagnosing cervicofacial actinomycosis [2]. However, in the previous reports of actinomycosis of the lip, five of six cases were not clinically considered a bacterial infection [7, 8]. Consistent with these reports, in the present case, the clinician initially suspected a benign submucosal tumor rather than an infection, and a bacterial culture was not performed. Moreover, it was reported that the results of culture tests may be negative in 50% of actinomycosis cases and suggested that a culture test has no role as a diagnostic aid in tongue actinomycosis [12].

Second, no considerable advantage in prescribing antibiotics may be obtained by treating actinomycosis with a small and limited lesion. Although it is known that actinomycosis can be treated with penicillin [2, 13], our patient was not prescribed antibiotics; because (a) the lesion was not clinically diagnosed as a bacterial infection and (b) the surgeon considered that the risk of postoperative infection was not high. The lesion was treated well by total excision only, and no evidence of recurrence was observed 6 months post-excision. The patient did not show any signs of a lowered immune system related to postoperative infection. It has been proposed that shorter courses of antibiotics are sufficient for small and localized cases with actinomycosis [3]. From the view of antibiotic resistance, it is important that dental clinicians use caution when prescribing antibiotics. The accumulation of further studies regarding the use of antibiotics in cases of small and localized actinomycosis is needed.

Third, we suspect that the lesion in our patient's case was due mainly to the bacterial infection via a duct of a minor salivary gland. Dental manipulation, soft tissue injury, odontogenic infection, poor oral hygiene, diabetes, immunosuppression, malnutrition, irradiation, and neoplasm have each been associated with cervicofacial actinomycosis [12]. Dental panoramic radiography did not reveal any significant findings that would seem to be associated with our patient's lesion, whereas microscopy demonstrated a colony of basophilic club-shaped bacteria arranged in a radiating pattern surrounded within a salivary duct, with normal squamous epithelium covering them. The patient had no history of trauma in the mucosa of her lower lip or at her presentation. Since the histological examination confirmed little reactive epithelial change plus inflammatory cell infiltration, the effects of trauma seem unlikely to apply in her case. The patient also had no history of the systemic conditions described above. However, although she had maintained good oral hygiene, an effect of dry mouth due to aging could not be ruled out. The lips can be mechanically cleaned by saliva, and we speculate that dry mouth caused the bacterial infection in our patient's case. In the dry condition of oral mucosa, bacteria may easily adhere to lip mucosa and invade a minor salivary duct. In fact, a case with the coexistence of actinomycosis and sialolithiasis in a submandibular gland caused by an oral dehydration condition has been reported [10].

In conclusion, a microscopic examination is essential to achieve an accurate diagnosis of actinomycosis involving the lip. Although oral antibiotic therapy may not be necessary for small and localized lesions, further studies are required to clarify this. Our patient's actinomycosis of the lower lip might have been caused by the bacterial infection via a duct of a minor salivary gland.

Authors' Contributions

M.S. was responsible for the manuscript drafting, literature search, and collection of clinical records. M.S. was responsible for the histological evaluation. D.T. was responsible for the collection of clinical records and the revision of the manuscript. M.A. supervised the work. All authors reviewed and accepted the final version of the manuscript.

Acknowledgments

We thank Prof. Tomoo Ito for the valuable discussions and histopathological suggestions and all technicians of the Division of Diagnostic Pathology, Department of Pathology, Kobe University for the excellent technical assistance.

References

[1] V. Kalioras, L. Thanos, S. Mylona, M. Pomoni, and N. Batakis, "Scalp actinomycosis mimicking soft tissue mass," *Dento Maxillo Facial Radiology*, vol. 35, no. 2, pp. 117–118, 2006.

[2] F. Valour, A. Sénéchal, C. Dupieux et al., "Actinomycosis: etiology, clinical features, diagnosis, treatment, and management," *Infection and Drug Resistance*, vol. 7, pp. 183–197, 2014.

[3] M. C. Lan, T. Y. Huang, T. Y. Lin, and M. Y. Lan, "Pathology quiz case 1: actinomycosis of the lip mimicking minor salivary gland tumor," *Archives of Otolaryngology Head & Neck Surgery*, vol. 133, no. 4, pp. 411–414, 2007.

[4] D. Kikiewicz, "A case of actinomycosis of the upper lip," *Czasopismo Stomatologiczne*, vol. 31, no. 2, pp. 187–189, 1978 (in Polish).

[5] S. Appiah-Anane and M. Tickle, "Actinomycosis – an unusual presentation," *The British Journal of Oral & Maxillofacial Surgery*, vol. 33, no. 4, pp. 248–249, 1995.

[6] J. Sánchez-Estella, M. T. Bordel-Gómez, E. Cardeñoso-Alvarez, and E. Garabito-Solovera, "Actinomycosis of the lip: an exceptional site," *Actas Dermo-Sifiliográficas*, vol. 100, no. 9, pp. 824–826, 2009 (in Spanish).

[7] Y. S. Lee, H. S. Sim, and S. K. Lee, "Actinomycosis of the upper lip," *Annals of Dermatology*, vol. 23, Suppl 1, pp. S131–S134, 2011.

[8] H. Kim, I. H. Park, W. K. Lee, J. E. Seol, S. Y. Jung, and H. Y. Wang, "Unusual clinical presentation of actinomycosis mimicking mucocele," *The Journal of Dermatology*, vol. 42, no. 7, pp. 746–747, 2015.

[9] I. Kolm, L. Aceto, M. Hombach, J. Kamarshev, J. Hafner, and M. Urosevic-Maiwald, "Cervicofacial actinomycosis: a long forgotten infectious complication of immunosuppression – report of a case and review of the literature," *Dermatology Online Journal*, vol. 20, no. 5, p. 22640, 2014.

[10] J. S. Kang, H. J. Choi, and M. S. Tak, "Actinomycosis and sialolithiasis in submandibular gland," *Arch Craniofac Surg*, vol. 16, no. 1, pp. 39–42, 2015.

[11] F. Palonta, G. Preti, N. Vione, and A. L. Cavalot, "Actinomycosis of the masseter muscle: report of a case and review of the literature," *The Journal of Craniofacial Surgery*, vol. 14, no. 6, pp. 915–918, 2003.

[12] R. Y. Al-Rawee, N. M. T. Jawhar, and M. M. Saeed, "Challenge dilemma of actinomycosis in the tongue: review and case report," *International Journal of Surgery Case Reports*, vol. 75, pp. 176–181, 2020.

[13] D. Patil, B. Siddaramappa, B. S. Manjunathswamy et al., "Primary cutaneous actinomycosis," *International Journal of Dermatology*, vol. 47, no. 12, pp. 1271–1273, 2008.

6

Active Peripheral Osteoma in the Mandibular Notch: A Longitudinal Clinical Report

Jun Sasaki,[1,2] Shogo Hasegawa,[1] Hitoshi Miyachi,[1] and Toru Nagao[1]

[1]*Department of Maxillofacial Surgery, School of Dentistry, Aichi-Gakuin University, 2-11 Suemori-Dori, Chikusa, Nagoya, Aichi 464-8651, Japan*
[2]*Department of Maxillofacial Surgery, Okazaki City Hospital, 3-1 Goshoai, Koryujicho, Okazaki, Aichi 444-8553, Japan*

Correspondence should be addressed to Shogo Hasegawa; shogo@dpc.aichi-gakuin.ac.jp

Academic Editor: Yasuhiro Morimoto

Osteomas are benign osteogenic tumors composed of mature compact or cancellous bone and are characterized by slow, painless growth. A peripheral osteoma located in the mandibular notch is extremely rare. Here, we describe the case of a 38-year-old woman with an active peripheral osteoma in the mandibular notch for long-term follow up. Surgical resection of the lesion was performed, which resulted in the improvement of the mandibular function and temporomandibular dysfunction. This is the first report of resection surgery after confirming the activity of peripheral osteoma by bone scintigraphy. Creating a three-dimensional model of the mandible promises an accurate surgical plan.

1. Introduction

Osteomas are benign tumors composed of mature compact or cancellous bone and are characterized by slow, painless growth [1–3]. They can be peripheral, central, or extraskeletal [4, 5]. Most peripheral osteomas are known to occur in the mandibular body, angle, condyle, or coronoid process [2, 4, 5]. The occurrence of a peripheral osteoma in the mandibular notch is extremely rare, with an incidence of 1.6% among mandibular peripheral osteoma cases [4, 5]. Although several studies have described peripheral osteomas of the jawbone, only eight cases of peripheral osteomas in the Sigmoid notch of the mandible have been reported.

We report the case of an active peripheral osteoma in the mandibular notch of a 38-year-old woman in whom we were able to clarify the temporal course of the disease.

2. Case Presentation

A 38-year-old woman with complaints of pain during mandibular movement was referred to our department by a dental clinic. She had no significant medical history, and she was not taking any medication. The patient was evaluated based on preoperative clinical manifestations, panoramic radiography, computed tomography (CT), magnetic resonance imaging (MRI), and radioisotope imaging (RI). Panoramic radiography revealed a circular radiopacity between the right mandibular condyle and the muscle process (Figure 1(d)). On reviewing the patient's panoramic radiograph taken at the age of 18 and 21 years, no osteoma was found in the mandibular notch (Figures 1(a) and 1(b)). At the age of 26, a bone bulge was found in the right mandibular notch (Figure 1(c)). CT showed a 13.3×12.8×10.0mm lesion showing Hounsfield units (HU) equivalent to that of the mandible, arising from the right mandibular notch (Figures 2(a) and 2(b)). MRI showed uniform hypointense trabecular bone, and there was no continuity of fat signals in the bone marrow, suggesting the exclusion of the lateral pterygoid muscle due to bone lesions (Figure 2(c)). RI showed significant uptake of Tc-99m (Figure 2(d)). Bone scintigraphy showed circular area of strong radioisotope accumulation with indistinct boundaries, consistent with lesion in right mandibular notch. No neurological symptoms of the

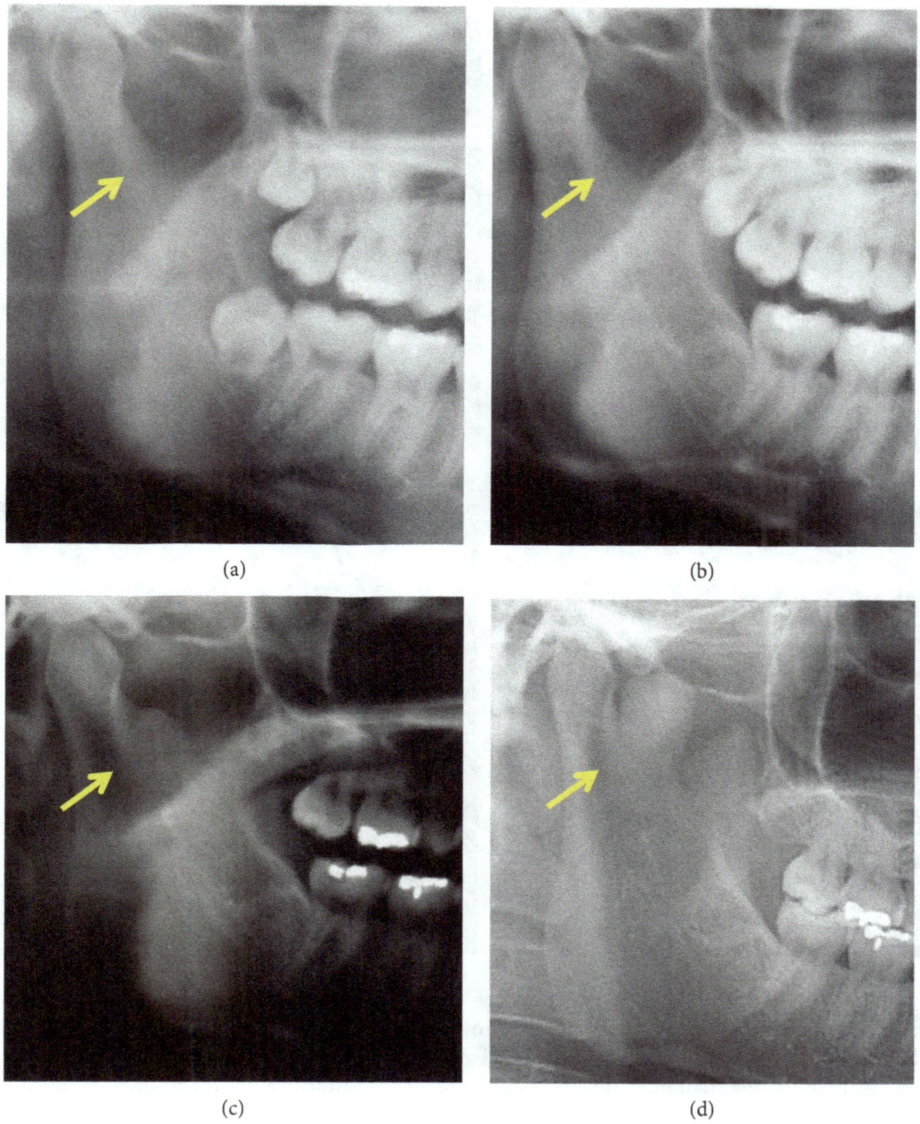

FIGURE 1: Time course of osteoma in the right mandibular notch by panoramic radiography. (a) At the age of 18, no osteoma was found in the right mandibular notch. (b) At the age of 21, no osteoma was found in the right mandibular notch. (c) At the age of 26, a bony bulge was found in the right mandibular notch. (d) At the age of 38, an oval radiodense mass was observed in the right mandibular notch.

mandible were observed, and there was no history of trauma or infection in the maxillofacial region. No abnormalities were found on blood or urine analysis. Based on these findings, the diagnosis of an active peripheral osteoma was suspected. Using the CT data and Mimics software® (version 23.0, Materialise, Leuven, Belgium), we created a three-dimensional (3D) model of the mandible (Figure 3) to facilitate an explanation to the patient. Resective surgery using an intraoral approach was planned. A fused deposition modeling 3D printer (da Vinci Mini w Plus, XYZ printing, Taiwan) and a thermoplastic resin (polylactic acid filament) were used to prepare the model.

On June 23, 2021, the entire tumor, including the portion that demonstrated Tc-99m uptake, was resected under general anesthesia. The myoprojection was temporarily dissected (Figure 4(a)), and the bone was repositioned and fixed with an absorbent plate (Super FIXSORB®) (Figure 4(b)). The excised mass measured 13×12.0×10.0mm with a weight of 2.7 g (Figure 4(c)). On histologic examination, osteomas are composed of dense, mature, predominantly lamellar bone. The osteoma was diagnosed an actively growing lesion ("hot") with radionuclide bone imaging, interosseous spaces composed of fibrous, fibrovascular, and lined by osteoblasts within a well-vascularized moderately cellular fibrous stroma (Figure 5). The case presented here was diagnosed as a compact osteoma because of its characteristic microscopical features, radiographic findings, and clinical features. Immediately after the operation, there was a slight trismus with no other complications. There were few functional changes and minimal temporomandibular joint dysfunction. The patient was followed-up for 5 months, and no recurrence was noted.

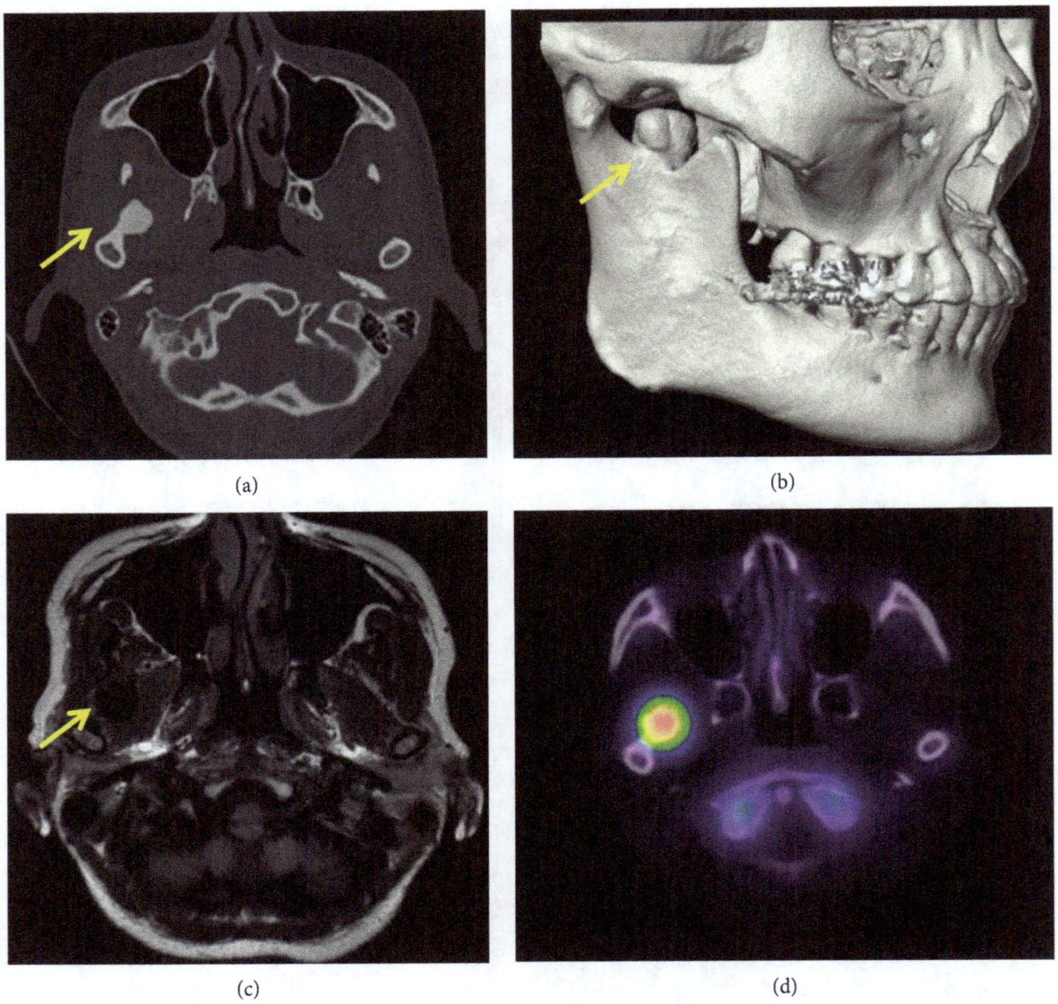

FIGURE 2: Preoperative examination. (a) Computed tomography showed a 13.3×12.8×10.0mm sized lesion showing Hounsfield units (HU) equivalent to that of the mandible, arising from the right mandibular notch. The CT values of osteoma ranged from 1480 to 1580 HU. (b) 3D-CT showed osteoma was found in the right mandibular notch. (c) Magnetic resonance imaging showed uniform hypointense trabecular bone, and there was no continuity of fat signals in the bone marrow, suggesting exclusion of the lateral pterygoid muscle because of bone lesions. (d) Radioisotope imaging showed significant uptake of Tc-99m by the osteoma in the right mandibular notch.

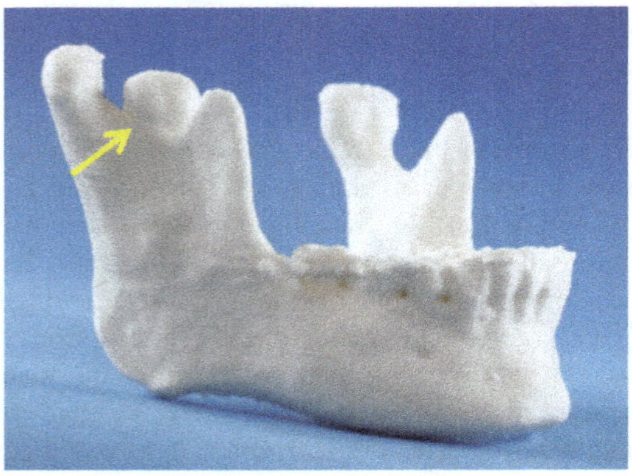

FIGURE 3: Three-dimensional model of the mandible. We created a three-dimensional model of the mandible to facilitate an explanation to the patient resection surgery using an intraoral approach was planned.

3. Discussion

Peripheral osteomas, also known as periosteal osteomas, most frequently involve the craniofacial bones and are the most common benign tumors of the paranasal sinuses. Peripheral osteomas of the jawbones are however uncommon [2]. The origin of peripheral osteoma onset is unknown, and it has been suggested that it results from a reaction to trauma and infection [2]. However, there was no history of infection or trauma in the present case. The osteoma may have slowly developed during the age of 21–26 years after the cessation of mandibular growth and development of secondary sexual characteristics. Surgery is considered for large, deforming osteomas [1, 6]. In the present case, surgical resection was considered owing to the progressive nature of the lesion confirmed by RI.

Only eight cases of osteomas in the mandibular notch have been reported so far [1, 6–10], and the present case is the ninth (Table 1). In the previous cases, the patients' age ranged from 16 to 78 years, with a male-to-female ratio of

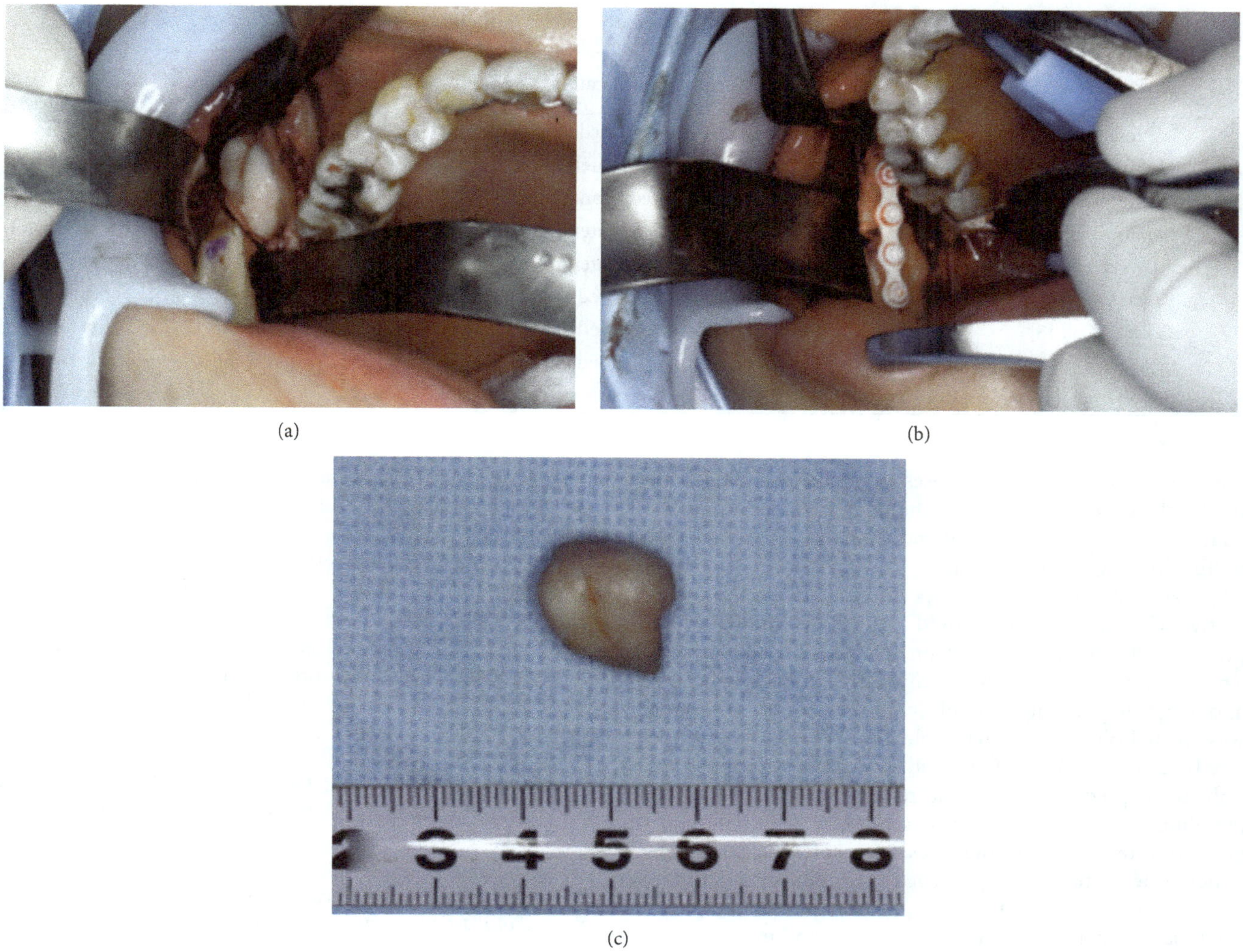

FIGURE 4: Intraoperative view. (a) The lesion was exposed by an intraoral approach. (b) The myoprojection was temporarily dissected, and the bone was repositioned and fixed with an absorbent plate. (c) Excised osteoma.

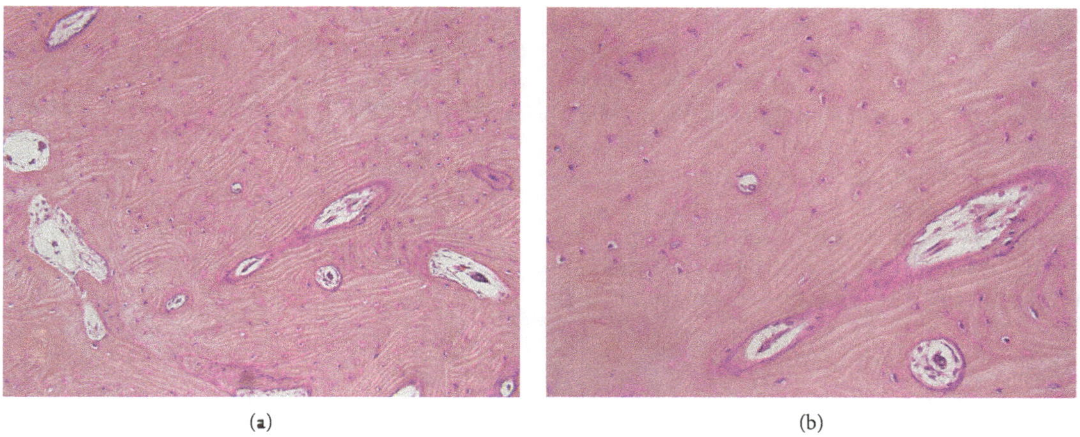

FIGURE 5: The histopathology of the peripheral osteoma. (a) Microscopic features of peripheral osteoma (hematoxylin-eosin, original magnification ×200). (b) Microscopic features of peripheral osteoma (hematoxylin-eosin, original magnification ×400).

1 : 3.5. The location of the osteoma was medial in four cases, lateral in four cases, and medial and lateral in one case. The lesion developed in the right mandibular notch in five cases and in the left mandibular notch in four cases. The patients displayed symptoms of swelling in four cases and pain in two, with no symptoms in three cases. Of

Table 1: Reported cases of peripheral osteoma in the mandibular notch.

No.	Reference	Year of publication	Age (years)	Sex	Location	Side	Size (in mm)	Symptoms	Treatment
1	Present case	2021	38	Female	Medial	Right	15×14×10	Pain	Surgery (intraoral)
2	*Nakayama* et al. [3]	2021	69	Female	Lateral	Left	25×20×15	Swelling	Surgery (extraoral)
3	*Bocchialini* et al. [1]	2018	37	Female	Medial and lateral	Left	15×13×11	Pain	Surgery (intraoral)
4	*Sasidharan* et al. [6]	2015	52	Female	Lateral	Left	30×25×20	Swelling	Surgery (intraoral)
5	*Rao* et al. [7]	2013	16	Female	Lateral	Right	30×30	Swelling	Surgery (intraoral)
6	*Iwai* et al. [4]	2013	78	Female	Medial	Right	36×35×30	None	Follow-up
7	*Sekerci* et al. [8]	2011	59	Male	Medial	Right	Not available	None	Follow-up
8	*Schulze* [9]	2008	73	Female	Medial	Left	30×30×27	Pain	Unknown
9	*Bessho* et al. [10]	1987	26	Male	Lateral	Right	34×29×17	Swelling	Surgery

the five surgically treated cases of osteoma, four were intraoral approaches. This is the first case to use RI to confirm the dynamic state of the osteoma; RI is therefore useful for diagnosing osteomas.

In addition, a 3D model was created based on the preoperative CT data using a fused deposition modeling 3D printer and a thermoplastic resin (polylactic acid filament). The 3D model is useful for preoperative patient education and surgical planning. In this case, because a 3D model was created only for the mandible, the surgery of the maxillary tuberosity and maxillary teeth was restricted, and it was difficult to predict. Among the reports of osteomas in the mandibular notch, there were descriptions of intraoral surgery in four cases. In the present case, considering the patient's aesthetics, we approached the lesion intraorally.

Currently, the number of reported cases of peripheral osteoma in the mandibular notch is small, and many aspects of this entity remain unclear, including the treatment method and prognosis. Further accumulation and examination of cases are expected.

4. Conclusions

We encountered a case of an active peripheral osteoma in the mandibular notch, which has rarely been reported in the literature. A dynamic diagnosis of peripheral osteoma was made possible using composite imaging. It was easy to obtain anatomical orientation in the surgical field through preoperative surgical simulation using a 3D model. An osteoma in the mandibular notch can be resected by an intraoral approach, in which case it is desirable to reposition the myoprojection.

References

[1] G. Bocchialini, A. B. Bolzoni Villaret, S. Negrini, A. Tironi, L. Salvagni, and A. Castellani, "The first case of osteoma of the mandibular notch located both medially and laterally and treated with a transoral endoscopy assisted approach. A case report," *International Journal of Surgery Case Reports*, vol. 49, pp. 70–73, 2018.

[2] I. Kaplan, S. Calderon, and A. Buchner, "Peripheral osteoma of the mandible: a study of 10 new cases and analysis of the literature," *Journal of Oral and Maxillofacial Surgery*, vol. 52, no. 5, pp. 467–470, 1994.

[3] A. Nakayama, R. Abe, M. Takahashi, H. Yamada, and Y. Takeda, "Peripheral osteoma in an unusual region of the mandible: a case report," *Oral and Maxillofacial Surgery Cases*, vol. 7, no. 1, article 100207, 2021.

[4] T. Iwai, T. Izumi, J. Baba, J. Maegawa, K. Mitsudo, and I. Tohnai, "Peripheral osteoma of the mandibular notch: report of a case," *Iranian Journal of Radiology*, vol. 10, no. 2, pp. 74–76, 2013.

[5] C. T. Chen and K. Adriane, "Endoscopic resection of a mandibular body and condylar osteoma," *Minimally Invasive Therapy & Allied Technologies*, vol. 17, no. 5, pp. 323–325, 2008.

[6] A. Sasidharan, A. Gohil, S. Koshy, and A. K. Gupta, "Bony tumour in an unusual location on the mandible," *Indian Journal of Plastic Surgery*, vol. 48, no. 2, pp. 200–203, 2015.

[7] S. Rao, S. Rao, and D. S. R. Pramod, "Transoral removal of peripheral osteoma at sigmoid notch of the mandible," *Journal of Maxillofacial and Oral Surgery*, vol. 14, Suppl. 1, pp. 255–257, 2015.

[8] A. E. Sekerci, H. Sahman, E. T. Ertas, and Y. Sisman, "An unusual peripheral osteoma of the mandibular notch: a case report with computed tomography evaluation," *Oral Radiology*, vol. 27, no. 1, pp. 78–82, 2011.

[9] D. Schulze, "Radiographic diagnostics: osteoma of the left mandibular notch," *Quintessence International*, vol. 39, no. 8, pp. 702-703, 2008.

[10] K. Bessho, K. Murakami, T. Iizuka, and T. Ono, "Osteoma in mandibular condyle," *International Journal of Oral and Maxillofacial Surgery*, vol. 16, no. 3, pp. 372–375, 1987.

7

A Full Computerized Workflow for Planning Surgically Assisted Rapid Palatal Expansion and Orthognathic Surgery in a Skeletal Class III Patient

Orazio Bennici,[1] Alessia Malgioglio,[2] Serena Moschitto,[2] Gianrico Spagnuolo,[3] Alberta Greco Lucchina,[4] Vincenzo Ronsivalle,[2] Gaetano Isola,[2] and Antonino Lo Giudice[2]

[1]*Private Practice, Catania 95123, Italy*
[2]*Department of Medical-Surgical Specialties, School of Dentistry, University of Catania, Policlinico Universitario "G. Rodolico-San Marco", Via Santa Sofia 78, Catania 95123, Italy*
[3]*Department of Neurosciences, Reproductive and Odontostomatological Sciences, University of Naples "Federico II", Naples, Italy*
[4]*Regenerative Medicine Research Laboratory, Saint Camillus University of Health Sciences, Rome, Italy*

Correspondence should be addressed to Gianrico Spagnuolo; gspagnuo@unina.it and Gaetano Isola; gaetano.isola@unict.it

Academic Editor: Jiiang H. Jeng

In the present case report, we present and discuss the digital workflow involved in the orthodontic/orthognathic combined treatment of a skeletal malocclusion correction in a 17-year-old male patient affected by a skeletal class III, facial asymmetry, sagittal and transversal deficiency of the medium third of the skull, dental crowding, and bilateral cross-bite. The first stage of the treatment involved surgically assisted rapid palatal expansion and occlusal decompensation, using fixed self-ligating appliance. An orthodontic software package (i.e., Dolphin 3D Surgery module) was used to perform virtual treatment objective evaluation by integrating data from cone beam computer tomography acquisition, intraoral scan, and extraoral photographs. The software allowed a comprehensive evaluation of skeletal, dento-alveolar, and soft-tissue disharmonies, qualitative and quantitative simulation of surgical procedure according to skeletal and aesthetic objectives, and, consequently, the treatment of the malocclusion. Using a specific function of the software, the surgical splint was designed according to the pre-programmed skeletal movements, and subsequently, the physical splint was generated with a three-dimensional (3D) printing technology. Once a proper occlusal decompensation was reached, a Le Fort I osteotomy of the maxilla and a bilateral sagittal surgical osteotomy of the mandible were executed to restore proper skeletal relations. The whole treatment time was 8 months. The orthodontic/orthognathic combined treatment allowed to correct the skeletal and the dental imbalance, as well as the improvement of facial aesthetics. Accordingly, the treatment objectives planned in the virtual environment were achieved. Virtual planning offers new possibilities for visualizing the relationship between dental arches and surrounding bone and soft structures in a single virtual 3D model, allowing the specialists to simulate different surgical and orthodontic procedures to achieve the best possible result for the patient and providing an accurate and predictable outcome in the treatment of challenging malocclusions.

1. Introduction

Conventional orthognathic surgery plan includes clinical examination and diagnostic tools, such as lateral cephalometric radiographs, plaster models, face-bow, articulators, and photographs [1]. However, traditional planning procedure based on plaster casts neglects the anatomical information of the whole skull, which, in patients with severe deformities, could leave a variation with unpleasant consequences that could lead to significant problems [2].

For these reasons, it would be useful to evaluate not only the occlusion but also the facial soft tissues, jaws, and the underlying skeleton. Three-dimensional (3D) virtual imaging and planning techniques offer the advantage of combining information from the soft tissues of the face, skeleton, and dentition [3]. This technology allows surgeons to design individually appropriate osteotomy plans and orthodontists to evaluate different therapeutic scenarios in a virtual computer environment. In particular, the possibility to integrate 3D models of maxillary and mandibular arches with the reconstruction of the skull form cone-beam computed tomography (CBCT) generates a virtual reliable patient's representation, with realistic reproduction of the skeletal and soft-tissue changes determined by the planned surgery [4].

In the present case report, we present and discuss the orthodontic/orthognathic combined treatment of a skeletal malocclusion correction in a 17-year-old male patient affected by a skeletal class III, facial asymmetry, sagittal and transversal deficiency of the medium third of the skull, dental crowding, and bilateral cross-bite. In particular, the present study will be focused on the effectiveness and advantages of integrating 3D digital technology, from virtual treatment plan to computer-aided design and computer-aided manufacturing (CAD-CAM) systems, in treating complex cases, such as malocclusion requiring orthognathic surgery.

2. Materials and Methods

2.1. Diagnosis and Etiology. A 17-year-old male patient attended an orthodontic consultation to evaluate his craniofacial dysmorphosis and to improve his smile and facial appearance. The extraoral examination showed a severe skeletal class III, a severe lower third facial lengthening with an aging appearance, thin lips with little represented vermillion, and an underdevelopment of the middle third. On a frontal view, the face was asymmetrical with the labial commissure tilted higher from the left side, the chin dislocated to the left, and emimandibular elongation on the right side (Figure 1). The intraoral examination revealed a class III with total reverse bite extending throughout the arch, a transversely reduced maxilla, and a dental crowding in both upper and lower arches. The superior median line was deviated to the right and the inferior median line to the left (Figure 2). No clinically evident signs or symptoms of temporomandibular dysfunction were reported.

The analysis of the 3D models (TRIOS 3Shape A/S, Copenhagen, Denmark) was performed to deeply investigate the occlusal characteristics and the presence of abnormal contacts (Figure 3).

Dental panorex showed impaction of both upper and lower third molars (Figure 4).

The cephalometric analysis confirms a severe class III malocclusion in a hyperdivergent type subject with the following values SNA 79.4°, SNB 85.3°, ANB −5.9°, WITS −17, FMA (MP-FH) 29°, IMPA 71.9°, MP-SN 37.9. A soft-tissue cephalometric analysis was also performed to investigate the vertical and anterior–posterior (AP) projection of the lips and soft-tissue components, according to Arnett. The analysis revealed a severe soft-tissue imbalance according to the following parameters: A' point −1.6, B' point 2.1, Pog′-Sn 3.9, naso-labial angle (Col-Sn′-ULA) 117.7°, upper lip length (Sn′-ULI)17.5 [5] (Figure 5).

CBCT examination was also performed to investigate the entity of the skeletal disharmony, facial imbalance, the location and extension of the mandibular asymmetry, and a preliminary integrated evaluation of soft-tissue imbalance with skeletal components. The CBCT scans were acquired using Scanora 3Dx (Soredex, Tuusula, Finland) equipment with the following machine settings: fold of view (FOV) 130 mm × 145 mm, 6.3 mA.

2.2. Treatment Goals. The objectives of the treatment were the correction of both maxillary and mandibular crowding, the correction of both sagittal and transverse skeletal dysmorphosis up to the achievement of class I, and obtaining an improvement in smile aesthetics and facial profile.

2.3. Treatment Alternatives. The first therapeutic option involved a multibracket orthodontic treatment with 3.4 and 4.4 extraction, space closure, and resolution of the superior dental crowding. However, this treatment would not allow to achieve an improvement in the profile and middle third aesthetic and the reduction of class III skeletal malocclusion as requested by the patient.

The second option included the miniscrew-assisted rapid maxillary expansion for correction of the transverse maxillary deficiency, supported by the application of miniplates in the lower arch to manage class III correction with the usage of inter-maxillary elastics. However, considering the amount of the sagittal discrepancy as well as the patient's age, this approach would have not assured to reach the aesthetic expectations of the patient. The third option involved a combined surgical-orthodontic treatment consisting on a first approach with multibrackets therapy to decompensate the dysmorphosis and a following maxillofacial surgery with LE FORT I and BSSO (bilateral sagittal surgical osteotomy) for the skeletal correction of the dysmorphosis. However, this path would not permit an adequate transverse expansion of the middle third, limiting the treatment of the skeletal imbalance to the sagittal and vertical component.

The fourth and last option involved a surgically assisted rapid palatal expansion (SARPE) to correct the transverse dimension of the upper jaw, followed by a combined orthodontic-surgical treatment with maxillofacial intervention. LE FORT I and BSSO as reported above.

The patient, supported by the parents, decided for the third option, in order to correct the dento-skeletal dysmorphosis, asymmetry, aesthetic appearance, crowding, and asymmetry. Patient signed an appropriate consent form for the treatment option chosen and for the availability of sensitive data.

2.4. Virtual Treatment Objectives (VTO). The virtual planning was performed with the orthodontic software Dolphin 3D Surgery module, according to the objectives defined by the orthodontist and surgeon. A comprehensive iconographic description of the digital workflow for orthognathic surgery performed with the Dolphin 3D Surgery software is fully documented in the Supplementary Materials.

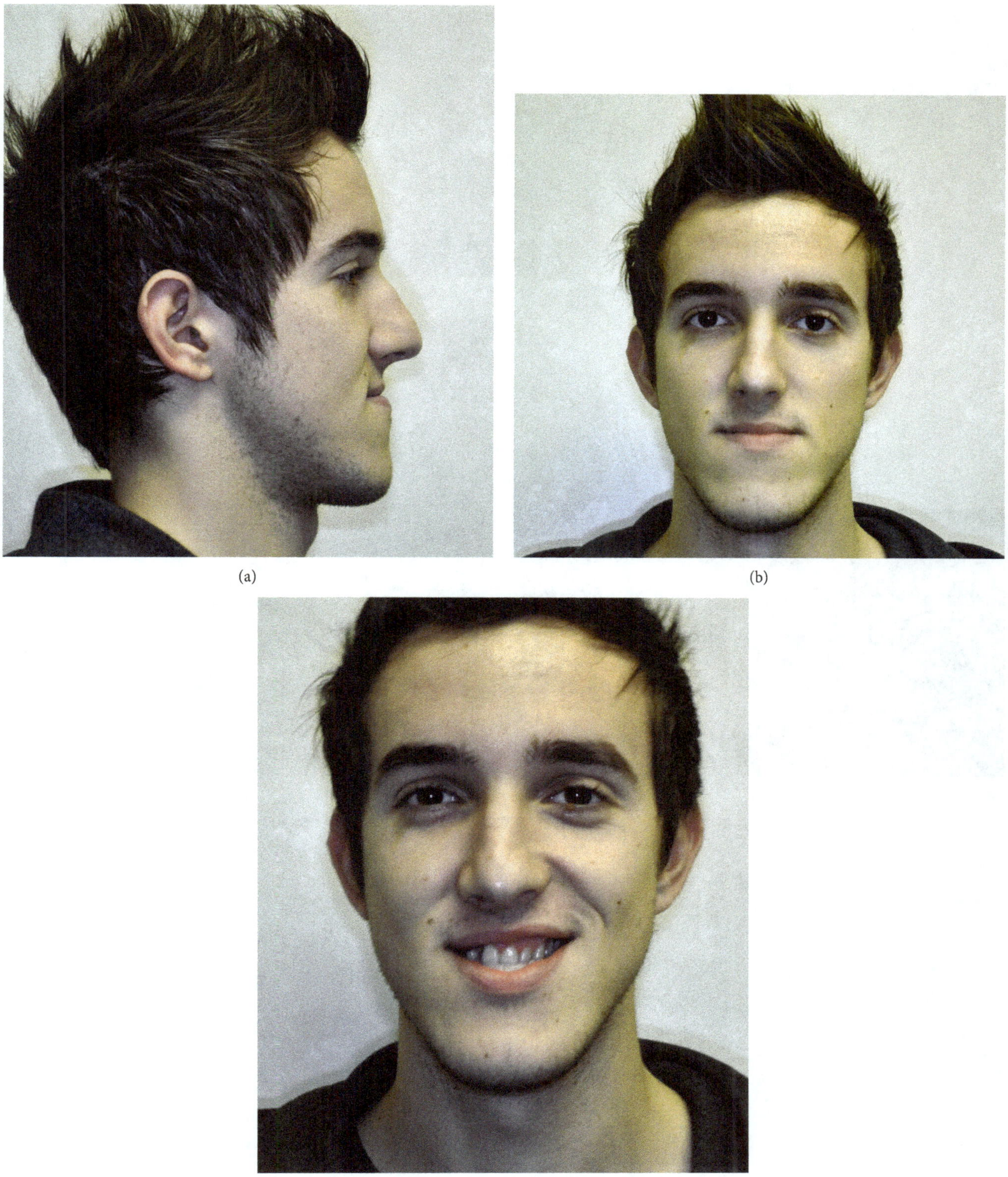

(a) (b) (c)

Figure 1: Pretreatment extraoral photographs: (a) right profile view, (b) full face, and (c) smiling.

In particular, the virtual skeletal movements were performed according to the following parameters: (1) correction of the midlines; (2) correction of the occlusal plane: downward pitch movement of the maxilla; (3) correction of AP position of the maxilla. In this regard, the software allows to monitor the changes of specific cephalometric parameters, the SNA angle in this case, during the simulation movement; (4) correction of the AP and vertical position of mandibular jaw; (5) correction of the anterior facial proportion; (6) achievement of soft-tissue balance [6, 7].

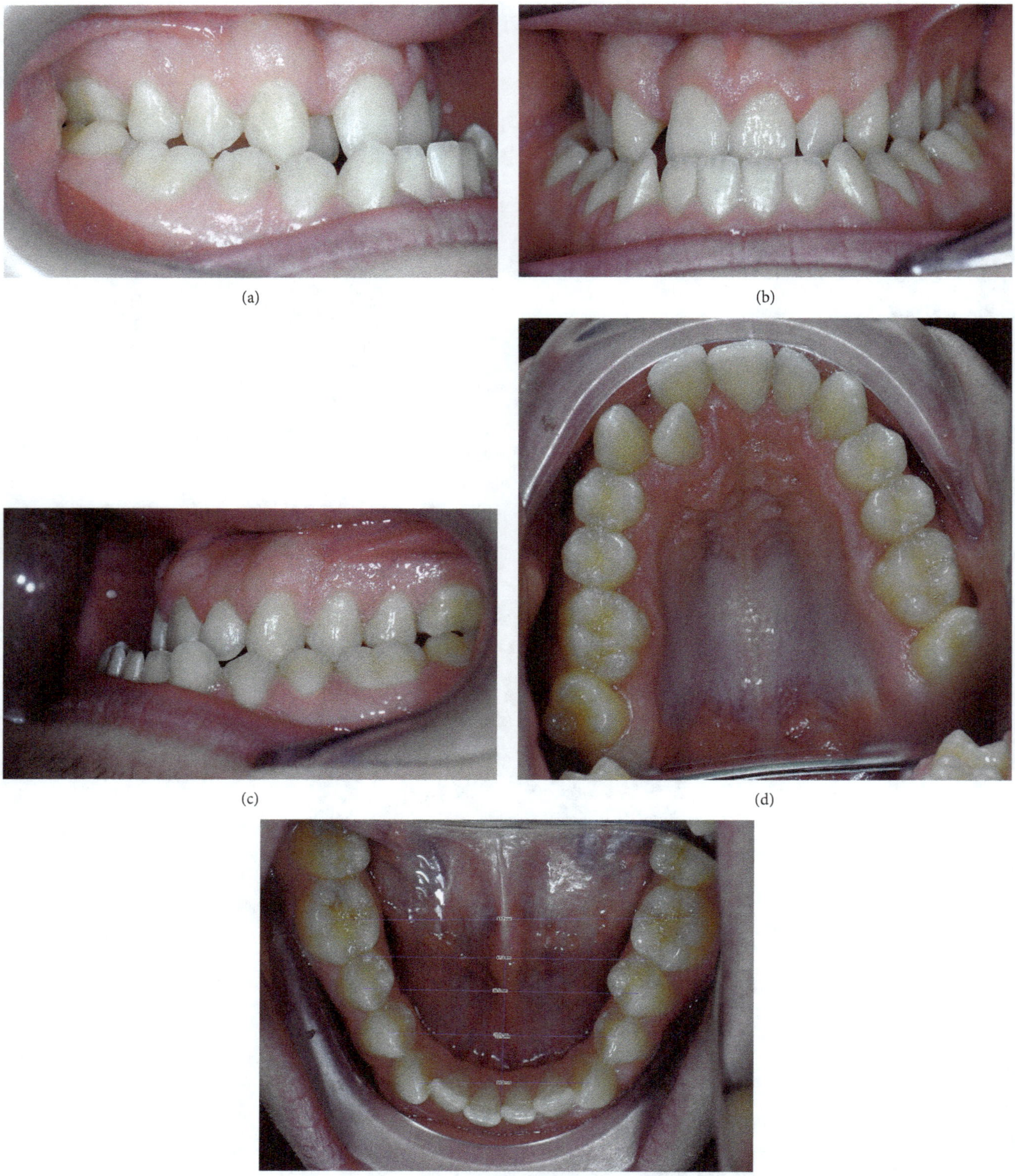

(a) (b) (c) (d) (e)

FIGURE 2: Pretreatment intraoral photographs: (a) right lateral, (b) anterior, (c) left lateral, (d) maxillary occlusal view, and (e) mandibular occlusal view.

2.5. Treatment Progress. First, the upper and lower third molars were extracted in order to facilitate osteotomic surgical maneuvers, as well as repositioning and osteosynthesis maneuvers [8].

The first phase involves maxillary expansion with SARPE, which consists of a surgical liberation of the sites of resistance combined using orthopedic forces. In this regard, intraoral scans (Trios 3Shape A/S, Copenhagen, Denmark) were sent to an orthodontic digital laboratory for the production of HYRAX maxillary expander, featuring bands on 1.6 and 2.6 and with arms extended to the second

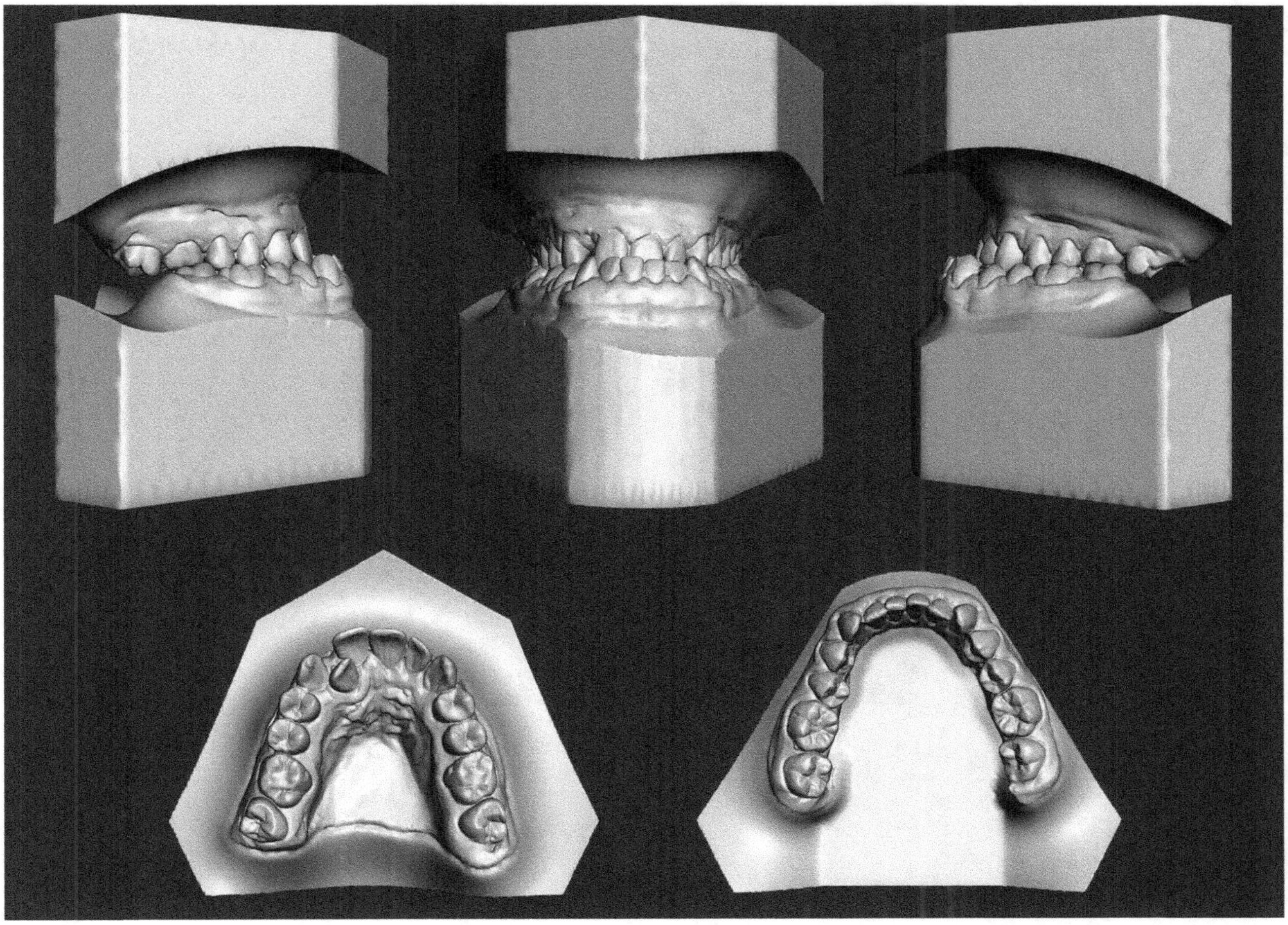

Figure 3: Pretreatment digital dental casts.

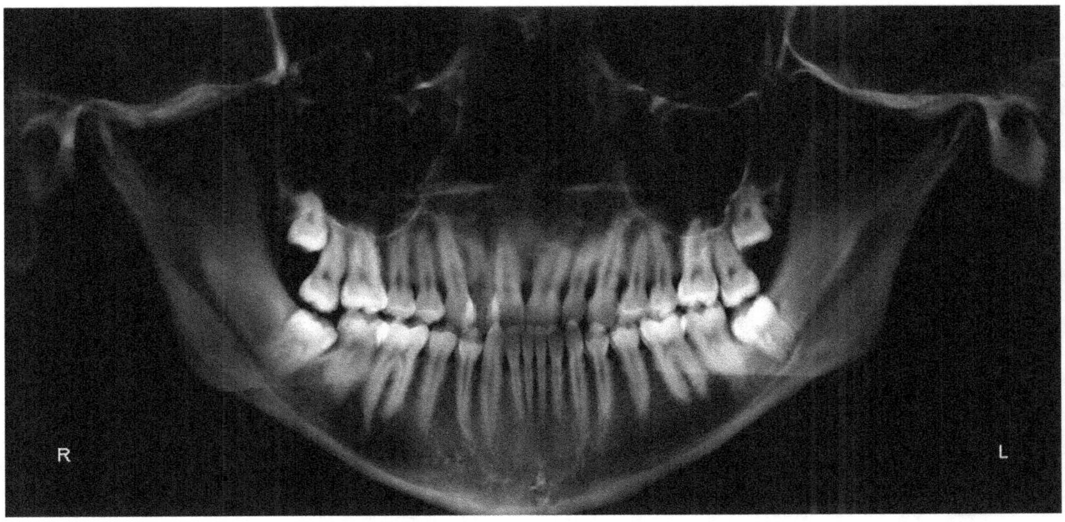

Figure 4: Pretreatment panorex.

molars 1 mm above the gingival margin. The appliance was cemented with glass ionomer cement (KETAC 3M, Saint Paul, MN, USA) 2 days before surgery (Figure 6).

The surgical procedure was performed in the surgery unit of private dental office in Catania; patient underwent conscious intravenous sedation, successfully managed by an experienced anesthetist, in order to reduce intraoperative stress. General anesthesia has been usually advocated for these procedures, with the concern that pterygomaxillary disjunction was too traumatic to be performed under sedation. However, recent

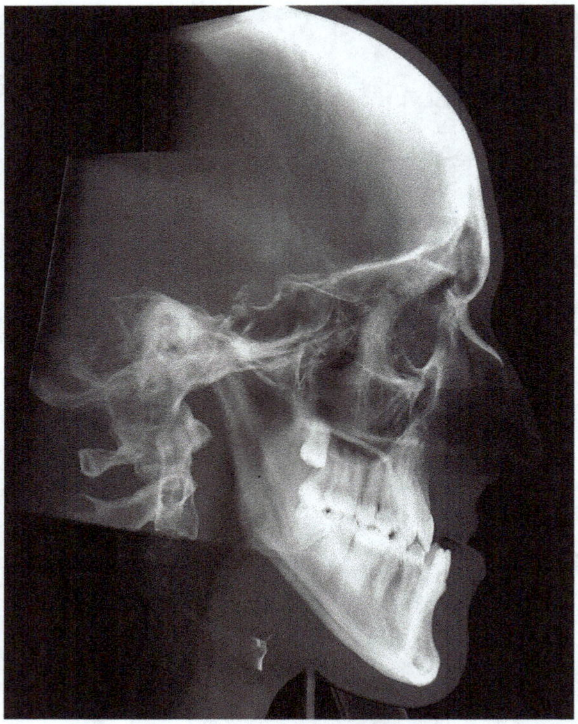

(a)

Group/Measurement	Value	Norm	Std Dev	Dev Norm
* HORIZONTAL SKELETAL *				
SNA (°)	79.4	82.0	3.5	-0.8
SNB (°)	85.3	80.0	3.0	1.8 *
ANB (°)	-5.9	2.0	2.4	-3.3 ***
Maxillary Skeletal (A-Na Perp) (mm)	-1.8	0.0	3.1	-0.6
Mand. Skeletal (Pg-Na Perp) (mm)	13.4	-4.0	5.3	3.3 ***
Wits Appraisal (mm)	-17.0	0.0	1.0	-17.0 ******
* VERTICAL SKELETAL *				
FMA (MP-FH) (°)	29.0	26.0	5.0	0.6
MP - SN (°)	37.9	33.0	6.0	0.8
Palatal-Mand Angle (°)	28.5	28.0	6.0	0.1
Palatal-Occ Plane (PP-OP) (°)	8.0	10.0	4.0	-0.5
Mand Plane to Occ Plane (°)	20.5	18.6	5.0	0.4
Mx occlusal plane (MxOP-Na Perp) (°)	98.5	95.0	1.4	2.5 **
* ANTERIOR DENTAL *				
IMPA (°)	71.9	95.0	7.0	-3.3 ***
U-Incisor Protrusion (U1-APo) (mm)	-1.7	6.0	2.2	-3.5 ***
U1 - NA (mm)	4.9	4.3	2.7	0.2
U1 - NA (°)	29.5	22.8	5.7	1.2 *
L1 - NA (mm)	11.6	4.0	2.0	3.8 ***
L1 - NA (°)	9.1	25.0	5.0	-3.2 ***
L1 Protrusion (L1-APo) (mm)	5.4	2.0	2.3	1.5 *
Interincisal Angle (U1-L1) (°)	141.4	135.0	6.0	1.1 *
U1 - Palatal Plane (°)	118.3	110.0	5.0	1.7 *
U1 - Occ Plane (°)	53.7	59.0	7.0	-0.8
Upper Lip to E-Plane (mm)	-13.1	-8.0	2.0	-2.6 **
Lower Lip to E-Plane (mm)	-4.9	-2.0	2.0	-1.5 *
L1 - Occ Plane (°)	87.7	72.0	5.0	3.1 ***
Nasolabial Angle (Col-Sn-UL)	140.3	N/A	N/A	N/A
Soft tissue A pt to SnV (mm)	5.2	-2.0	N/A	N/A
Soft tissue B pt to SnV (mm)	-4.1	-5.0	N/A	N/A
Upper lip anterior (ULA - Sn Vertical) (mm)	-1.1	3.0	1.0	-4.1 ****
Lower lip anterior (LLA - Sn Vertical) (mm)	1.1	1.0	1.0	0.1
Soft tissue B pt to SnV (mm)	-4.1	-5.0	N/A	N/A
Soft tissue Pogonion - Sn-7 (mm)	115.9	N/A	N/A	N/A
Soft tissue Lower lip - Sn-7 (mm)	81.0	N/A	N/A	N/A

(b)

FIGURE 5: Pretreatment cephalometric analysis (value, norm, standard, deviation, and deviation norm).

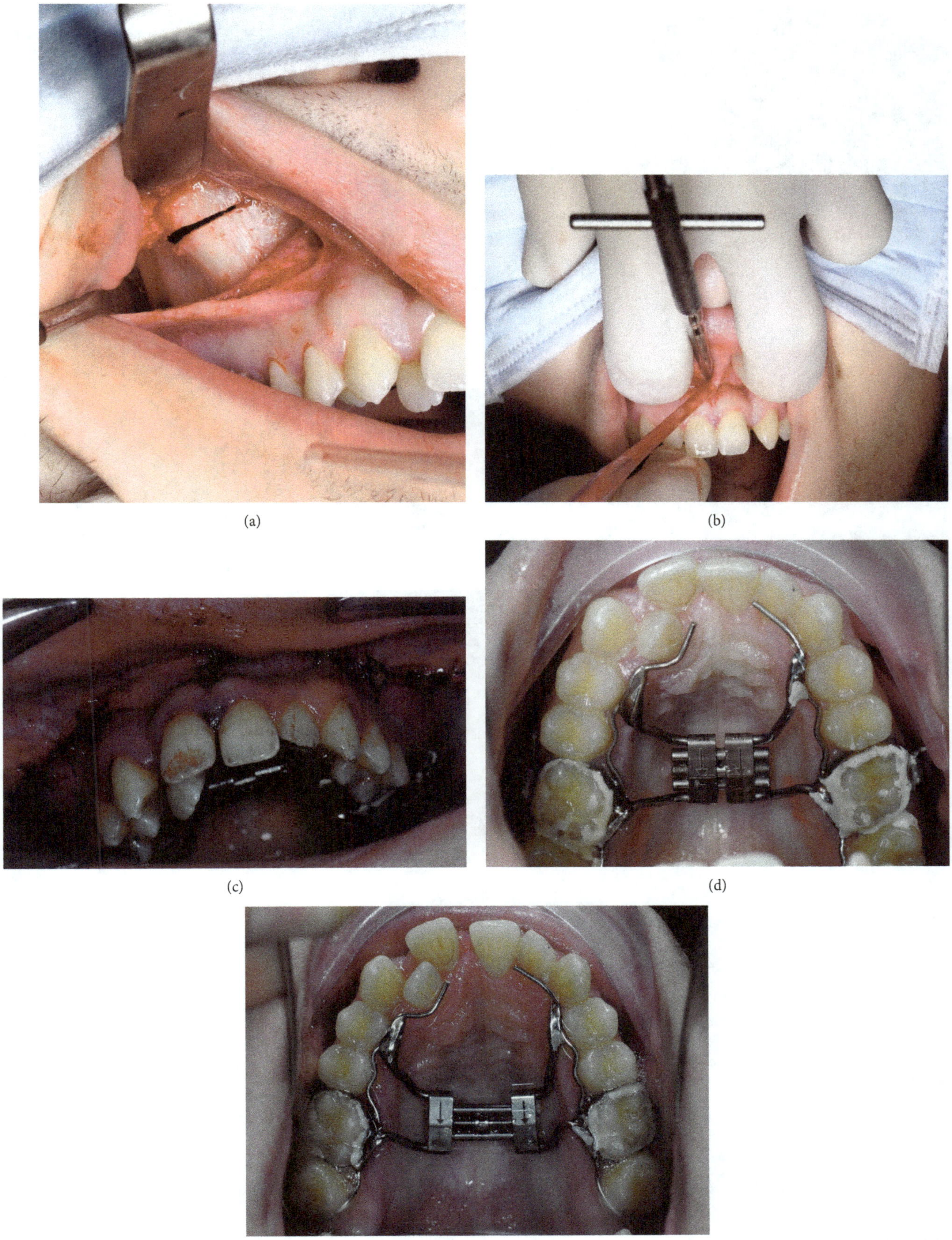

FIGURE 6: Surgical procedures: (a) osteotomy underneath the zygomatic process bilaterally, (b) osteotomy in the anterior median region, (c) suture, and (d and e) HYRAX maxillary expander pre- and post-activations.

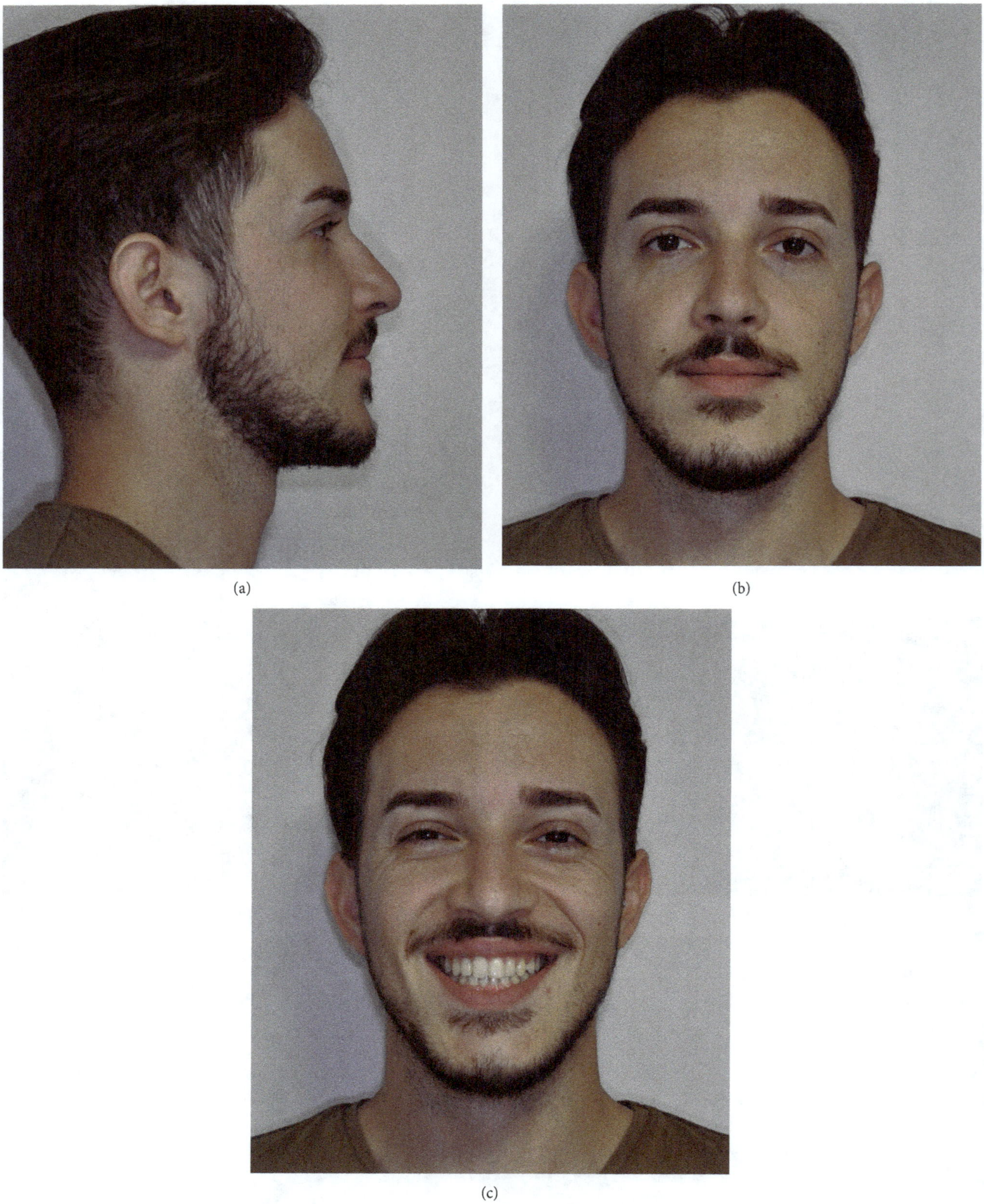

FIGURE 7: Pre-surgery extraoral photographs: (a) right profile view, (b) full face, and (c) smiling.

evidences have suggested that conscious intravenous sedation is adequate to avoid patient stress experience during SARPE [9].

Infiltration anesthesia (articaine) was administered throughout the upper maxilla at the fornix level; afterward, skeletonization (mucoperiosteal incision and dissection) of the right and left alveolar processes was executed. Osteotomy margins were executed (1) underneath the zygomatic process bilaterally and (2) in the anterior median region, in

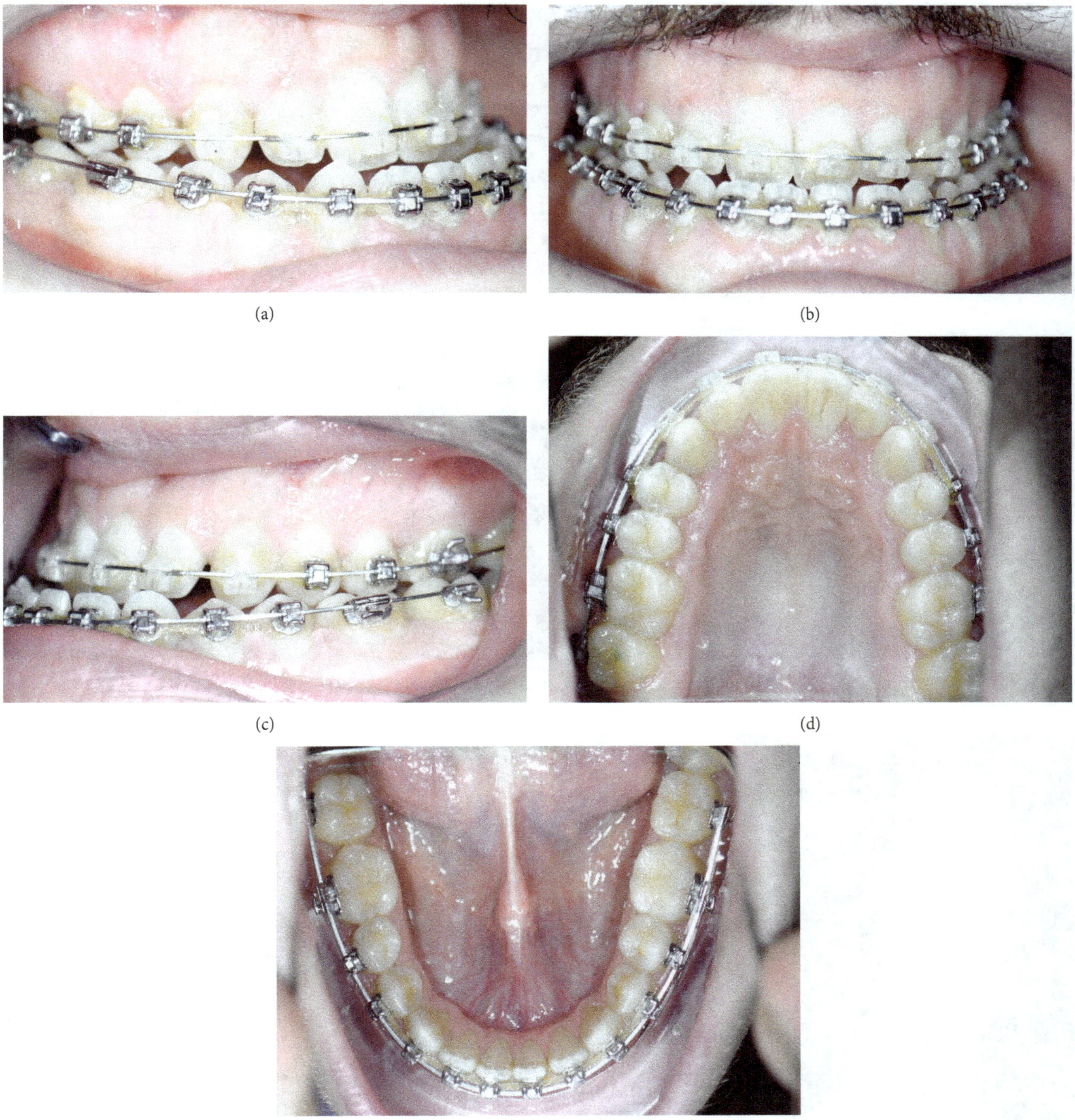

(a) (b) (c) (d) (e)

Figure 8: Pre-surgery intraoral photographs: (a) right lateral, (b) anterior, (c) left lateral, (d) maxillary occlusal view, and (e) mandibular occlusal view.

proximity to the anterior nasal spine, exactly 1 cm above the interproximal contact point between central upper incisors (Figures 6(a)–(c)). A straight dental elevator was used to perform paramedian surgical distraction of the maxilla. The surgical technique used sought to attain a balance between maximum mobilization of the maxilla with a complete liberation of all the buttresses and minimum morbidity to avoid further complications.

Afterwards, 10 activations of the expander screw were administered (Figures 6(d) and 6(e)). Two activations per day were performed until the screw was completely open (10 mm); once the activations were completed, the screw was blocked with passive stainless steel (SS) 0.010 mm. After 6 months of retention, a fixed 0.022 self-ligating appliance with the Damon prescription (Ormco, Orange, CA, USA) was bonded on the buccal surface of all erupted teeth.

Both maxillary and mandibular arches were treated with the same arch-wire sequences, that is, 0.014 Cu 155 NiTi, 0.018 Cu NiTi, 0.014×0.025 Cu NiTi, 0.018×0.025 NiTi, 0.017×0.025 TMA, and 0.019×0.025 SS posted. This

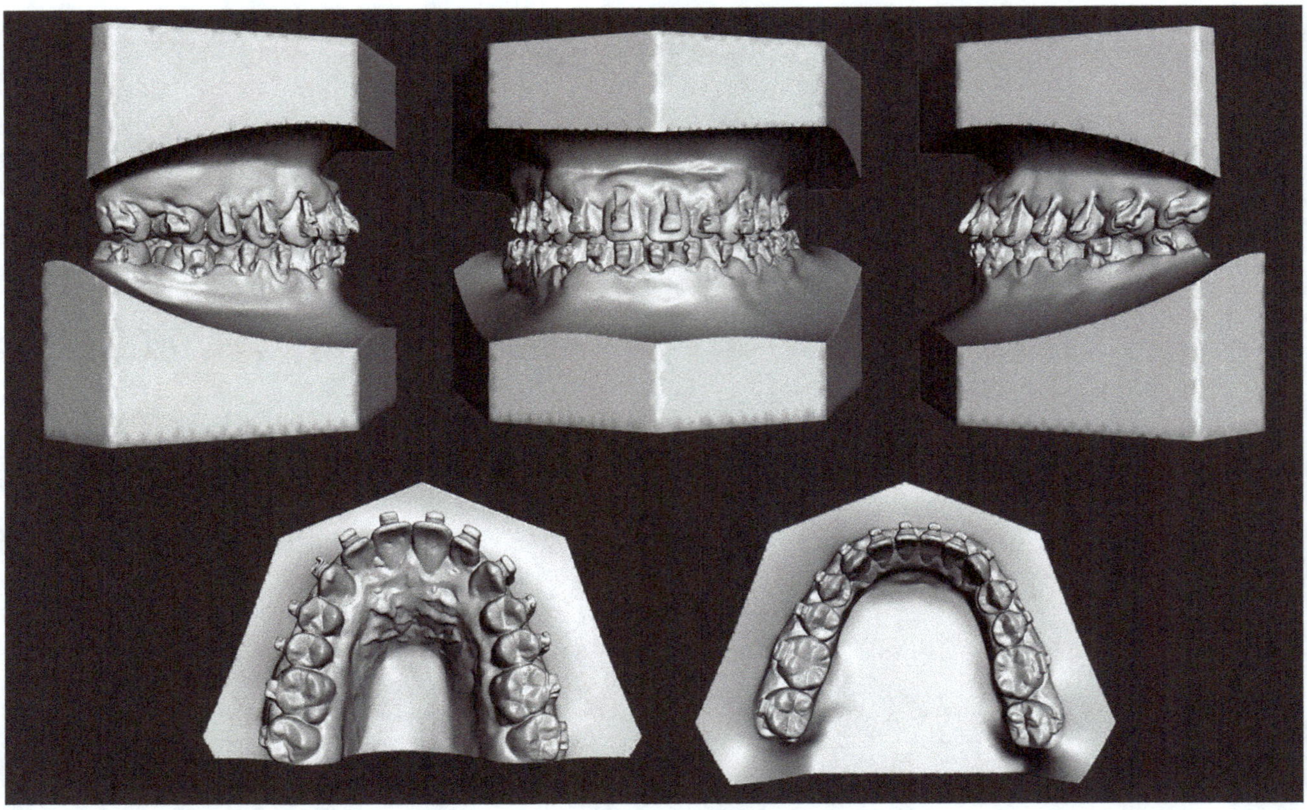

Figure 9: Digital casts oriented according to the planned surgical movements.

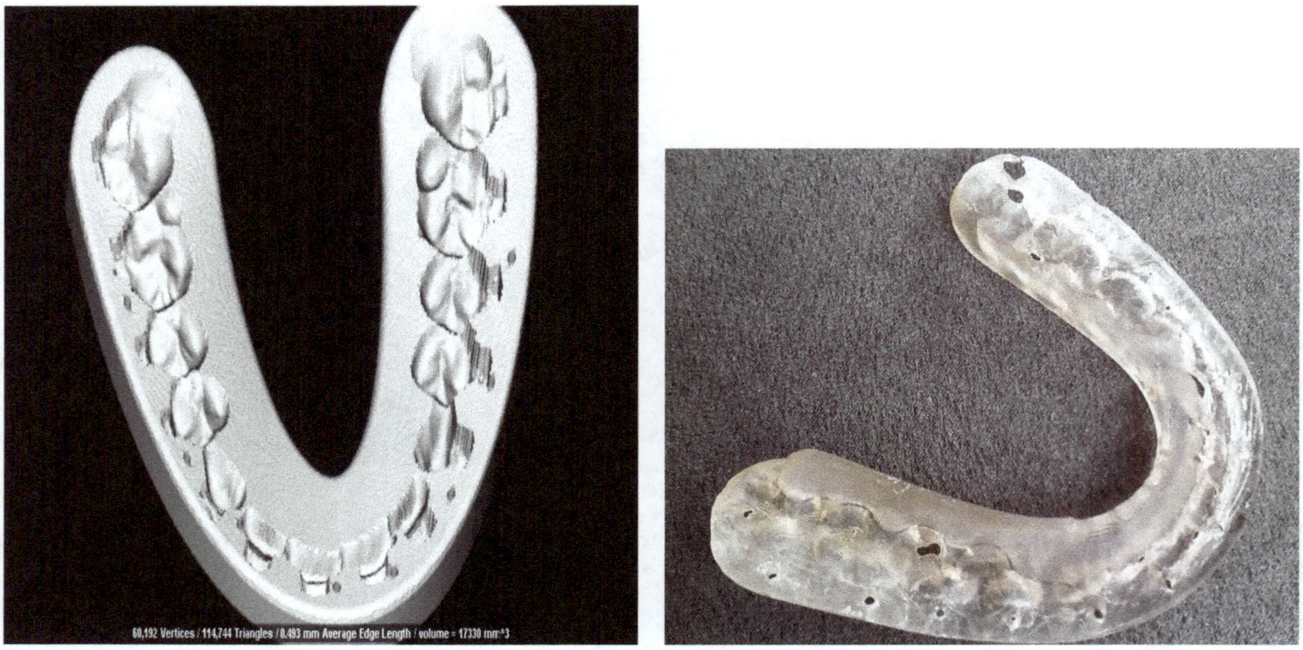

(a)

(b)

Figure 10: Final splint: (a) STL files and (b) transparent biocompatible resin.

arch-wire sequence allowed to achieve alignment, leveling, and coordination of the arches, up to pre-surgical preparation with SS rigid arches. In particular, the combination of self-ligating brackets and thermal NiTi arch-wires generates a low-force range biomechanics system, which allow the correction of the dento-alveolar discrepancy without causing periodontal iatrogenic damage [10, 11].

Once the arch-wire sequence was completed (with fully transmission of brackets prescription) and dento-alveolar transverse and sagittal compensation eliminated, a pre-

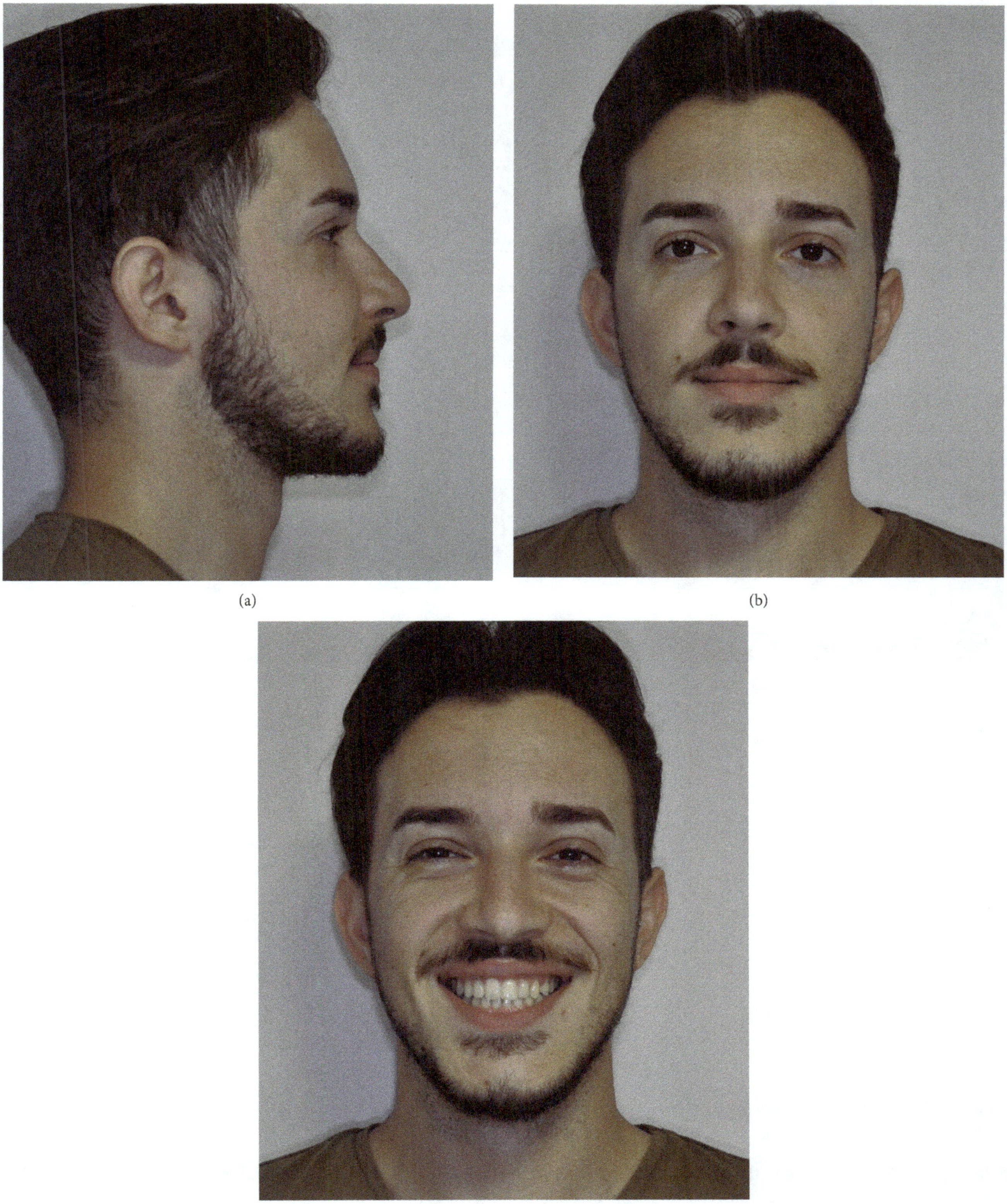

(a) (b) (c)

FIGURE 11: Post-treatment extraoral photographs: (a) right profile view, (b) full face, and (c) smiling.

surgery diagnostic check-up was performed, including the acquisition of new extraoral and intraoral photographs (Figures 7 and 8; Supplementary Figure 1), intraoral scans (Figure 9), and CBCT scans with large FOV [12]. The intraoral and CBCT scans were imported into Dolphin 3D Surgery module and matched in order to obtain a virtual model of the patient's skull with the dental arches in high definition. Moreover, the software allows to integrate the extraoral patient

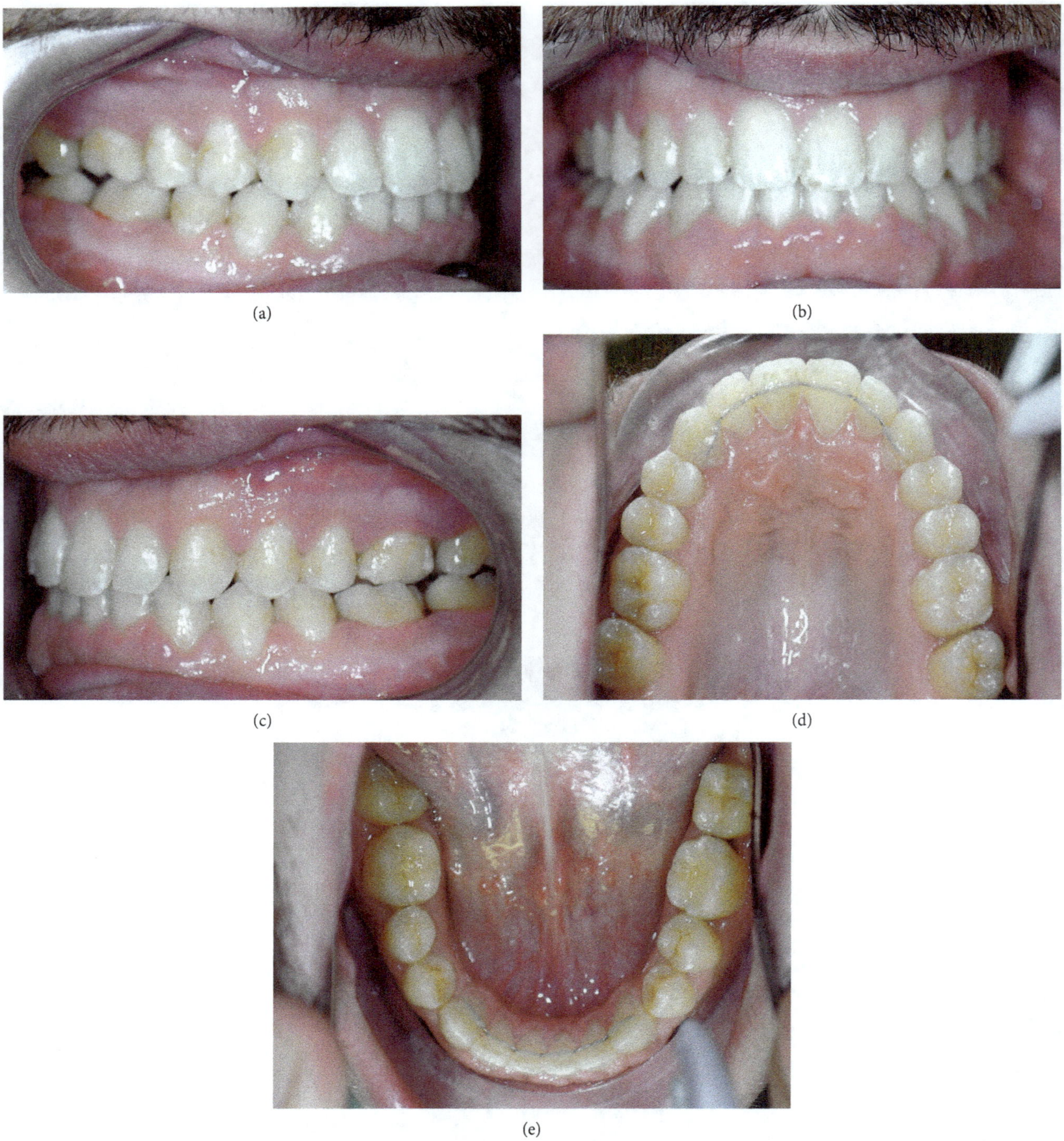

Figure 12: Post-treatment intraoral photographs: (a) right lateral, (b) anterior, (c) left lateral, (d) maxillary occlusal view, and (e) mandibular occlusal view.

photographs in frontal view with the surface of the 3D rendered skull model, allowing a comprehensive evaluation of patient skeletal and soft-tissue characteristics before planning virtual surgical jaw movement (Supplementary Figures 2–4).

Once the final position of both jaws was defined, the "Splint tool" function of the 3D Dolphin software was used to design a digital intermediate splint and final splints with the insertion of the holes for intermaxillary fixation (Figure 10(a)). In particular, the tool allows selecting the width, thickness, and other parameters of the splint based on your treatment plans. All splint data files were generated in industry-standard STL files* to be exported for final prototyping process.

The splints (file .STL) were prototyped with FORMLAB 3D printer (SLA technology, FORMLAB, Somerville, MA, USA) in transparent biocompatible resin (Surgical Guide Resin) with 50 μm of layer thickness (Figure 10(b)). The post-curing process was managed according to the manufacturer's instructions.

The surgical procedure follows the pre-planned settings for LE FORT I and BSSO approaches for the skeletal

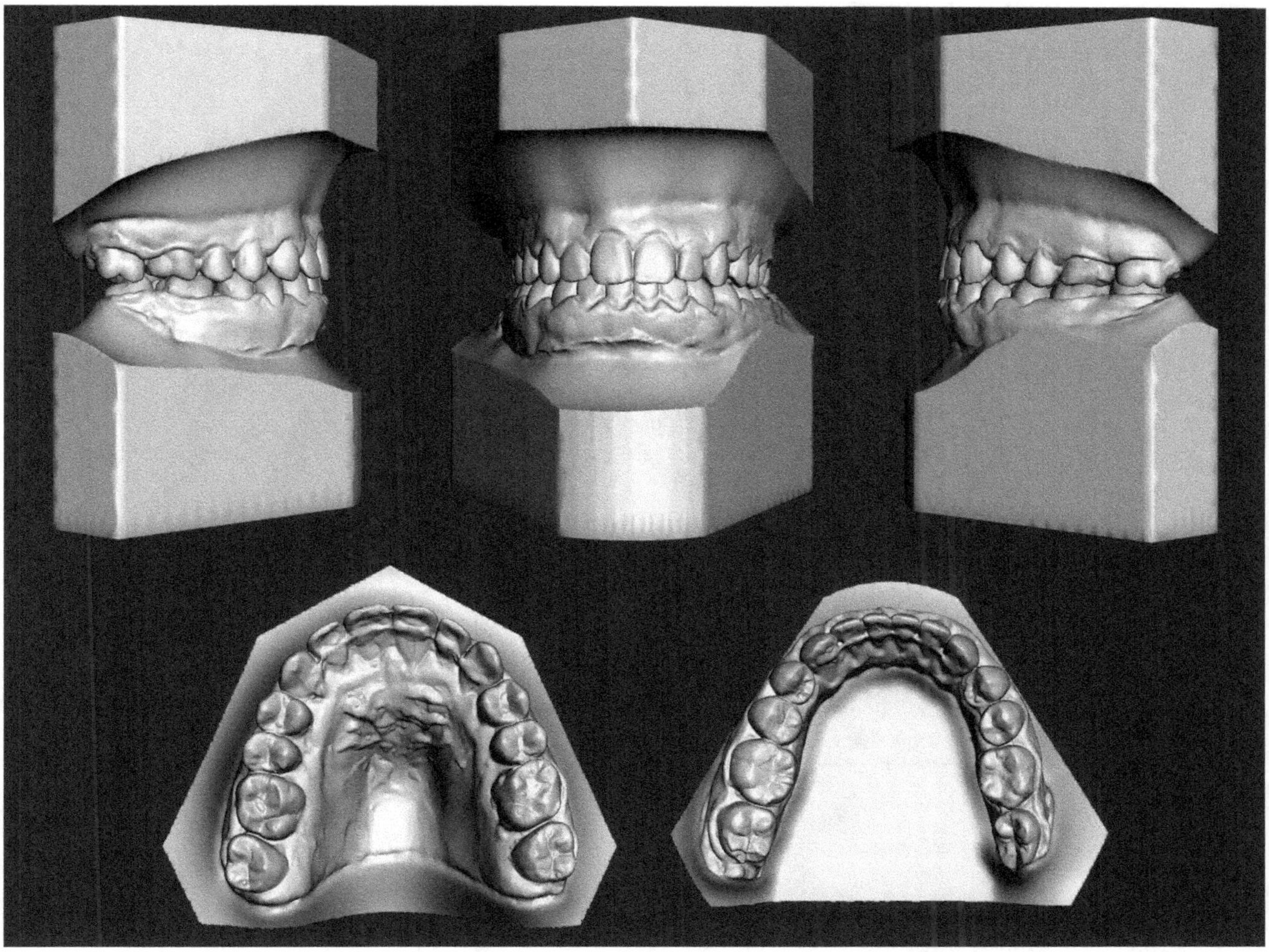

FIGURE 13: Post-treatment digital casts.

correction of the dysmorphosis, and finalized with osteosynthesis plates and screws. After the healing of soft tissues, an 8-week home physiotherapy is scheduled to increase speech, chewing, and joint mobility. 10 months after maxillofacial surgery, the case is concluded with rubber bands to increase the intercuspation and finishing arches. The restraint is carried out with upper and lower permanent splint and Essix® appliance during the night.

3. Results

The post-treatment records showed a significant enhancement of both skeletal and dento-alveolar parameters; in particular, facial photographs showed a remarkable improvement in the patient smile and facial aesthetics (Figures 11–15). The comparison between post-treatment and pre-treatment lateral cephalogram revealed that hyperdivergent skeletal pattern (long face) was corrected to normo-divergency on the sagittal plane, with a significant improvement in the ratio between anterior and posterior facial heights, while on the frontal plane, the facial proportions follow the golden proportions of the face (Figure 16, Supplementary Figures 5–7) (Figure 17).

The final cephalometric analysis illustrates the changes achieved by the orthodontic and the surgical treatment. In this regard, it was obtained a correction and normalization of the previous cephalometric values: SNA 83.2° (79.4°), SNB 82.3° (85.3°), ANB 1° (−5.9°), WITS −5.7 (−17), FMA (MP-FH) 30.1° (29°), IMPA 84.5° (71.9°), MP–SN 38.6° (37.9°). The improvement involved not only the skeletal part but also all the aspects related to aesthetics and soft tissues, which now appear very well proportionate in line with the current benchmarks: A' 210 point −2.4 (−1.6), B' point −10.7 (2.1), Pog$'$-Sn −5.8 (3.9), naso-labial angle (Col-Sn$'$-ULA) 122° (117.7°°), upper lip length (Sn$'$-ULI) 20.5 (17.5; Figure 14). The superimposition of pre-treatment and post-treatment cephalograms show the effectiveness of the combination of orthognathic surgery and orthodontic treatment in this patient (Figure 17).

The final orthopantomography shows adequate parallelism and absence of significant root resorption (Figure 15). The final models and intraoral photos show a class I canine with normalization of overjet and overbite, with the achievement of an incisive and canine guide. However, the crowding correction did not predispose to the proinclination of the incisors or periodontal problems (Figures 12 and 13).

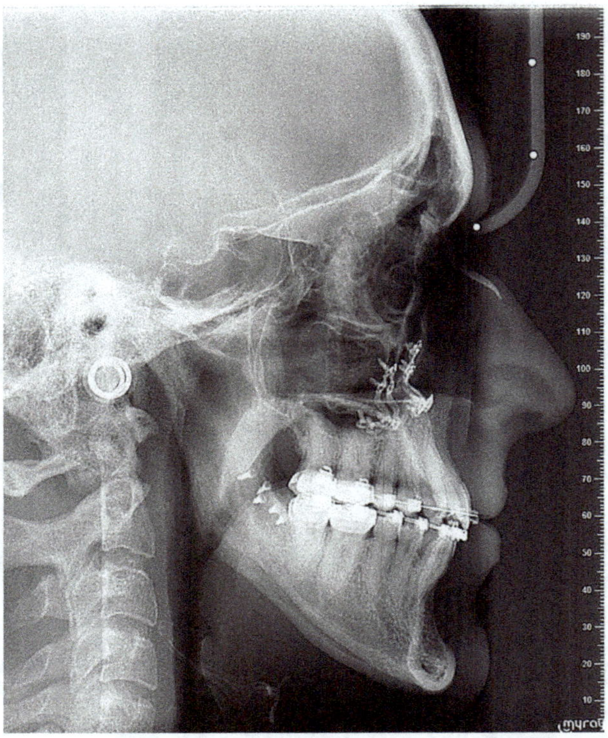

(a)

Group/Measurement	Value	Norm	Std Dev	Dev Norm
* HORIZONTAL SKELETAL *				
SNA (°)	82.6	82.0	3.5	0.2
SNB (°)	81.6	80.0	3.0	0.5
ANB (°)	1.1	2.0	2.4	-0.4
Maxillary Skeletal (A-Na Perp) (mm)	1.6	1.0	3.1	0.2
Mand. Skeletal (Pg-Na Perp) (mm)	7.5	-2.0	5.3	1.8 *
Wits Appraisal (mm)	-6.9	-1.0	1.0	-5.9 *****
* VERTICAL SKELETAL *				
FMA (MP-FH) (°)	30.3	26.0	5.0	0.9
MP - SN (°)	39.3	33.0	6.0	1.0 *
Palatal-Mand Angle (°)	32.6	28.0	6.0	0.8
Palatal-Occ Plane (PP-OP) (°)	11.2	10.0	4.0	0.3
Mand Plane to Occ Plane (°)	21.5	18.6	5.0	0.6
Mx occlusal plane (MxOP-Na Perp) (°)	98.8	95.0	1.4	2.7 **
* ANTERIOR DENTAL *				
U-Incisor Protrusion (U1-APo) (mm)	4.9	6.0	2.2	-0.5
L1 Protrusion (L1-APo) (mm)	2.3	1.0	2.3	0.6
U1 - Palatal Plane (°)	112.4	110.0	5.0	0.5
U1 - Occ Plane (°)	56.5	59.0	7.0	-0.4
L1 - Occ Plane (°)	73.9	72.0	5.0	0.4
IMPA (°)	84.7	95.0	7.0	-1.5 *
Subnasale - ST Menton	77.1	N/A	N/A	N/A
Soft tissue A pt to SnV (mm)	6.2	-2.0	N/A	N/A
Soft tissue B pt to SnV (mm)	-10.9	-5.0	N/A	N/A
Upper lip anterior (ULA - Sn Vertical) (mm)	-1.2	3.0	1.0	-4.2 ****
Lower lip anterior (LLA - Sn Vertical) (mm)	-3.2	1.0	1.0	-4.2 ****
Soft tissue Lower lip - Sn-7 (mm)	83.5	N/A	N/A	N/A
Soft tissue Pogonion - Sn-7 (mm)	110.5	N/A	N/A	N/A

(b)

FIGURE 14: Post-treatment cephalometric analysis (value, norm, standard, deviation, and deviation norm).

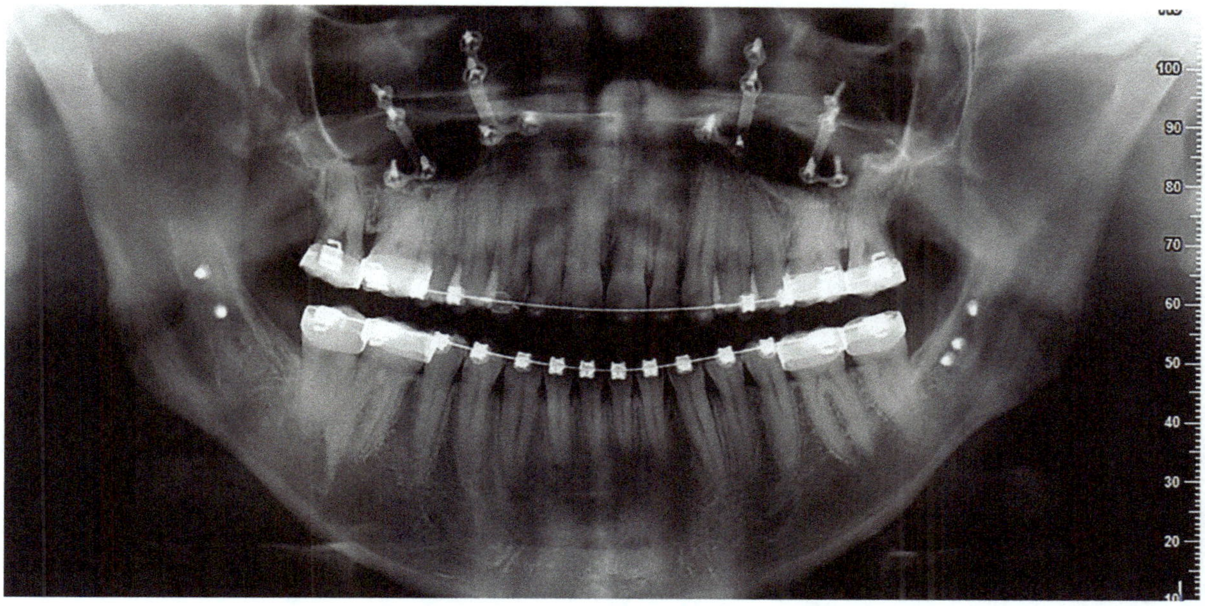

Figure 15: Post-treatment panorex.

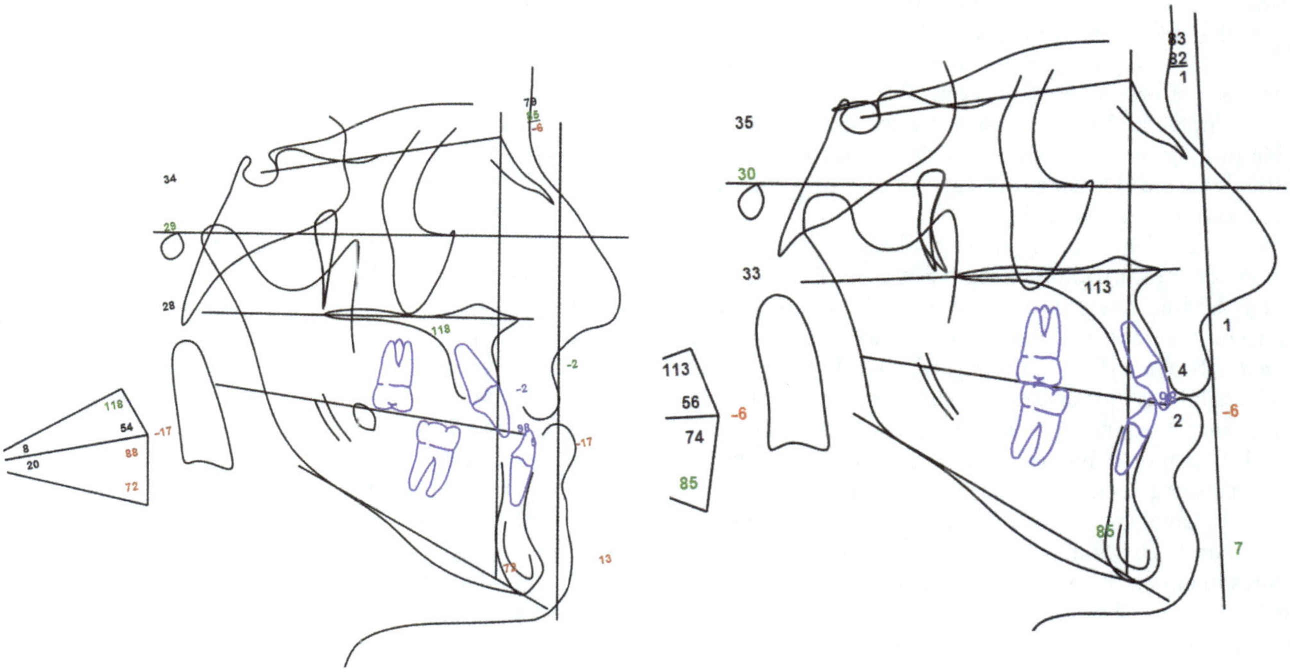

(a) (b)

Figure 16: Post-treatment and pre-treatment lateral cephalogram.

The new position of the upper jaw has improved the frontal exposure of the incisal group, restoring muscle tone to the upper lip, which appears well balanced both in frontal and lateral views with a preserved and improved labial competence.

The choice of the combined treatment has achieved all the objectives set, and the patient is satisfied of the aesthetic, functional, and chewing results obtained. The total treatment time was 34 months.

4. Discussion

The present case report shows a patient with severe dysmorphosis, in which non-surgical treatment would have not be able to achieve the correction of the dento-facial objectives. Orthognathic surgery allows the correction of skeletal jaws and facial disharmonies and the associated malocclusion, ensuring also aesthetic changes and other benefits, such as chewing, breathing, and speech improvement.

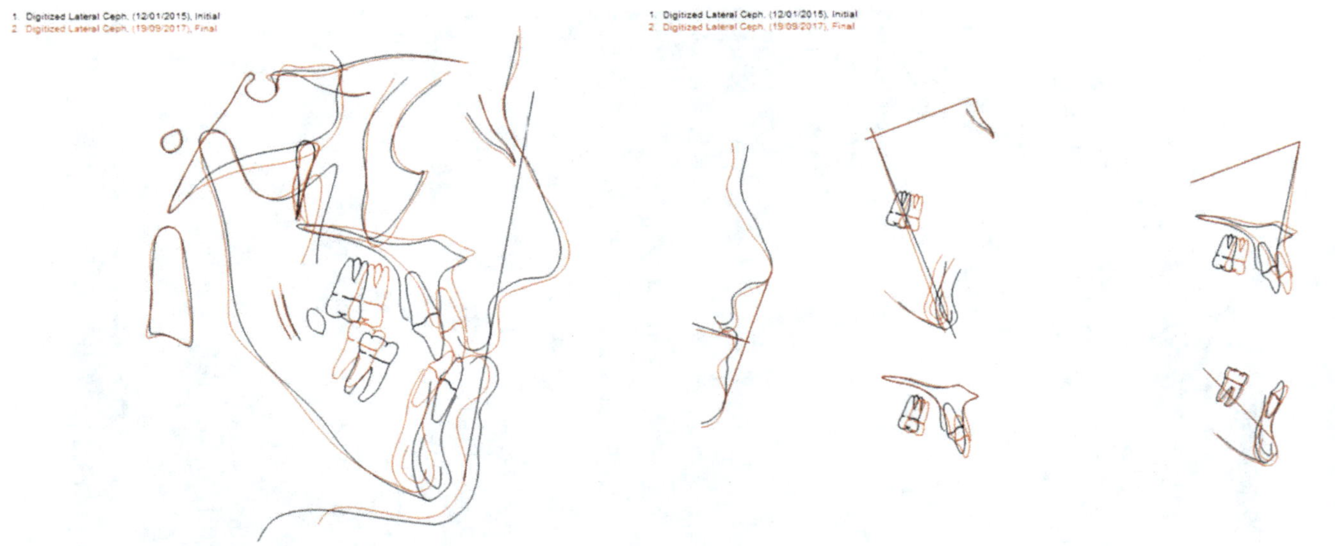

FIGURE 17: Comparison between post-treatment and pre-treatment lateral cephalogram by anatomical superimposition.

The first treatment phase involved the SARPE, according to the diagnosis of maxillary transverse skeletal discrepancy. In this regard, it could be argued that microimplant assisted rapid palatal expansion would have provided skeletal opening of the midpalatal suture with less invasive procedure [13, 14], increasing the skeletal and dento-alveolar maxillary diameters. However, SARPE, even if it is associated with more complex and longer post-operative stage, is the most stable procedure in the long term since it favors an expansion only of the alveolar processes, not affecting other adjacent maxillary sutures [15].

The second treatment phase involved the orthognathic surgery for the correction of sagittal/vertical skeletal malocclusion, and we referred to digital technology and 3D imaging techniques for preliminary evaluation of the surgical movements of the jaws. In this regard, virtual planning offers new possibilities to visualize the relationship between dental arches and surrounding bone structures in a single virtual model. This approach offers several advantages over conventional planning, including a diagnostic evaluation performed on a 3D virtual model [3]. Virtual 3D planning allows the surgeon and orthodontist to simulate different surgical procedures to obtain the best possible result for the patient, taking into account both skeletal and soft-tissue components, which is fundamental for predicting and achieving adequate aesthetic results [4]. 3D virtual planning facilitates the assessment and correction of the centric relationship in the temporomandibular joint, limiting pre-contacts and post-surgical dislocations; virtual 3D planning is a valuable educational information tool for both the patient and the clinical area [16–18].

For the present case report, we used the Dolphin 3D Surgery software to perform virtual treatment planning. In this regard, the virtual positioning method of the jaws for surgery determines intraoperative success, especially in the prediction of displacement, compared with classic VTO systems and management of gypsum models for several reasons. In fact, this tool permits both planning and presentation of the case showing the patient's skeletal and facial changes in real time and providing a precise surgical guidance [19].

Comparing the photo of the 3D simulation with the final result obtained after the orthodontic-surgical treatment, a significant correspondence of the lateral profile is evident. This is an example of how virtual treatment planning can be reliable in a clinical setting; future studies are warmly encouraged to comparatively assess the planned and post-treatment craniometric and photographic parameters as well as the 3D radiographic parameters.

In computer-aided surgical simulation systems, the virtual occlusal plane is transferred to the patient using surgical splints, which can be fabricated directly using CAD-CAM techniques [20]. In this case, we used 3D printed surgical splints since prototyping technology has been found to be accurate in producing occlusal devices [21–24]. One of the main advantages of prototyped splints is the possibility to select the width, thickness, and other parameters of the splint based on the treatment plans. Afterward, an intermediate splint can be created for the positioning of the maxilla or mandible, according to the order of surgery preferred, and finally, a final splint is generated.

All splint data files are generated in dental and non-dental industry standard .STL files, in order to be produced by the printing process with certified and biocompatible resins. The possibility to directly prototyping surgical splints streamlines the entire digital workflow as well as assures comfortable and accurate occlusal appliance.

5. Conclusions

The orthodontic/orthognathic combined treatment allowed to correct the skeletal and the dental imbalance, as well as the improvement of facial aesthetics. Virtual planning allows visualizing the relationship between dental arches and surrounding bone and soft tissues in a single virtual 3D model; thus, the specialists can simulate different surgical and orthodontic maneuvers to achieve predictable outcomes in the treatment of challenging malocclusions.

Abbreviations

SARPE: Surgically assisted rapid palatal expansion
VTO: Virtual treatment objectives
CBCT: Cone beam computer tomography
BSSO: Bilateral sagittal split osteotomy
3D: Three-dimensional
CAD-CAM: Computer-aided drafting-computer-aided manufacturing
FOV: Field of view
AP: Anterior–posterior
SS: Stainless steel
MARPE: Microimplant assisted rapid palatal expansion.

Supplementary Materials

Supplementary Figure 1. On the 3D Surgery module, the first step consists in delimiting the reference areas on the virtual OPT: right and left maxilla, right and left body and mandibular branch. Supplementary Figure 2. The software generates the STL file of this anatomical areas that must be cleaned (eliminating the external areas) in order to have an anatomical section of the part that have to be moved. Supplementary Figure 3. Mandibular and maxillary. STL file with teeth in high definition. Supplementary Figure 4. Once the virtual anatomical pieces have been obtained, the desired osteotomy lines are determined: in this case is made a Le Fort I for the maxilla and a BSSO for the mandible. Supplementary Figure 5. At this point, it is necessary to have the software recognize the cephalometric points by assigning skeletal and soft-tissue points by performing the 3D cephalometry, the software producing the traces and it is possible to start managing. Malocclusion. Supplementary Figure 6. Now everything is ready to plan the displacements. In this clinical case, the upper jaw is first moved as it would be done during the surgery; the software in the associated screen shows the real-time result of the movement performed and determines the three-dimensional parameters by recording them, including the variation in the soft tissues. Then the mandibular position is corrected too. This step can be managed manually or with the automatic function PIGGY BACK: the intraoral scan can also be done on the models and acquired in post correction centric occlusion. The software drags the teeth and the mandible according to the previously recorded occlusion. This system seems to be the best for having the most reliable and predictable guidance of case management. Supplementary Figure 7. Digital design (CAD) of prototyped surgical splint, according to the simulated surgical movements. *(Supplementary Materials)*

References

[1] Z. Chen, S. Mo, X. Fan, Y. You, G. Ye, and N. Zhou, "A meta-analysis and systematic review comparing the effectiveness of traditional and virtual surgical planning for orthognathic surgery: based on randomized clinical trials," *Journal of Oral and Maxillofacial Surgery*, vol. 79, pp. 471 e471–471 e419, 2021.

[2] F. Baan, E. M. van Meggelen, A. C. Verhulst, R. Bruggink, T. Xi, and T. J. J. Maal, "Virtual occlusion in orthognathic surgery," *International Journal of Oral and Maxillofacial Surgery*, vol. 50, no. 9, pp. 1219–1225, 2021.

[3] A. Alkhayer, J. Piffko, C. Lippold, and E. Segatto, "Accuracy of virtual planning in orthognathic surgery: a systematic review," *Head & Face Medicine*, vol. 16, no. 1, p. 34, 2020.

[4] R. H. Tonin, L. Iwaki Filho, A. L. Yamashita et al., "Accuracy of 3D virtual surgical planning for maxillary positioning and orientation in orthognathic surgery," *Orthodontics & Craniofacial Research*, vol. 23, no. 2, pp. 229–236, 2020.

[5] G. W. Arnett, J. S. Jelic, J. Kim et al., "Soft tissue cephalometric analysis: diagnosis and treatment planning of dentofacial deformity," *American Journal of Orthodontics and Dentofacial Orthopedics*, vol. 116, no. 3, pp. 239–253, 1999.

[6] M. H. Elnagar, S. Aronovich, and B. Kusnoto, "Digital workflow for combined orthodontics and orthognathic surgery," *Oral and Maxillofacial Surgery Clinics of North America*, vol. 32, no. 1, pp. 1–14, 2020.

[7] J. M. Plooij, T. J. Maal, P. Haers, W. A. Borstlap, A. M. Kuijpers-Jagtman, and S. J. Berge, "Digital three-dimensional image fusion processes for planning and evaluating orthodontics and orthognathic surgery. A systematic review," *International Journal of Oral and Maxillofacial Surgery*, vol. 40, no. 4, pp. 341–352, 2011.

[8] D. M. Steinbacher and K. L. Kontaxis, "Does simultaneous third molar extraction increase intraoperative and perioperative complications in orthognathic surgery?," *The Journal of Craniofacial Surgery*, vol. 27, no. 4, pp. 923–926, 2016.

[9] F. Hernandez-Alfaro, J. Mareque Bueno, A. Diaz, and C. M. Pagés, "Minimally invasive surgically assisted rapid palatal expansion with limited approach under sedation: a report of 283 consecutive cases," *Journal of Oral and Maxillofacial Surgery*, vol. 68, no. 9, pp. 2154–2158, 2010.

[10] S. Tecco, D. Di Iorio, G. Cordasco, I. Verrocchi, and F. Festa, "An in vitro investigation of the influence of self-ligating brackets, low friction ligatures, and archwire on frictional resistance," *European Journal of Orthodontics*, vol. 29, no. 4, pp. 390–397, 2007.

[11] M. Cozzani, D. Sadri, L. Nucci, P. Jamilian, A. P. Pirhadirad, and A. Jamilian, "The effect of Alexander, Gianelly, Roth, and MBT bracket systems on anterior retraction: a 3-dimensional finite element study," *Clinical Oral Investigations*, vol. 24, no. 3, pp. 1351–1357, 2020.

[12] J. B. Ludlow, R. Timothy, C. Walker et al., "Effective dose of dental CBCT-a meta analysis of published data and additional data for nine CBCT units," *Dentomaxillofacial Radiology*, vol. 44, no. 1, p. 20140197, 2015.

[13] C. Carlson, J. Sung, M. C. RW, A. W. Machado, and W. Moon, "Microimplant-assisted rapid palatal expansion appliance to orthopedically correct transverse maxillary deficiency in an adult," *American Journal of Orthodontics and Dentofacial Orthopedics*, vol. 149, no. 5, pp. 716–728, 2016.

[14] H.-S. Baik, Y.-G. Kang, and Y. J. Choi, "Miniscrew-assisted rapid palatal expansion: a review of recent reports," *Journal of the World Federation of Orthodontists*, vol. 9, no. 3S, pp. S54–S58, 2020.

[15] P. H. A. Carvalho, L. B. Moura, G. S. Trento et al., "Surgically assisted rapid maxillary expansion: a systematic review of complications," *International Journal of Oral and Maxillofacial Surgery*, vol. 49, no. 3, pp. 325–332, 2020.

[16] R. Leonardi, K. Aboulazm, A. Lo Giudice et al., "Evaluation of mandibular changes after rapid maxillary expansion: a CBCT study in youngsters with unilateral posterior crossbite using a sur-face-to-surface matching technique," *Clinical Oral Investigations*, vol. 25, no. 4, pp. 1775–1785, 2021.

[17] A. Lo Giudice, V. Ronsivalle, C. Spampinato, and R. Leonardi, "Fully automatic segmentation of the mandible based on convolutional neural networks (CNNs)," *Orthodontics & Craniofacial Research*, vol. 24, no. S2, pp. 100–107, 2021.

[18] R. Leonardi, S. Muraglie, A. Lo Giudice, K. S. Aboulazm, and R. Nucera, "Evaluation of mandibular symmetry and morphology in adult patients with unilateral posterior crossbite: a CBCT study using a surface-to-surface matching technique," *European Journal of Orthodontics*, vol. pii, p. cjz106, 2020.

[19] D. Schneider, P. W. Kammerer, M. Hennig, G. Schon, D. G. E. Thiem, and R. Bschorer, "Customized virtual surgical planning in bimaxillary orthognathic surgery: a prospective randomized trial," *Clinical Oral Investigations*, vol. 23, no. 7, pp. 3115–3122, 2019.

[20] S. J. Chin, F. Wilde, M. Neuhaus, A. Schramm, N. C. Gellrich, and M. Rana, "Accuracy of virtual surgical planning of orthognathic surgery with aid of CAD/CAM fabricated surgical splint-a novel 3D analyzing algorithm," *Journal of Cranio-Maxillo-Facial Surgery*, vol. 45, no. 12, pp. 1962–1970, 2017.

[21] H.-H. Lin, D. Lonic, and L.-J. Lo, "3D printing in orthognathic surgery—a literature review," *Journal of the Formosan Medical Association*, vol. 117, no. 7, pp. 547–558, 2018.

[22] F. d'Apuzzo, G. Minervini, V. Grassia, R. P. Rotolo, L. Perillo, and L. Nucci, "Mandibular coronoid process hypertrophy: diagnosis and 20-year follow-up with CBCT, MRI and EMG evaluations," *Applied Sciences*, vol. 11, no. 10, p. 4504, 2021.

[23] F. Lerario, M. Roncati, A. Gariffo et al., "Non-surgical periodontal treatment of peri-implant diseases with the adjunctive use of diode laser: preliminary clinical study," *Laser in Medical Science*, vol. 31, no. 1, pp. 1–6, 2016.

[24] M. E. De Felice, L. Nucci, A. Fiori, C. Flores-Mir, L. Perillo, and V. Grassia, "Accuracy of interproximal enamel reduction during clear aligner treatment," *Progress in Orthodontics*, vol. 28, no. 21, p. 28, 2020.

8

Persistent Necrotizing Mediastinitis after Dental Extraction

Eugênia Leal de Figueiredo,[1] Carolina Chaves Gama Aires,[1] Bruno José Carvalho Macêdo Neres,[1] Bruna Luna de Araújo,[1] José Alcides Almeida de Arruda,[2] and Ricardo José de Holanda Vasconcellos[1]

[1]*Department of Oral and Maxillofacial Surgery, School of Dentistry, Universidade de Pernambuco, Camaragibe, PE, Brazil*
[2]*Department of Oral Surgery and Pathology, School of Dentistry, Universidade Federal de Minas Gerais, Belo Horizonte, MG, Brazil*

Correspondence should be addressed to José Alcides Almeida de Arruda; alcides_almeida@hotmail.com

Academic Editor: Jiiang H. Jeng

Mediastinitis is a rare, progressive, and destructive infectious process due to cervical or odontogenic infections, which, if not diagnosed early, may lead to several complications, including airway involvement and even an imminent risk of death. Herein, we report an unusual case of a 37-year-old male with a bilateral submandibular hard swelling after the left third molar extraction. After surgical intervention with submandibular drainage and antibiotic therapy, the infection persisted without explanation, since the patient was not hypertensive, did not have diabetes mellitus or sexually transmitted infections such as HIV or syphilis, and did not smoke or drink alcoholic beverages. A thoracic surgeon then intervened, treating the mediastinitis surgically by drainage, thus obtaining a significant improvement of the patient's health. Mediastinitis is a serious condition. Clinicians and maxillofacial surgeons should be alert to make an immediate diagnosis and select the appropriate treatment in order to prevent worsening of the patient's clinical condition.

1. Introduction

Odontogenic infections are among the most common conditions affecting the oral and maxillofacial region and can lead to severe complications, including airway obstruction, such as Ludwig's angina, septic thrombosis of the cavernous sinus, necrotizing fasciitis, and mediastinitis [1, 2]. They are usually limited to the etiology of origin; however, under certain circumstances involving vascular obliteration with microthrombosis around the locus of infection, accompanied by acute inflammation of subcutaneous tissue and swelling of the underlying tissues with progression of the condition, there is no local intravascular coagulation and the infected tissue becomes necrotic. Thus, the infectious process may spread and overcome bone, muscle, and mucosal barriers, coming into contact with adjacent facial spaces and resulting in severe infections in cavities of the body [2].

Mediastinitis is a rare, progressive, and destructive disease that may often lead to an imminent risk of death [3]. It originates from an infection in a deep cervical space. Sixty to 70% of reported cases are due to odontogenic infections, especially those involving extractions of mandibular third molars [3, 4]. Epidemiological data estimate a mortality rate of 4.8 per 1,000,000 per year, with higher incidence rates among African, Hispanic, and American-Indian populations [4]. In contrast, a lower incidence has been documented among Asians [4]. Due to the robust blood supply, infection in the head and neck region is uncommon, accounting for 1% to 10% of cases [5].

Mediastinitis has a fulminating course with a potential risk of sepsis, pericarditis, and multiple organ failure. The main reasons cited as crucial factors in the poor prognosis of the disease are a late diagnosis and inappropriate surgical approaches. The complications resulting from odontogenic infections are uncommon, and therefore, it is important to use a well-directed anamnesis and to choose responsibly the appropriate treatment for these infections [6]. Immediate diagnoses with aggressive surgical treatment and careful

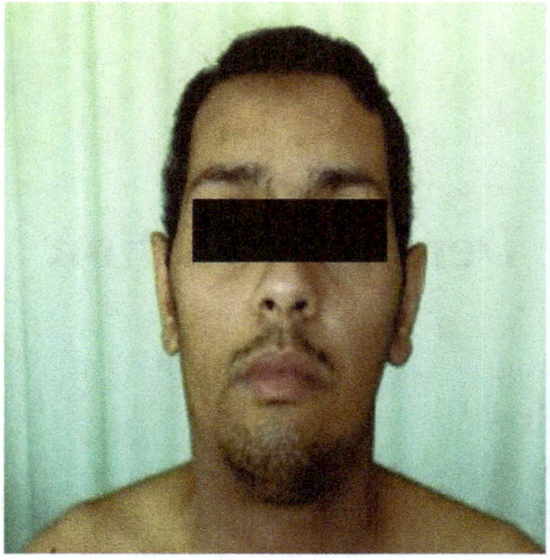

(a)

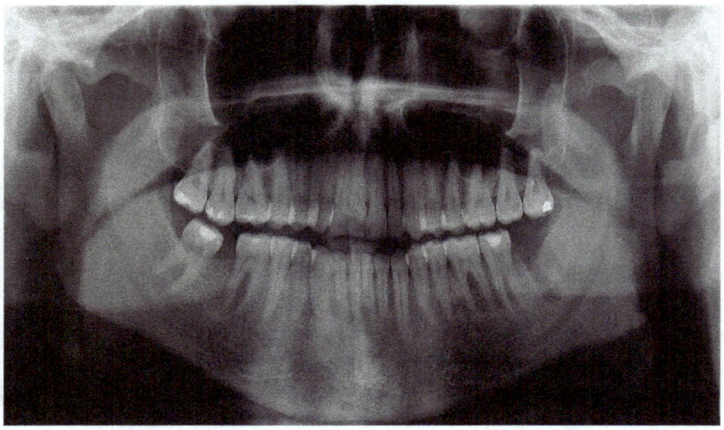

(b)

FIGURE 1: (a) Initial clinical aspect showing swelling in the submandibular region. (b) Panoramic radiograph taken after removal of the left mandibular third molar.

surveillance may limit the progression of the disease [7, 8]. Thus, the aim of the present report was to present an unusual case of a young adult with persistent necrotizing mediastinitis after dental extraction. This article provides information that could help clinicians and maxillofacial surgeons with the diagnosis and management of this condition.

2. Case Presentation

A 37-year-old male patient presented at the emergency service of oral and maxillofacial surgery of a private hospital in Recife, Brazil, with complaints of a painful hard swelling in the submandibular region (Figure 1(a)). He had undergone extraction of the left third molar seven days before presentation (Figure 1(b)). He has noncontributory medical or socioeconomic history, since he was not hypertensive, did not have diabetes mellitus or sexually transmitted infections such as HIV or syphilis, and did not smoke or drink alcoholic beverages.

A computed tomography revealed a hypodense image in the submandibular region accompanied by the presence of gas in their interior (Figure 2). Respiratory rate and blood pressure changes were not observed. On extraoral examination, the skin of the submandibular region was tender bilaterally and of normal color. Intraoral examination revealed maximal interincisal opening (<20 mm), as well as absence of the left mandibular third molar. Blood cultures were performed, and intravenous Metronidazole (500 mg, 8/8 hours) and Rocefin (1 g, 12/12 hours) were empirically started.

On the third day, there was a slight hyperemia in the cervical region and in the thorax, and the patient reported dysphagia and dysphonia. Due to the persistence of the infection, the antibiotic was changed and a new cycle was started with 1.5 g Tazocin injected intravenously every 6 hours. To monitor the clinical status of the patient, daily laboratory tests were carried out, which showed that the body continued to exhibit marked leukocytosis (15,290). There was also positivity and an increase in the 7.32 reference value for C-reactive protein, indicating that there was still a significant infection in the body.

A new contrast-computed tomography of the face, neck, and chest clearly showed the presence of a purulent collection in pharyngeal spaces, with a descending path to the mediastinum and marked deviation of the trachea (Figure 3). In view of the emergency situation, after antisepsis of the region, bilateral drainage of the submandibular and submental regions, and tissue divulsion, irrigation with copious amounts of 0.9% saline solution to serve as drainage orifices was performed on the 5th day of hospitalization (Figure 4). Next, two No. 2 Penrose drains were installed in drainage holes, and the patient was also referred to the intensive care unit (ICU) for 5 days due to the severity of his condition and the need for daily care. The patient underwent orotracheal intubation and, because of severe limitation of mouth opening, the aid of a bougie, an artifact used for intubation of a difficult airway, was selected. During the intensive care period, an investigation was carried out in search of data that could explain the poor evolution of the patient, since he had no comorbidities. A chest tomography revealed the presence of purulent collection in the region above the sternal furcula.

Due to a clinical presentation without significant improvement, the thoracic surgery team intervened six days after the procedure performed by the maxillofacial surgeons. The decision was made to perform tracheostomy and suprasternal cervicotomy, which revealed the presence of necrotic tissues mainly consisting of omohyoid musculature. A large pseudocyst extending from the submandibular region to the sternal furcula and containing secretion was also detected. A tracheal aspiration culture was performed and revealed *Pseudomonas aeruginosa* and *Klebsiella pneumoniae ssp pneumoniae*. Opening of the mediastinum revealed no devitalized tissues and very few purulent collections. A Penrose drain was installed in the furcula, and at the end of the procedure, the patient underwent a tracheostomy and returned to the ICU.

During the postoperative period, the patient was kept on antibiotic therapy with 1 g Meropenem 8/8 hours and 400 mg Targocid 12/12 hours intravenously, showing significant improvement with sudden falls in leukocytosis and C-reactive protein, as well as improvement of general clinical

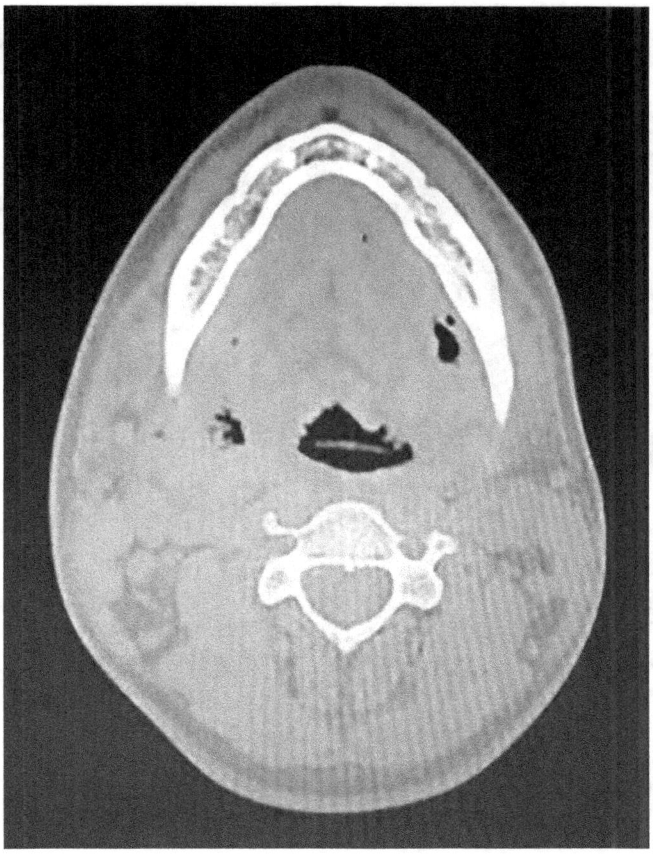

FIGURE 2: Computed tomography axial view showing the initial aspect of the patient's face.

status. After 1 year of treatment, the patient was invited by telephone to follow-up; however, he did not return to our service and only reported no symptomatology.

3. Discussion

Mediastinitis is defined as inflammation of mediastinal tissues and is often characterized by rapidly progressive bacterial infection on multiple tissue planes, leading to vascular, muscular, and airway involvement. In the present case, the infection originated due to tooth extraction. The infectious process reached submandibular, cervical, and mediastinal regions, in agreement with Fukuchi et al.'s explanation [9], i.e., odontogenic infections of the oropharynx can expand to the mediastinum through respiratory movements and negative intrathoracic pressure.

The literature suggests a higher prevalence of males in the development of deep cervical infections, possibly due to less care with oral hygiene [6]. According to Qu et al. [3], submandibular and pterygomandibular spaces were those most involved in the disease. This fact can be explained by anatomical reasons, since 75% of the odontogenic infections were due to extractions of mandibular molars, which eventually drain bacteria into these spaces. This is what happened to the present patient, with the infection evidently involving the submandibular space bilaterally.

Regarding the radiographic characteristics, the image is a diffuse and often well-defined area, demonstrating the increase in volume of the affected region. In the lateral radiograph of the neck, it is common to observe a displacement of the posterior wall of the pharynx with the presence of gas. When the infection progresses towards the mediastinum and the thorax, as observed in the anteroposterior radiograph of the thorax, an increase of the mediastinal space occurs, with air accumulating in this region [10].

Among the main signs and symptoms, the presence of dysphagia, pain, and edema in the cervical region, chest pain, and airway involvement should draw attention [3]. In addition to all the signs and symptoms mentioned, the present patient had a necrotic tissue region, which explains the severity of his infection. Furthermore, elevated levels of C-reactive protein, i.e., concentrations between 1.47 and 7.29, have indicated the need for surgical intervention in a number of cases of documented severe odontogenic infections [10–12]. This also applied to the current patient. Thus, the maxillofacial surgeon should always request laboratory tests, analyzing the number of leukocytes and C-reactive protein levels, since high values show that the patient has an odontogenic infection.

Regarding patient management, Martins et al. [11] showed that penicillin is the most used and therefore the first-choice drug, which may be associated with β-lactamase inhibitors if necessary. However, in the event of failure or allergy, clindamycin and the macrolide class of drugs, particularly azithromycin, are viable alternatives, along with moxifloxacin, which has shown promising results in clinical trials.

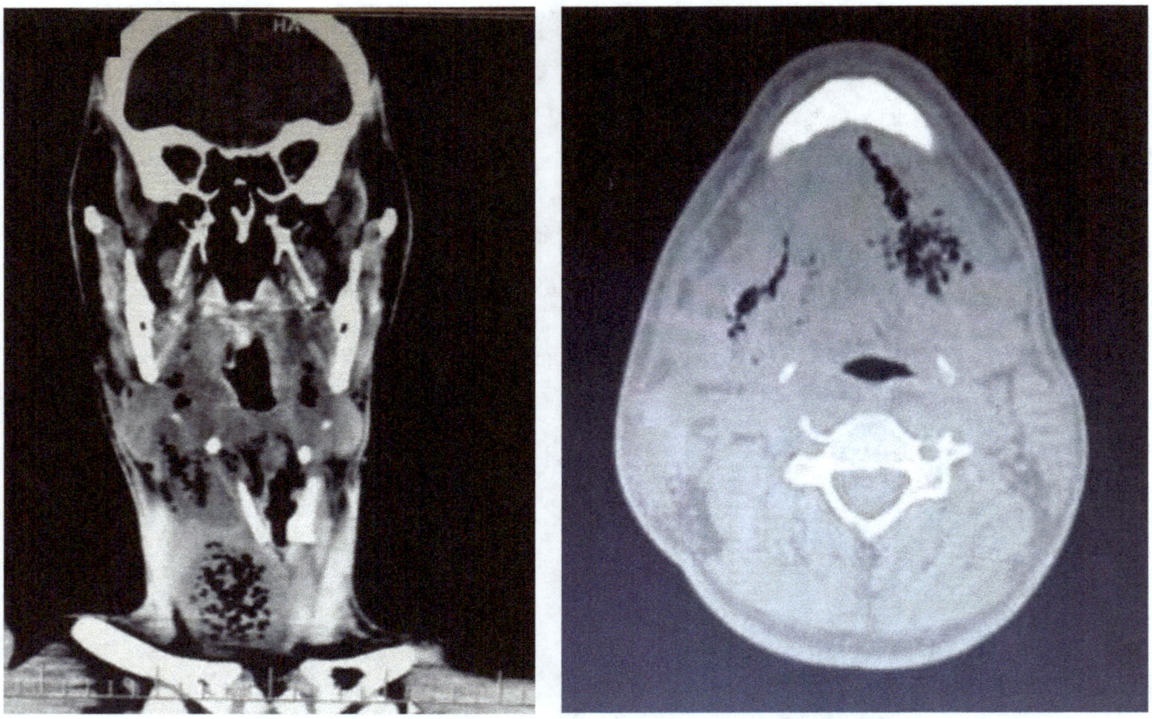

(a) (b)

FIGURE 3: (a, b) Computed tomography of the face and cervical region revealing soft tissue enlargement associated with subcutaneous emphysema between muscular planes. Purulent mediastinal collections with gaseous contents and tracheal deviation can be seen.

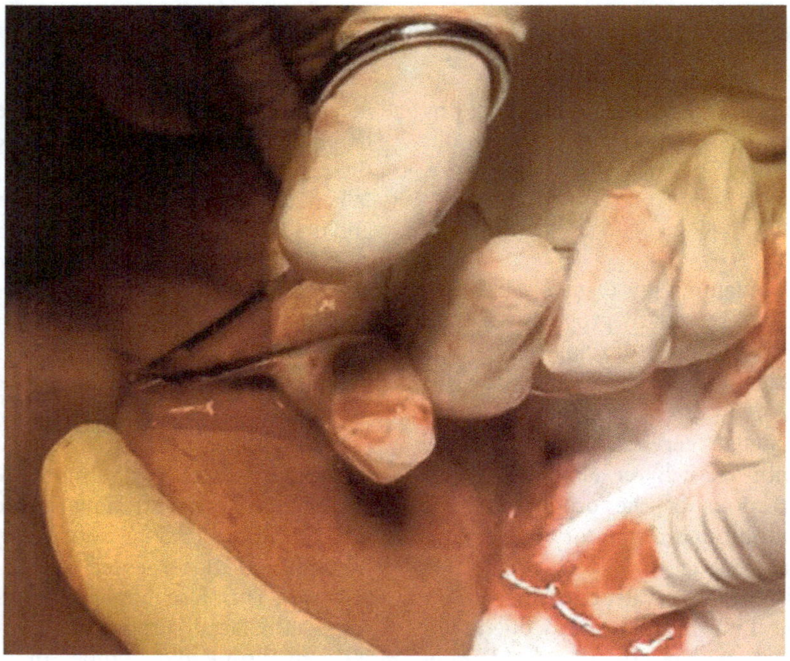

FIGURE 4: Submandibular incision and purulent collection drainage.

Here, the antibiotic therapy used was Metronidazole and Rocefin at the beginning, with a later switch to Tazocin and then to Meropenem and Targocid after drainage.

Considering the severity and rapid spread of the infection in the present case, it became clear that the maxillofacial surgeon should not underestimate its occurrence and should always be prepared for the appearance of deep infections, analyzing the case quickly for diagnosis and treatment and thus protecting the life of the patient. Therefore, in the presence of a severe odontogenic infection, we emphasize the importance of a multidisciplinary team consisting of a thoracic surgeon, general practitioner, and infectologist for better handling of the case and greater chances of successful treatment.

In summary, early diagnosis, a surgical approach involving drainage, and adequate antibiotic therapy are three key factors in the successful treatment of mediastinitis, a condition with a rapid and destructive course which can lead to death.

Acknowledgments

We would like to thank Coordenação de Aperfeiçoamento de Pessoal de Nível Superior (CAPES, Finance Code 001), Brazil. J.A.A.A. is the recipient of a postgraduate fellowship. Mrs. E. Greene provided English editing of the manuscript.

References

[1] H. M. Prado-Calleros, E. Jiménez-Fuentes, and I. Jiménez-Escobar, "Descending necrotizing mediastinitis: systematic review on its treatment in the last 6 years, 75 years after its description," *Head Neck*, vol. 38, no. S1, pp. E2275–E2283, 2016.

[2] J. A. Arruda, E. Figueiredo, P. Álvares et al., "Cervical necrotizing fasciitis caused by dental extraction," *Case Reports in Dentistry*, vol. 2016, Article ID 1674153, 5 pages, 2016.

[3] L. Qu, X. Liang, B. Jiang, W. Qian, W. Zhang, and X. Cai, "Risk factors affecting the prognosis of descending necrotizing mediastinitis from odontogenic infection," *Journal of Oral and Maxillofacial Surgery*, vol. 76, no. 6, pp. 1207–1215, 2018.

[4] D. A. Gunaratne, E. A. Tseros, Z. Hasan et al., "Cervical necrotizing fasciitis: systematic review and analysis of 1235 reported cases from the literature," *Head Neck*, vol. 40, no. 9, pp. 2094–2102, 2018.

[5] H. Hidaka, D. Ozawa, S. Kuriyama et al., "Risk factors for delayed oral dietary intake in patients with deep neck infections including descending necrotizing mediastinitis," *European Archives of Oto-Rhino-Laryngology*, vol. 274, no. 11, pp. 3951–3958, 2017.

[6] A. Adoviča, L. Veidere, M. Ronis, and G. Sumeraga, "Deep neck infections: review of 263 cases," *Otolaryngologia Polska*, vol. 71, no. 5, pp. 37–42, 2017.

[7] T. Sarna, T. Sengupta, M. Miloro, and A. Kolokythas, "Cervical necrotizing fasciitis with descending mediastinitis: literature review and case report," *Journal of Oral and Maxillofacial Surgery*, vol. 70, no. 6, pp. 1342–1350, 2012.

[8] M. R. Gore, "Odontogenic necrotizing fasciitis: a systematic review of the literature," *BMC Ear, Nose and Throat Disorders*, vol. 18, no. 1, p. 14, 2018.

[9] M. Fukuchi, O. Suzuki, D. Nasu et al., "Descending necrotizing mediastinitis treated with tooth extractions following mediastinal and cervical drainage," *Case Reports in Gastroenterology*, vol. 9, no. 3, pp. 311–316, 2015.

[10] Y. Jiménez, J. V. Bagán, J. Murillo, and R. Poveda, "Odontogenic infections. Complications. Systemic manifestations," *Medicina oral, patología oral y cirugía bucal*, vol. 9, no. 143-147, pp. 139–143, 2004.

[11] J. R. Martins, O. L. Chagas Jr., B. D. Velasques, Â. N. Bobrowski, M. B. Correa, and M. A. Torriani, "The use of antibiotics in odontogenic infections: what is the best choice? A systematic review," *Journal of Oral and Maxillofacial Surgery*, vol. 75, no. 12, pp. 2606.e1–2606.e11, 2017.

[12] S. Ylijoki, R. Suuronen, H. Jousimies-Somer, J. H. Meurman, and C. Lindqvist, "Differences between patients with or without the need for intensive care due to severe odontogenic infections," *Journal of Oral and Maxillofacial Surgery*, vol. 59, no. 8, pp. 867–872, 2001.

Preprosthetic Management of "Flabby Ridge" on Edentulous Patient

Amani Mizouri,[1] Oumaima Tayari,[1] AlaEddine Mahfoudhi,[1] Adel Bouguezzi,[2] and Jamila Jaouadi[1]

[1]*Complete Removable Prosthodontic Department, Research Laboratory LR12ES11, Faculty of Dental Medicine, University of Monastir, Monastir, Tunisia*
[2]*Oral Surgery Department, Research Laboratory LR12ES11, Faculty of Dental Medicine, University of Monastir, Monastir, Tunisia*

Correspondence should be addressed to Oumaima Tayari; oumaimatayari0@gmail.com

Academic Editor: Asja Celebic

For edentulous patients, the integrity of the osteomucosal-bearing surface is a significant factor for the balance of the future removable prosthesis. The supporting tissues are influenced by several factors. Physiological bone resorption, senescence, and changes caused by systemic diseases and polypharmacy lead to modifications in these tissues. Similarly, trauma caused by an ill-fitted prosthesis influences the degree of bone resorption and the development of hyperplastic tissue. The etiology of bone resorption is multifactorial and complex, with continuous individual variations that are often unexplained. Although, no study has been able to establish the importance of the different factors in relation to each other, it is often reported that chronic excessive mechanical pressure in relation to occlusal constraints is responsible for the appearance of local resorption's areas. The aim of this work is to present, through three clinical cases, the various factors involved in the alteration of the osteomucous-bearing surface and eventually, possible therapeutic attitude to deal with.

1. Introduction

The use of an ill-fitting or very old complete prosthesis leads to deep changes of the ecosystem, in the oral cavity, and can cause tissue damage [1].

Among the many injuries related to wearing a misadjusted removable prosthesis, prosthetic stomatitis, angular cheilitis, disinserted fibromucosa or "floating ridge," and fibrous hyperplastic lesion are included [2, 3].

An impression taken on altered or deformed tissue usually leads to the realization of an unstable prosthesis which will accelerate bone resorption.

This is why restoring a healthy state of osteomucous support appears as an indispensable preliminary condition for a consistent and efficient prosthetic treatment [3].

The success of prosthodontic treatment in edentulous patients depends closely on the state of the osteomucous surface that supports the prosthesis and requires a quantitative and qualitative evaluation of the bone and mucosal components [3, 4].

For the bone support, several parameters are evaluated, such as the degree of resorption: in fact, a residual bone represents a favorable factor to the prosthetic balance.

In case of significant resorption compromising the prosthetic retention, treatment with implant can be envisaged after a preimplant assessment [4].

Mucous membrane, due to its anatomical and histological particularities, can interfere with the use of prosthesis. Mucosal lesions induced by the complete prosthesis can be classified according to their etiology in the following:

(i) Traumatic injuries, especially anterior occlusal overload, caused by a defective and traumatic complete prosthesis for the underlying osteomucous-bearing surfaces, such as the case of flabby ridges and epulis fissuratum [1, 3, 5–8]

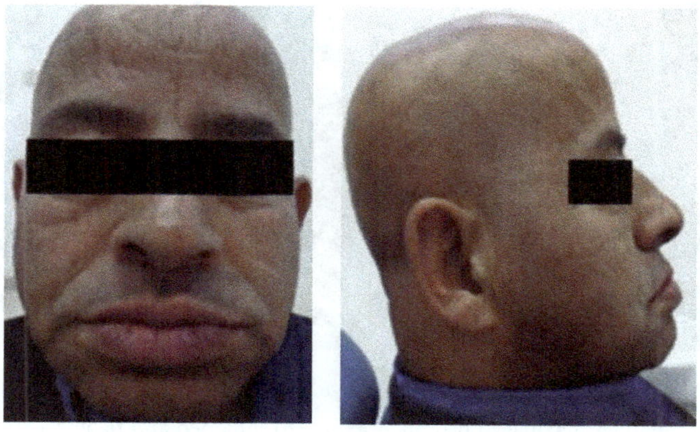

(a) (b)

FIGURE 1: Extraoral appearance: (a) front view and (b) side view.

(ii) Prosthetic stomatitis which is defined as a chronic inflammatory condition of the oral mucosa supporting a removable prosthesis. Its etiology is multifactorial, mainly, the trauma caused by ill-fitting prostheses associated to an infectious factor, oral and prosthetic deficient hygiene, continuous prosthetic use, salivary dysfunction, and smoking [1, 4, 9–11]

Management of prosthesis inducing mucosal lesions depends on the type of the lesion and its etiology. The treatment consists of several phases, either separately or concomitantly: tissue conditioning, special impression techniques for compromised ridges, and surgical option.

The purpose of this paper is to present various preprosthetic management techniques of hyperplastic soft tissue on edentulous patient.

2. Case Report 1

A 60-year-old man, with no medical history, was referred to the department of prosthodontics of the faculty of dental medicine of Monastir, Tunisia, requesting a new set of complete prosthesis.

The extraoral examination revealed the decrease of occlusal vertical dimension (OVD) (Figures 1(a) and 1(b)).

An intraoral examination allowed the evaluation of the existing prosthesis for which the occlusal plane was correctly oriented in the maxillary prosthesis obeying to esthetic and phonetic guidelines; the centric relation (CR) was faulty: the patient was used to make a protrusive occlusion so it was so difficult to guide him in correct CR because of his acquired occlusal memory, and the border extensions of maxillary and mandibular complete prostheses were correctly situated (Figure 2).

The maxillary and mandibular edentulous ridges showed a significant bone resorption, covered by inflamed fibromucosa.

A flabby tissue in the anterior mandibular ridge extending from the canine to canine region was noticed (Figures 3(a) and 3(b)).

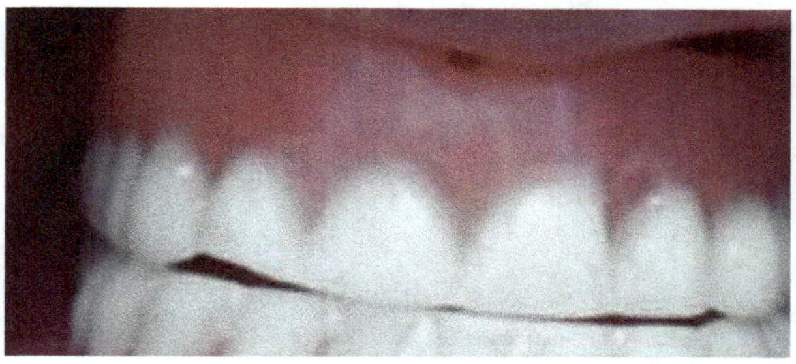

FIGURE 2: Prosthesis examination.

According to the data obtained, a diagnosis of a flabby ridge of the anterior mandibular region and a generalized prosthetic stomatitis due to the excessive and continuous mechanical pressure imparted by the faulty prosthesis's occlusion were performed.

A new complete prosthesis was planned for this patient concomitantly with an occlusal conditioning treatment followed by a vestibuloplasty to restore anterior alveolar ridge height.

The patient was informed in detail about the procedure, and his consent was obtained.

At the first appointment, a modification of the mandibular prosthesis using self-cured acrylic resin over the artificial teeth served to restore the vertical dimension and centric relation provisionally until fabricating new prostheses in order to break up with old protrusive reflex.

The procedure was to wrap two strands of wax and place them over teeth occlusal surfaces and record the new mandibular position (TENCH articulating); the purpose of this step is to guide the patient to close in CR that has been validated by finding the coincidence of the interincisal midpoint.

Then, the wax on the left side was replaced with self-cured acrylic resin and the same operation was repeated. Finally, eliminate the excess of resin, polish the prostheses, and recheck accuracy of previously made centric relation record (Figures 4(a)–4(h)). The same procedure was repeated on the right side.

This new occlusal situation will serve as a guide for manufacturing new complete dentures.

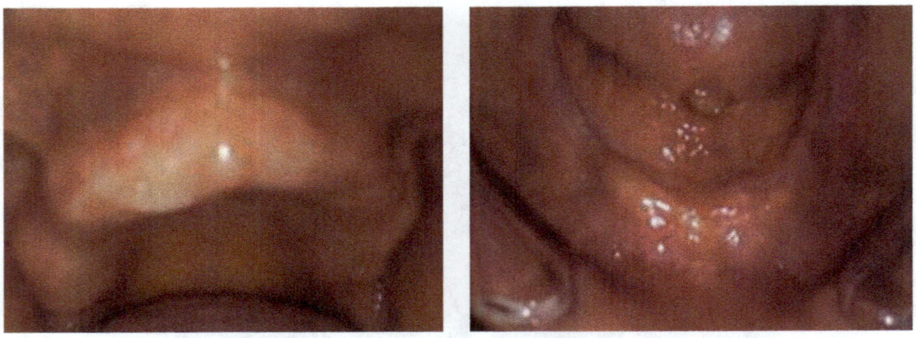

(a) (b)

Figure 3: Intraoral examination: (a) inflamed maxillary fibromucosa and (b) inflamed and flabby tissue in the mandibular anterior region.

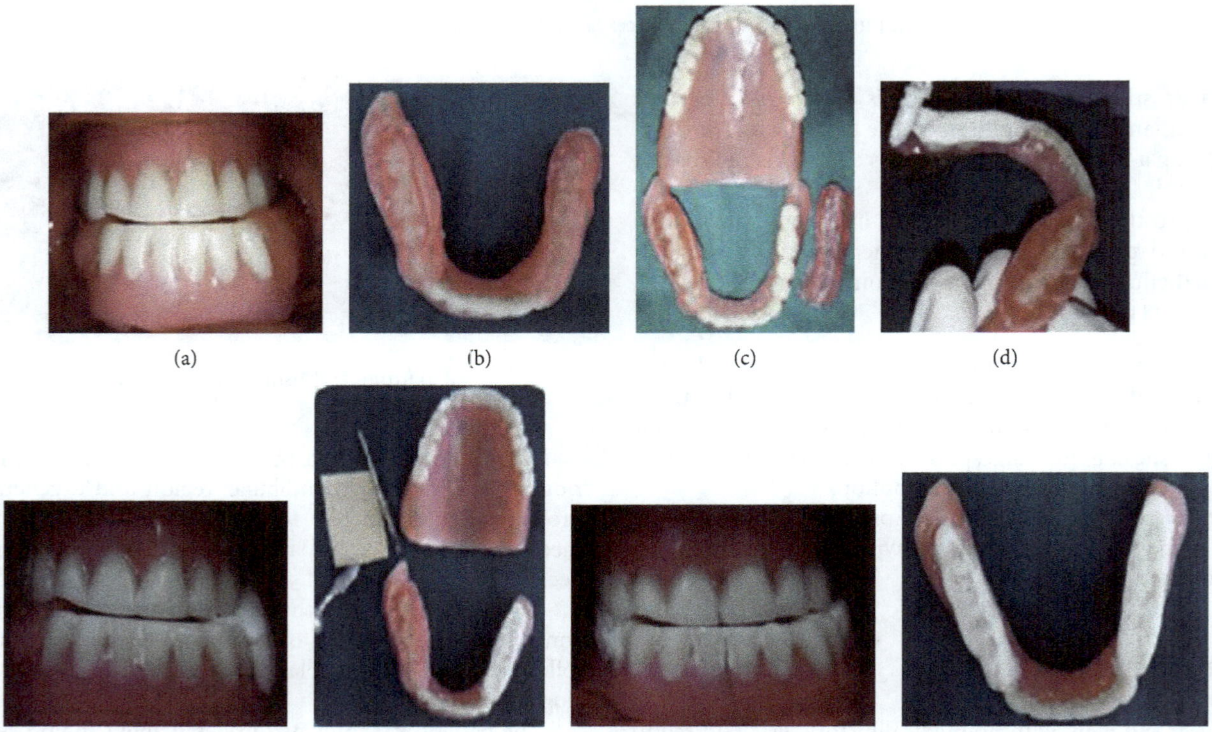

(a) (b) (c) (d)

(e) (f) (g) (h)

Figure 4: TENCH articulated technique. (a, b) Interocclusal record using wax. (c, d) Replacing the wax with chemopolymerized resin on the right side. (e) Centric relation. (f) Prosthesis polishing. (g, h) Procedure on the right side.

The fibromucosa status was evaluated in one and 2 weeks after the occlusal conditioning treatment; there was a significant regression of the inflammation (Figures 5(a)–5(c)). However, there was a persistent hyperplastic ridge that established an unfavorable bearing surface for the new prosthesis. During the next appointments, the clinical procedures for the new complete prosthesis were initiated following the conventional technique.

After manufacturing the final prostheses, surgical procedures were planned starting with vestibuloplasty, followed by placing an epithelioconnective palatal flap.

For this, an infiltrative local anesthesia technique (2% lidocaine) was necessary before performing soft tissue surgery. A deep incision was carried from the canine to canine region on the labial surface of the mandibular arch; then, the vestibule was deepened by a supraperiosteal dissection. The mucosal flap was turned downward from its attachment and placed directly against the periosteum to which it was sutured with interrupted ones.

The newly exposed periosteum was covered by the epithelial-connective tissue graft using a palatal flap (Figures 6(a)–6(f)).

Postsurgical prosthesis withdrawal was beneficial to not irritate the graft.

Antibiotics (amoxicillin 2 g per day for 7days), an anti-inflammatory drug (ibuprofen 600 mg every eight hours for 4 days), an analgesic (Paracetamol 650 mg every eight hours for 4days), and 0.12% chlorhexidine mouthwashes (used from the second day postsurgery) were prescribed.

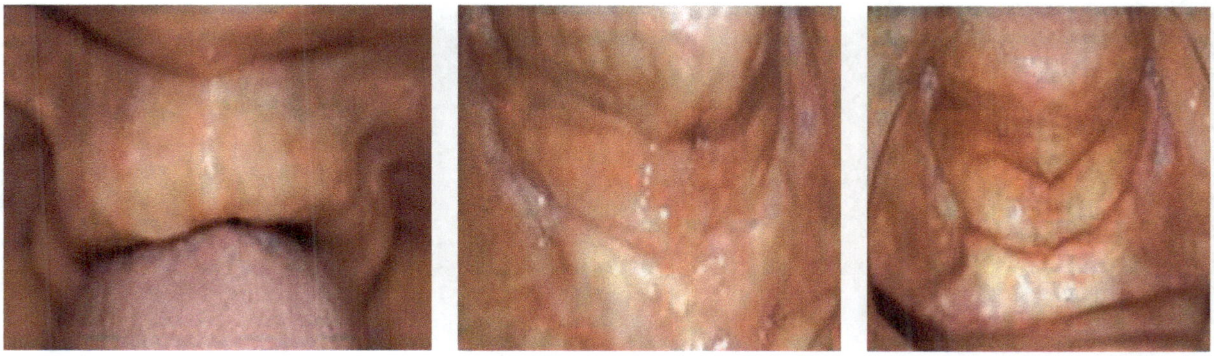

(a) (b) (c)

FIGURE 5: Regression of the inflammation of the maxillary and mandibular fibromucosa after occlusal conditioning treatment: (a, b) one week and (c) two weeks.

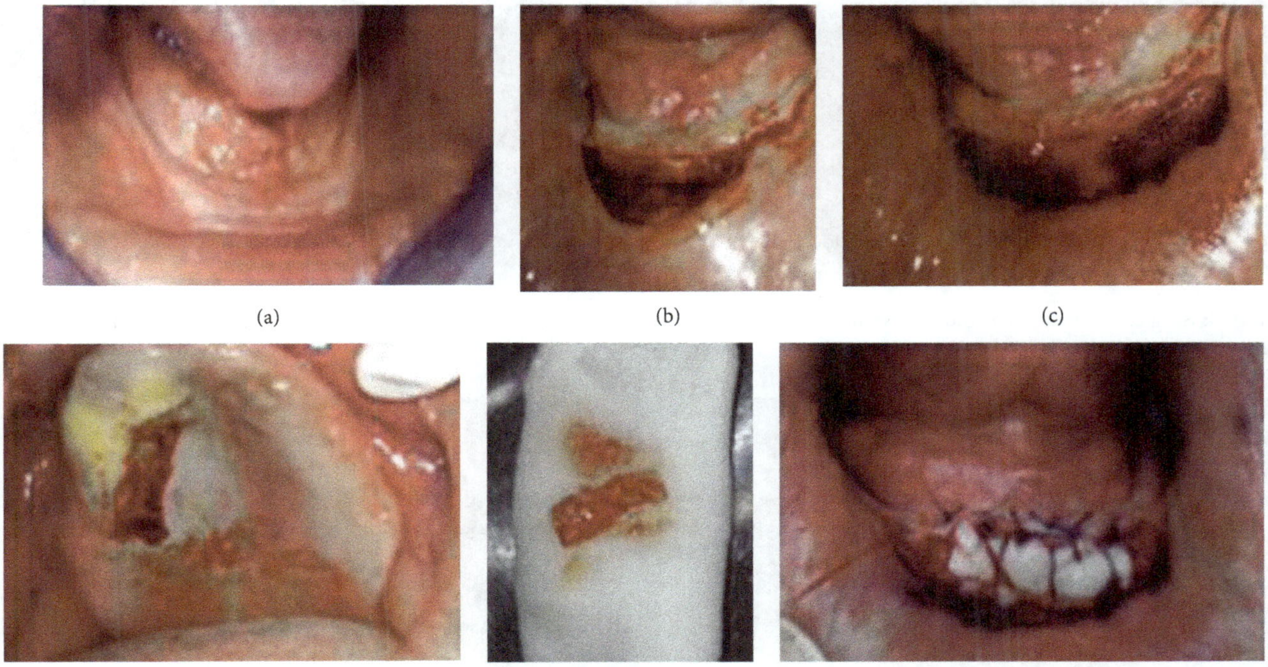

(a) (b) (c)

(d) (e) (f)

FIGURE 6: The surgical procedure: (a) preoperative view, (b) horizontal semilunar incision followed by Supra periosteal dissection deepening the vestibule, (c) suturing of the mucosal flap, (d, e) epithelioconnective palatal flap, and (f) immediate postoperative view.

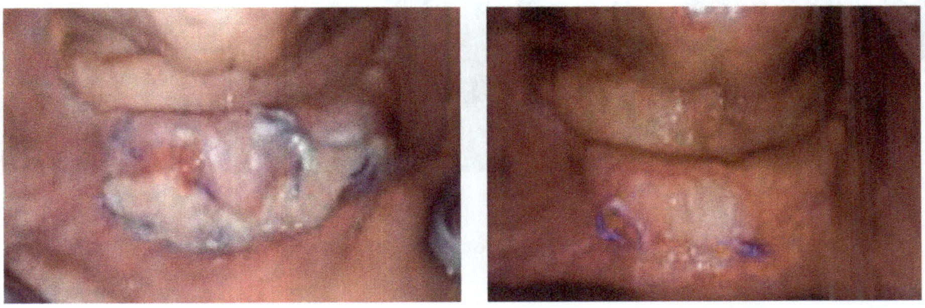

(a) (b)

FIGURE 7: Healing process of the treated area: (a) 7 days and (b) 14 days.

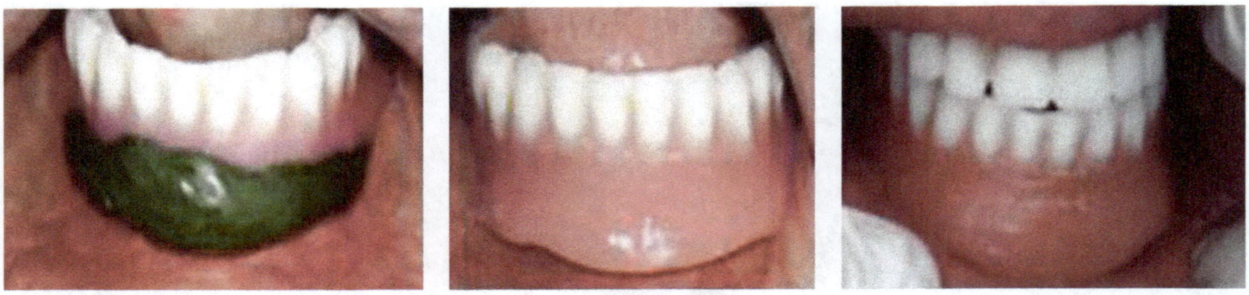

(a) (b) (c)

FIGURE 8: Prostheses adjustments: (a) border molded mandibular prosthesis, (b) chemopolymerized resin molding, and (c) occlusal adjustments.

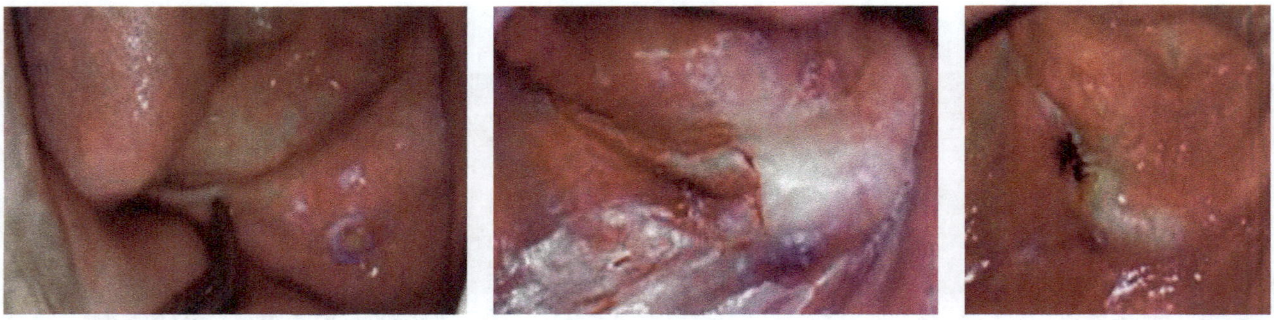

(a) (b) (c)

FIGURE 9: Surgical correction of the disinserted fibromucosa: (a) clinical examination of the disinserted fibromucosa and (b, c) surgical treatment.

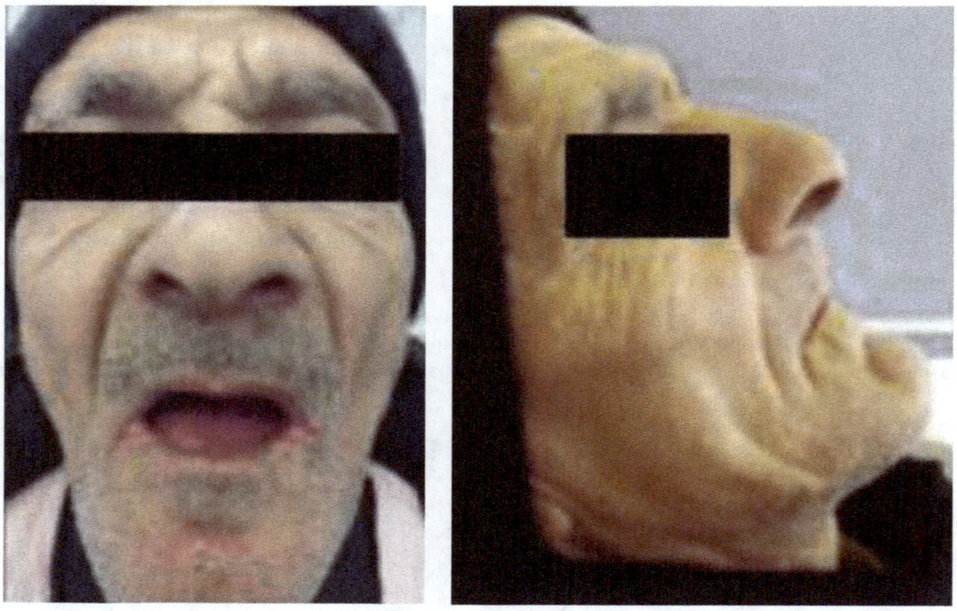

(a) (b)

FIGURE 10: Extraoral examination: (a) front view and (b) side view.

The patient was recalled for follow-up (7 days and 14 days) (Figures 7(a) and 7(b)).

Once healing was complete, the anterior edge of the mandibular prosthesis must be adjusted to the new vestibular height. The lack was adjusted by a border-molded impression compound that was replaced later with chemopolymerized resin. Finally, occlusal adjustments were performed (Figures 8(a)–8(c)).

In addition, a surgical correction of the disinserted fibromucosa at the posteromandibular ridge is necessary and

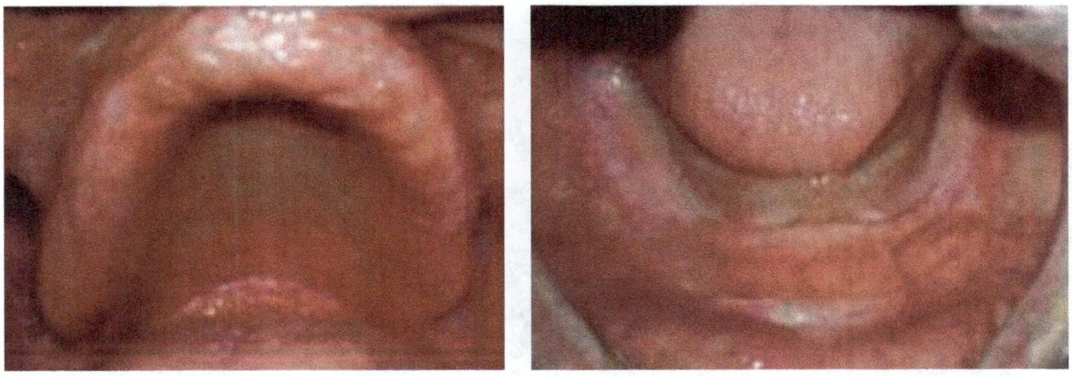

(a) (b)

FIGURE 11: Intraoral examination: (a) flabby tissue in the maxillary anterior region and (b) fibrous hyperplastic mass.

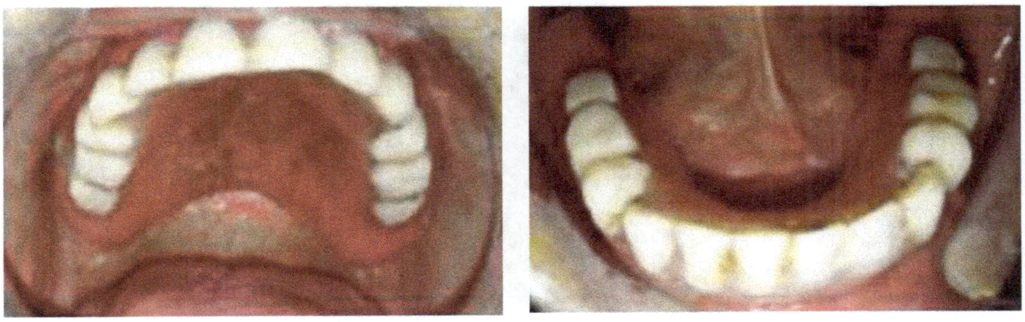

(a) (b)

FIGURE 12: Prosthesis examination: (a) old maxillary prothesis and (b) old mandibular prosthesis.

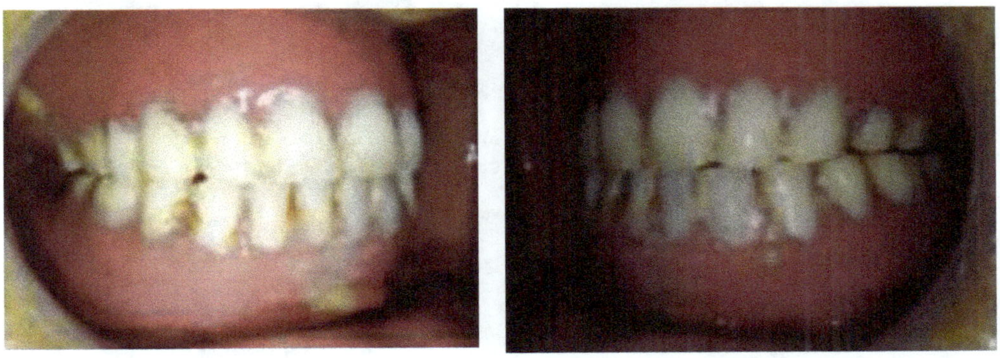

(a) (b)

FIGURE 13: Misadjusted occlusion: (a) right side and (b) left side.

managed by a surgical correction which includes simple trimming of the excessive tissue but not disturbing the attached fibromucosa (Figures 9(a)–9(c)).

3. Case Report 2

A 64-year-old-male patient consulted the prosthodontic department of the faculty of dental medicine of Monastir requesting new prostheses. His complaints were mainly about esthetic appearance and ill-fitting prostheses causing discomfort while it is used. He had been wearing the current prostheses for more than 10 years.

Extraoral examination revealed a decrease of the occlusal vertical dimension which caused angular cheilitis (Figures 10(a) and 10(b)).

Intraoral examination showed edentulous maxillary and mandibular resorbed ridges covered with an inflamed fibromucosa. An area of flabby tissue in the maxillary anterior region and a fibrous hyperplastic mass in relation with the anterior mandibular vestibule were found (Figures 11(a) and 11(b)).

Both maxillary and mandibular covering tissues presented an extensive inflammatory lesion due to traumatic occlusion and prosthetic stomatitis confirmed by oral mycological analysis. A preliminary tissue conditioning treatment

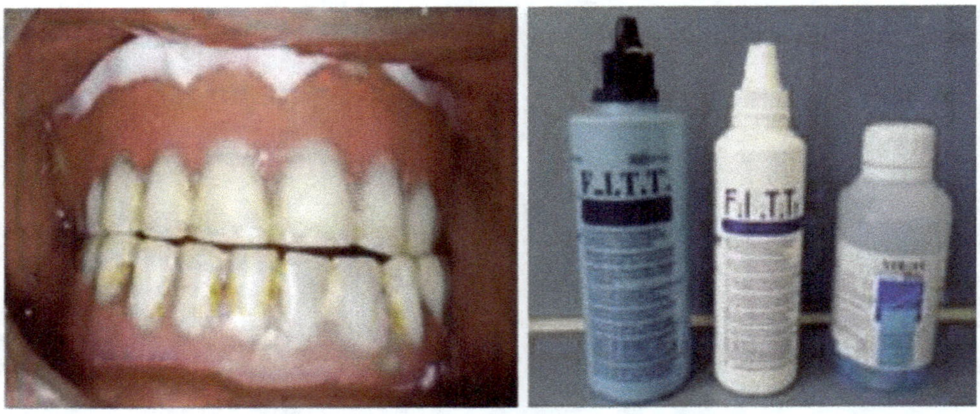

FIGURE 14: Tissue conditioning using soft tissue conditioner mixed with an anti-inflammatory mouthwash.

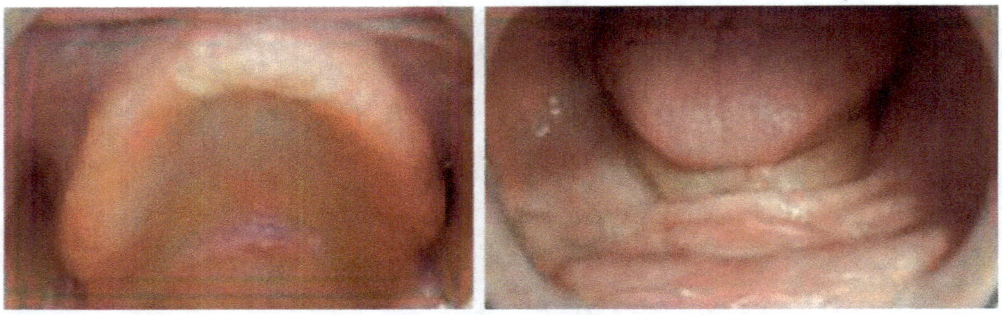

FIGURE 15: Healthy oral fibromucosa further to a tissue conditioning treatment.

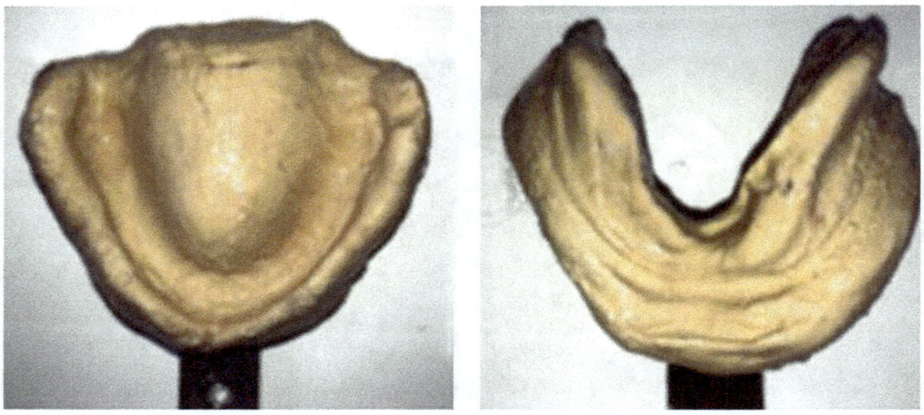

(a) (b)

FIGURE 16: (a) Preliminary impression. (b) The epulis fissuratum area's delineation on the mandibular preliminary impression.

associated to antifungal agent (0.2% chlorhexidine mouthwash) was indispensable.

Prosthesis examination revealed teeth abrasion, insufficient prosthesis hygiene, and misadjusted occlusion causing trauma to the area during swallowing and mastication (Figures 12 and 13).

A clinical diagnosis of an epulis fissuratum due to chronic irritation from the ill-fitting prosthesis was evoked. The oral patient consent was obtained in order to fabricate a new complete prosthesis followed by a surgical excision of the lesion and vestibuloplasty to avoid recurrence.

At the first appointment, the patient's existing prostheses were evaluated for fit and occlusion. Then, prostheses were relined according to the present residual ridges using the temporary soft resin (FITT Kerr®) to improve the state of the soft tissues before manufacturing new prostheses. The procedure is repeated every 2-3 weeks until the soft tissues recovery (Figures 14 and 15).

The patient is now ready for the fabrication of new prostheses.

The preliminary impressions were made using impression plaster to record hyperplastic tissues in the uncompressed state (Figures 16(a) and 16(b)). This negative record was meticulously taken so that the compression was minimized; no major pressure spots were found. The impression was poured using a white dental plaster.

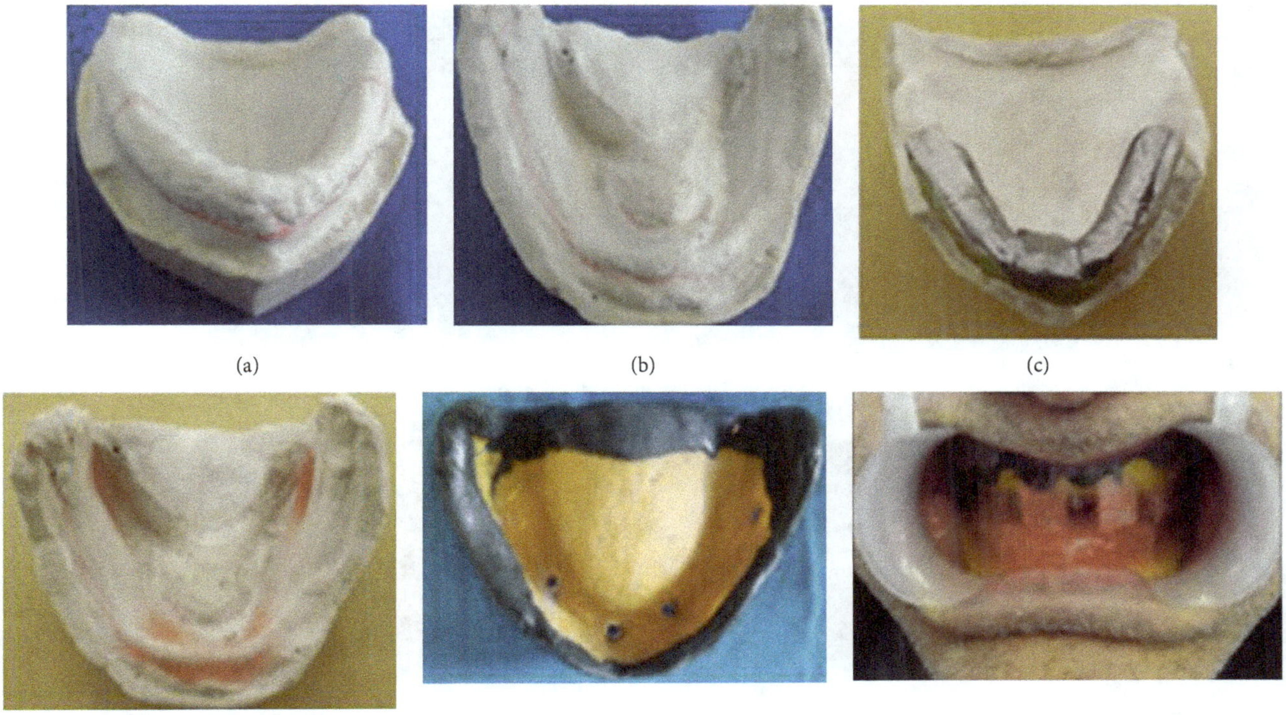
(a) (b) (c)
(d) (e) (f)

FIGURE 17: Prerequisites to the final impression. (a, b) The hyperplastic maxillary and mandibular area delineation scribed on the preliminary cast. (c) Dental tin foil over the maxillary hyperplastic area. (d) Blocking out the undercut as well as redundant tissue on the cast with wax. (e) Perforations corresponding to the hyperplastic area. (f) Final impression under occlusal pressure.

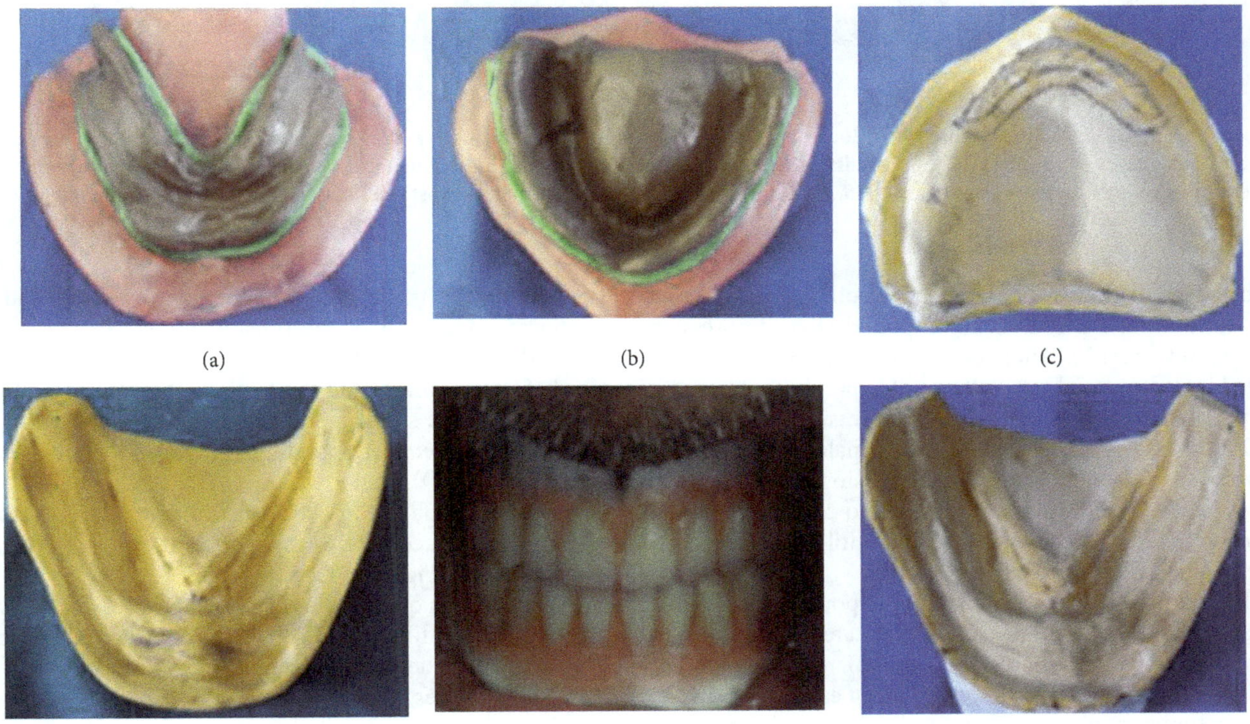
(a) (b) (c)
(d) (e) (f)

FIGURE 18: (a, b) Boxing impression. (c, d) The secondary casts. (e) Teeth arrangement try-in. (f) Surgery simulation.

The floating tissue is perfectly defined by palpation and scribed on the cast (Figures 17(a) and 17(b)). Then, it was blocked out by applying a 3 mm thick layer of dental tin foil over the maxillary hyperplastic area (Figure 17(c)). The special tray was made using a self-curing resin. Two occlusion rims were contoured and adjusted to record centric relation

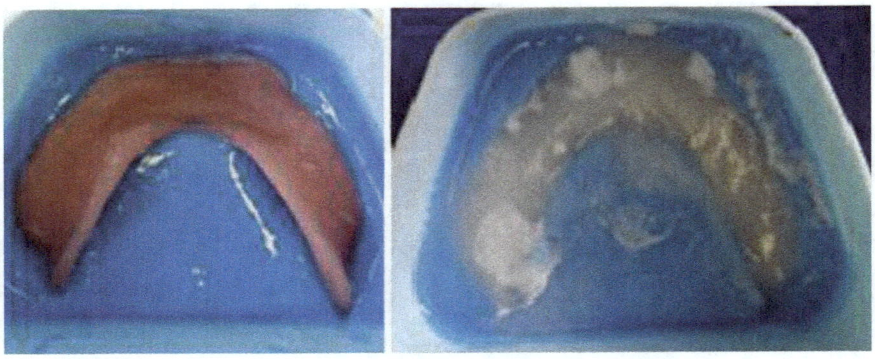

Figure 19: Prosthesis duplication.

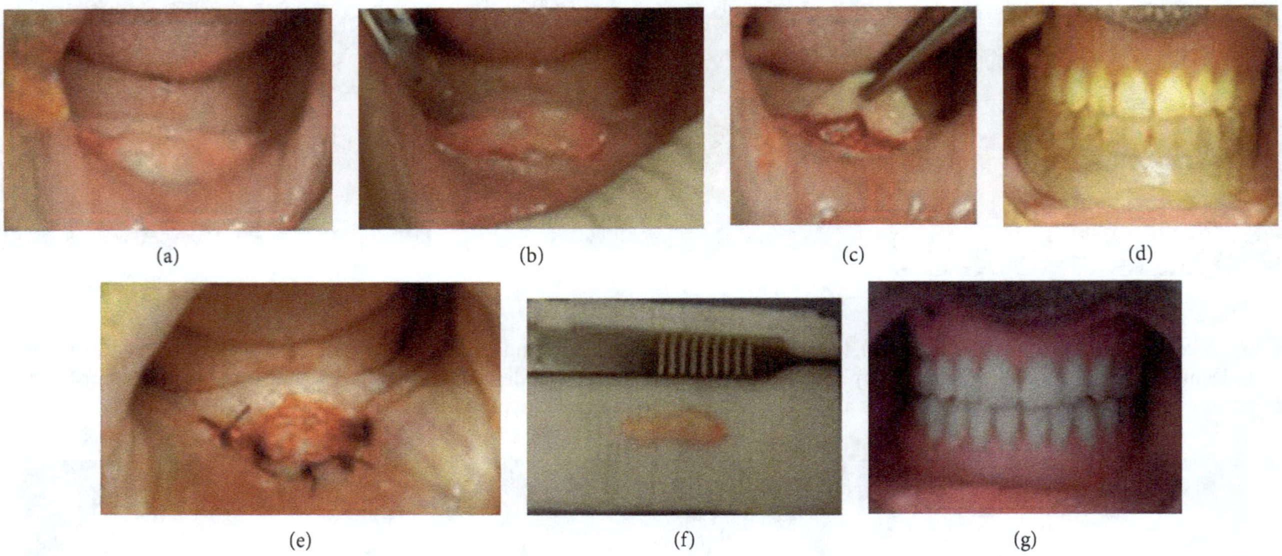

Figure 20: Surgical procedure: (a) infiltrative local anesthesia, (b) semilunar incision, (c) total excision using conventional scalpel surgery, (d) surgery control using surgical guide, (e) immediate aspect of the treated area: suture preserving the depth of the buccal side in the mandible. (f) operatory specimen of the mandibular lesion. and (g) frontal view after immediately prostheses insertion and occlusal adjustment.

at the adequate occlusal vertical dimension. Border molding was done using a green stick compound (Kerr Impression Compound Green®). After testing the retention, holes were drilled into the special tray, in front of hyperplastic area, with a round bur to remove the excess of impression material. The final impression was taken with Permalastic Polysulfide Impression Material, Kerr Dental®, using the functional pressure; the patient was gently guided to centric relation at the correct vertical occlusal dimension until the material setting (Figures 17(d)–17(f)).

Final impressions were boxed and poured to get final casts on which record bases were fabricated and occlusion rims were prepared (Figures 18(a)–18(d)).

The occlusal plane was oriented using esthetic, phonetic, and anatomic guidelines. Then, occlusal vertical dimension was established using the physiological rest position associated with phonetic and esthetic techniques. Finally, the centric relation recording was done followed by the transfer of jaw relation to a semiadjustable articulator. Maxillary cast was mounted using facebow record, while mandibular cast was mounted using interocclusal record.

During the try-in appointment, the occlusion and the aesthetic integration of the prosthetic reconstruction were verified and accomplished (Figure 18(e)).

Before manufacturing the final prostheses, surgical procedures must be simulated on the final cast by scarping the amount of plaster corresponding to the ulterior removed tissue (Figure 18(f)).

After manufacturing, the final mandibular prosthesis must be duplicated with transparent resin which served as a surgical guide (Figure 19).

The excision of the epulis fissuratum was performed with the conventional surgical procedure that was controlled by the surgical guide until obtaining the wanted width of the vestibule (Figures 20(a)–20(d)).

The depth of the vestibule was preserved. Bleeding control by compression and primary closure was performed with interrupted sutures (Figure 20(e)). All specimens obtained from the patient were sent for histopathological examination to confirm the diagnosis.

Healing was done by secondary intention (Figures 20(f) and 20(g)).

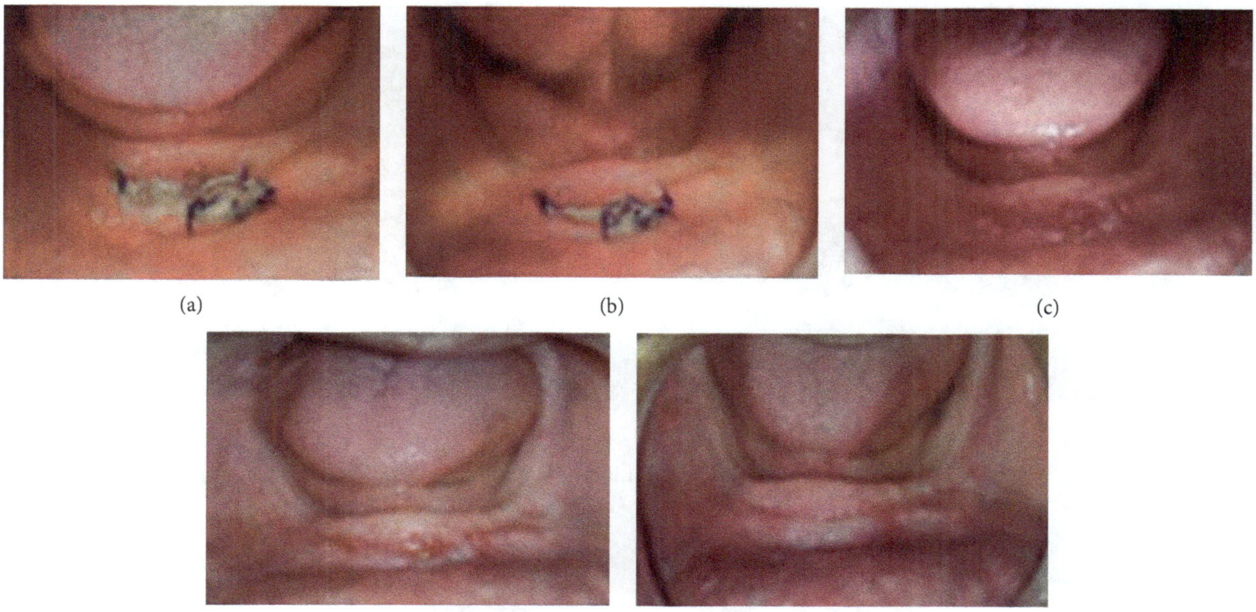

(a) (b) (c) (d) (e)

FIGURE 21: Healing process of the treated area: (a) 3 days, (b) 1 week, (c) 2 weeks, (d) 3 weeks, and (e) 4 weeks.

Minor occlusal adjustments were performed immediately after surgery and prostheses should be kept in place continuously during the first 2-3 days. Patient was recommended to start rinsing with a chlorhexidine mouthwash, the second day after surgery, three times a day during the postoperative first week. Amoxicillin and paracetamol were prescribed. Postoperative controls were performed 3 days and 1, 2, 3, and 4 weeks for the assessment of wound healing (Figures 21(a)–21(e)).

4. Case Report 3

A 57-year-old hypertensive male reported to the prosthodontic department with the chief complaint of an ill-fitting of his complete prostheses delivered about 7 years ago.

In addition, patient complained of pain and discomfort during mastication.

Extraoral examination revealed a decrease in the occlusal vertical dimension (Figure 22).

The clinical exam showed that the upper prosthesis was ill-fitting because of its multiple reparations and teeth replacement (Figures 23(a) and 23(b)).

On visual inspection, a fibrous hyperplastic mass in relation with the anterior maxillary vestibule was noticed. It extended to the anterior crest of the residual ridge (Figure 24).

A lateral frenulum on the right maxillary vestibule was noticed and which could impair the retention and stability of the future prosthesis (Figure 25).

Considering this clinical situation and the medical history (bleeding risk), the immediate confection of appropriate new prostheses and surgical removal with laser radiation was proposed and the patient was informed in detail about the surgical procedure.

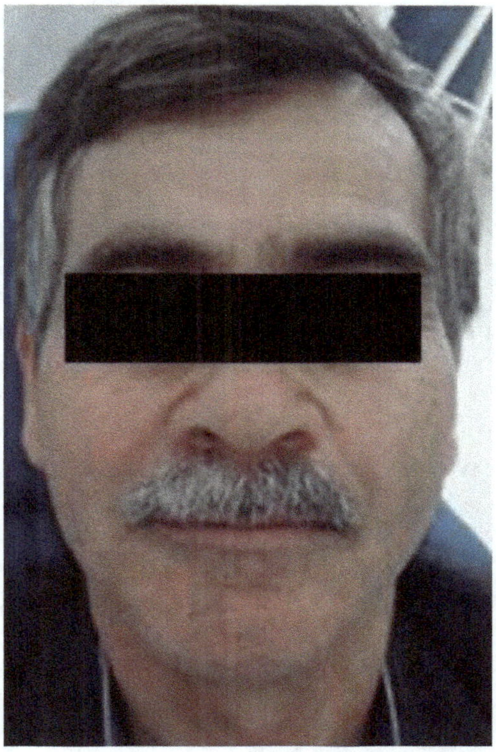

FIGURE 22: Extraoral view.

A habitual procedure for the confection of a complete prosthesis was followed; then, the surgery was proceeded.

The lesion removal was made using a diode laser with a wavelength of 810 nm.

.Additionally, a partial vestibuloplasty was performed in the maxillary sulcus and about 3 mm depth extension was

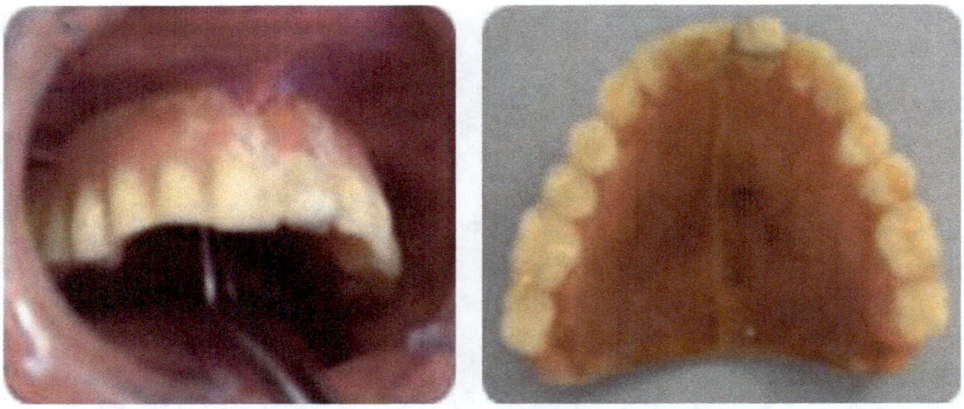

(a) (b)

FIGURE 23: (a, b) Prosthesis examination: an ill-fitting prostheses.

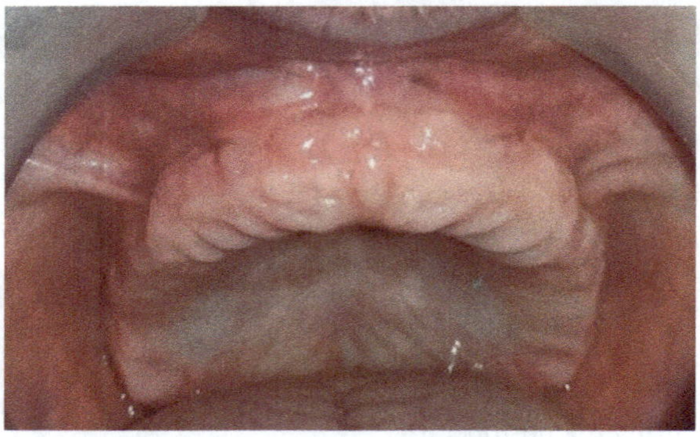

FIGURE 24: Intraoral view: right lateral frenulum.

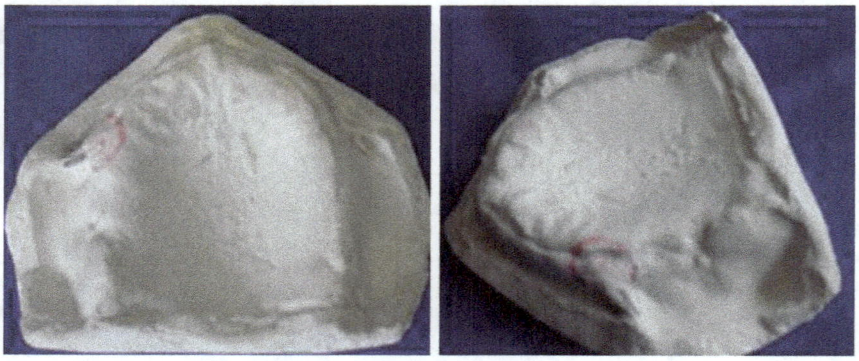

FIGURE 25: Lateral frenulum scribed on the preliminary cast.

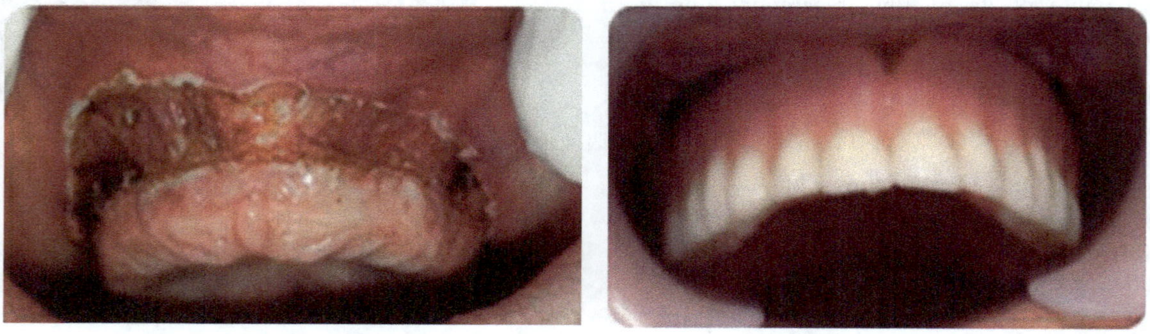

(a) (b)

FIGURE 26: (a) Vestibuloplasty using laser. (b) Surgery control using prosthesis.

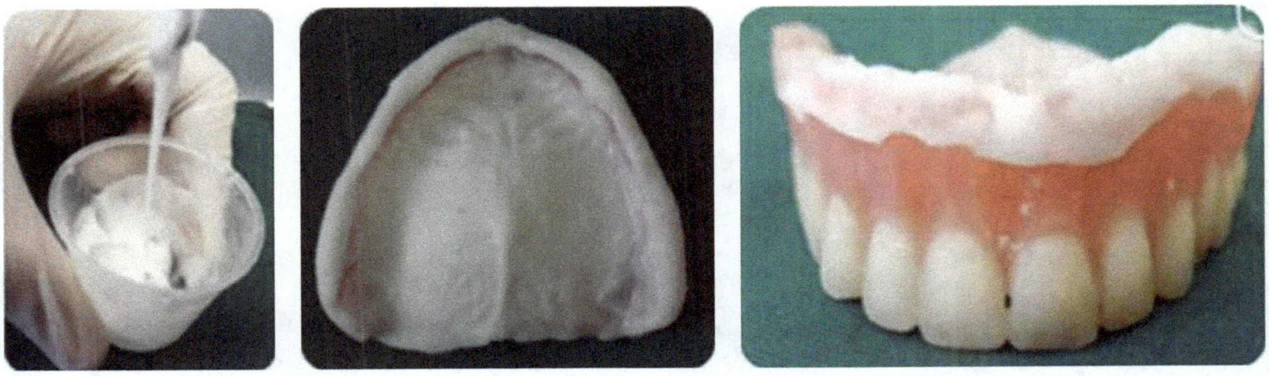

(a) (b) (c)

Figure 27: (a) Tissue conditioner consistency. (b) Molded soft tissue conditioner. (c) Soft tissue conditioner border.

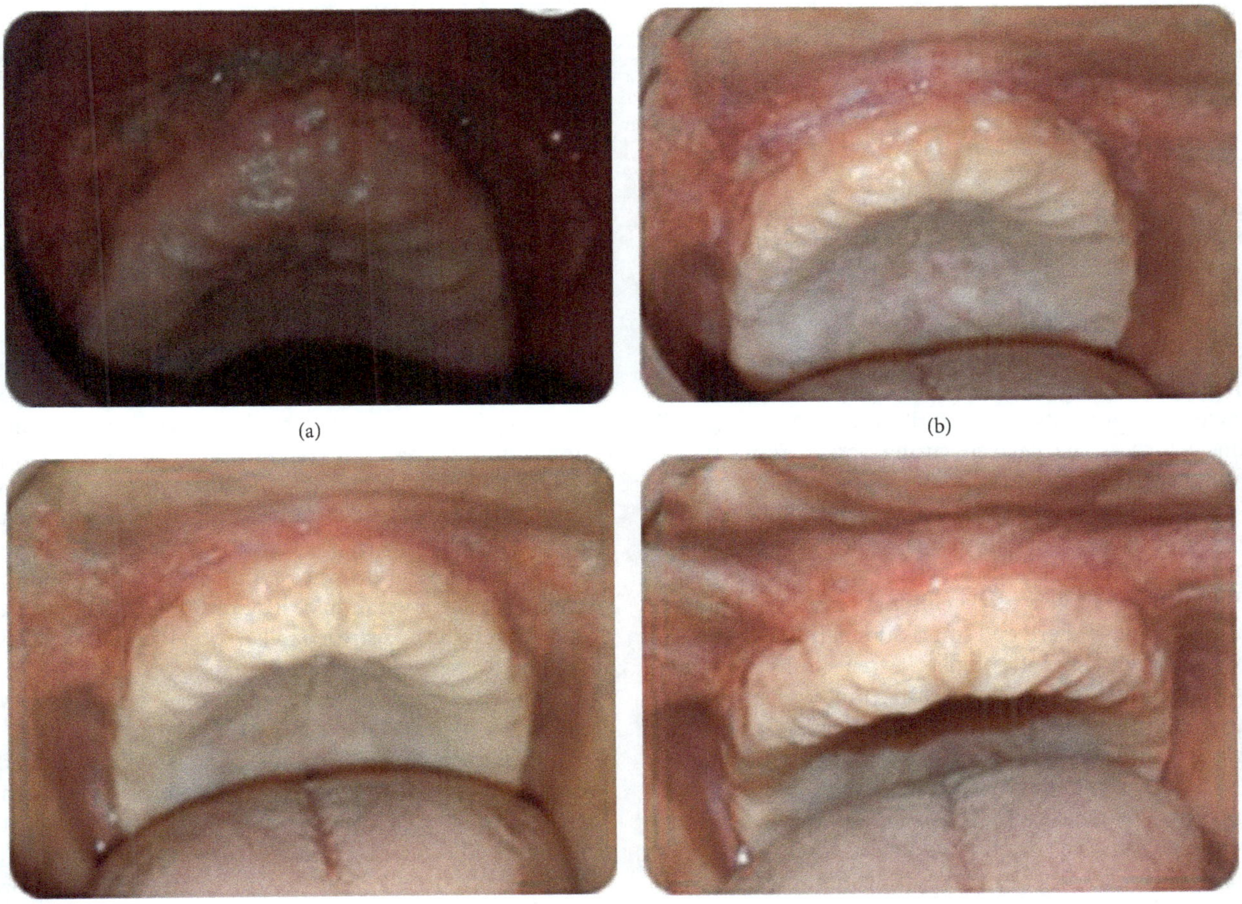

(a) (b) (c) (d)

Figure 28: Healing process: (a) 3 days, (b) 1 week, (c) 2 weeks, and (d) 1 month.

gained. The section was extended laterally to eliminate the frenulum (Figure 26(a)).

The treated area was clinically evaluated to verify the absence of bleeding or residual hyperplastic tissue. The maxillary prosthesis served as a guide to evaluate the intervention (Figure 26(b)).

Immediately, prostheses were positioned, and the upper one was carefully relined with a soft tissue conditioner (Fitt, Kerr ®) to stabilize the prosthesis and facilitate wound healing (Figures 27(a)–27(c)).

Patient was prescribed with antibiotics and analgesics for 3 days. The postoperative period was asymptomatic, and healing was satisfactory.

The patient was recalled after 3 days, 7 days, and 2 weeks for observation. The healing was good, and no postoperative pain or edema was reported (Figures 28(a)–28(c)).

After 1 month, there was no recurrence of the lesion (Figure 28(d)).

The patient was satisfied with the prosthesis fit, comfort, and phonetics, so the maxillary prosthesis was rebased with

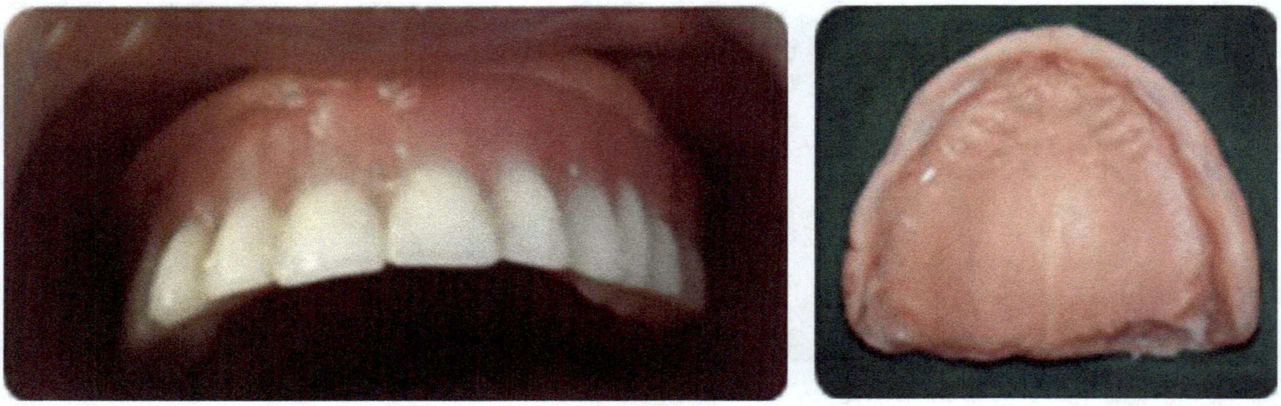

(a) (b)

FIGURE 29: (a, b) Chemopolymerized resin molding.

permanent tissue conditioner (DuraBase®) to stabilize the postoperative state (Figures 29(a) and 29(b)).

5. Discussion

When supporting tissues are altered, the practitioner must think at first to restore their physiological, histological, and anatomical behavior favorable to a qualitative prosthetic rehabilitation thanks to tissue conditioning. As shown in the three cases, preliminary preparation, defined as all procedures destined to improve the properties of osteomucos-bearing surfaces in contact with complete prosthesis, is indispensable associating the temporarily use of a tissue conditioning, which is the delayed curing acrylic resin and an antifungal agent prescription [4–6, 12–16].

In some cases, when there are no contraindications to surgery, a surgical procedure may be necessary to improve the prognosis of complete prosthesis [17].

Preprosthetic surgery target eliminating certain lesions or abnormalities of the hard and soft tissues of the jaws in edentulous patients such as alveoloplasty, frenectomy, vestibuloplasty, and reduction of hyperplastic mucosa, so that the replacement of the prostheses will be easier and with better prognosis, as it is done to all illustrated patients [15, 17].

According to the stage of the lesion and the general condition of the patient, excision can be performed by either conventional surgical approach that was used in the first and second clinical cases or by laser technique, as we chose to treat the third hypertensive patient.

In fact, since about twenty years, and thanks to a plethora of benefits, laser can be used by dentists, as an effective surgical technique, for the treatment of oral tissue pathologies to improve prosthetic status among elderly. It is a precise and effective treatment modality used to generate both hard and soft tissues and considered an enhancement to a traditional procedure providing a reduced need of anesthesia during surgery and a minimal postoperative edema and pain, making faster the healing process and easier the patient experience.

These advantages are very interesting when treating edentulous elderly patients suffering from systemic health problems that interfere with the therapeutic conduct and the healing process (diabetes, blood hypertension, cardiovascular disease, etc.).

Various types of lasers are used in the surgery of the soft oral tissues such as CO2 laser, ER : YAG laser, ND : YAG laser, diode laser, argon laser, and KTP laser [2, 18–20].

For geriatric patients, the transitional prosthesis is a procedure that can present real advantages and can be recommended with confidence.

Former prostheses may be refitted, vertical dimension corrected, occlusion reconstructed, as well as it being used, after rebasing, as an interim prosthesis, able to serve as a treatment denture until the healing and resorption process of inflamed traumatized tissues is complete, especially in presurgical procedures, as it was illustrated on cases 1 and 2.

On a physiological level, the adaptation is easier with minimal changes for the tongue space, perioral musculature and eating habits [21].

The transitional prosthesis may be used, also, as a postsurgical device to minimize trauma of the operated zone while healing process, to stabilize obtained surgical results and to allow a measured transition to new complete prosthesis status when function and aesthetics are satisfactory, while retaining a good quality of life [21].

When the former prostheses are not suitable for exploitation, the manufacturing of new ones before surgery is indispensable to be used after the preprogrammed intervention. Prosthesis adjustments, either of the occlusal contacts (case 2) or the prosthetic border (case 1), are needed immediately after the surgery to avoid trauma in the area of the wound then reinserted over the surgical bed, after being covered with tissue conditioner in some cases, permitting the maintenance of the new vestibular sulcus depth and width obtained by surgery [22, 23].

An evaluation of the clinical situation of the hard or soft oral tissues is decisive to the prosthetic treatment success. It is the responsibility of the practitioner to establish the right diagnosis and start the coherent treatment plan, as needed, leading to a functional and perfectly integrated complete prosthesis [4, 17].

The outcome of a successful treatment depended not only on the result but also on the way in which it was achieved. Fear and anxiety remain one of the most important barriers for the treatment of the elderly patient, but the transitional denture system can help overcome some of these difficulties.

6. Conclusion

Restoring a healthy state of the covering tissues is the first guarantee of a correct registration of the bearing surface, good adaptation of the prosthesis underside surface, and consequently, a satisfactory stability of the complete prostheses.

Management of the bearing surface, by fibromucous tissue cover sanitation, appears as the preliminary decisive step in the therapeutic success leading to functional and perfectly integrated stable complete prosthesis.

References

[1] A. Jones and J. B. Bridgman, "Case report: a patient who had not removed her full lower denture for 54 years," *New Zealand Dental Journal*, vol. 112, 2016.

[2] O. Tayari, S. Jemli, and J. Jaouadi, *Prosthetic management and diode laser sugery for the treatment of Epulis Fissuratum on endentulous patients*, Dental News, 2019.

[3] L. Fajri, F. Benfdil, N. Merzouk, B. El Mohtarim, and A. Abdedine, "Diagnosis and treatment of mucous lesions induced by complete denture," *Actualites Odonto Stomatologiques*, vol. 62, pp. 225–238, 2008.

[4] L. Fajri, S. Berrada, and A. Abdedine, "Clinical examination contributing to selection and orientation of prosthodontic treatments in completely edentulous patients," *Revue D Odontostomatologie-Paris*, vol. 37, pp. 91–107, 2008.

[5] J. Slaoui Hasnaoui, A. Sefrioui, O. Fromentin, and A. Abdedine, "Management of edentulous maxillae with an anterior flabby ridge," *AOS*, vol. 251, pp. 225–237, 2010.

[6] R. Bansal, R. Garg, S. Kaushala, M. Kumar, and R. Saini, "Prosthodontic rehabilitation of patient with flabby ridges with different impression techniques," *Indian Journal of Dentistry*, vol. 5, no. 2, pp. 110–113, 2014.

[7] E. M. Canger, P. Celenk, and S. Kayipmaz, "Denture-related hyperplasia: a clinical study of a Turkish population group," *Brazilian Dental Journal*, vol. 20, no. 3, pp. 243–248, 2009.

[8] P. Kafas, T. Upile, C. Stavrianos, N. Angouridakis, and W. Jerjes, "Mucogingival overgrowth in a geriatric patient," *Dermatology Online Journal*, vol. 16, no. 8, p. 7, 2010.

[9] A. Bilhan, O. Geckili, S. Ergin, O. Erdogan, and G. Ates, "Evaluation of satisfaction and complications in patients with existing complete dentures," *Journal of Oral Science*, vol. 55, no. 1, pp. 29–37, 2013.

[10] G. Mandali, I. D. Sener, S. Begum Turker, and H. Ulgen, "Factors affecting the distribution and prevalence of oral mucosal lesions in complete denture wearers," *Gerodontology*, vol. 28, no. 2, pp. 97–103, 2011.

[11] E. Emami, M. Kabawat, and L. Koninck, "Denture stomatitis: new perspective," *Journal De L'ordre Des Dentistes Du Québec 7*, vol. 50, no. 4, 2013.

[12] M. Bagui, L. Fajri, B. El Mohtarime, and N. Merzouk, "Instead of conditioning tissue in complete denture," *AOS*, vol. 275, 2016.

[13] V. Jain, P. Prakash, R. Vijay Kumar, and V. Udayshankar, "Impressing for excellence: special impression techniques for compromised ridges: case report," *International Journal of Contemporary Medical Research [IJCMR]*, vol. 6, no. 7, 2019.

[14] A. Regragui, A. Abdedine, and N. Merzouk, "Biofunctional space and tissular preparation: what perspectives in complete removable prosthesis?," *AOS*, vol. 255, pp. 197–206, 2011.

[15] S. Rahman, K. Mattoo, and T. Qassadi, "Vestibuloplasty as an aid to enhance complete denture stability," *JMSCR*, vol. 8, no. 4, pp. 331–334, 2020.

[16] Y.-T. Hsu, "Consequences of relining on a maxillary complete denture: a clinical report," *The Journal of Prosthetic Dentistry*, vol. 114, no. 1, pp. 13–16, 2015.

[17] H. Chari and K. Vali Shaik, "Preprosthetic surgery: review of literature," *IJSS Case Reports & Reviews*, vol. 3, no. 4, p. 10, 2016.

[18] R. Mekayssi, B. Taleb, N. Merzouk, and F. Benfdil, "The prosthetic management of a case of epulis fissuratum by a novel technique," *Odovtos - International Journal of Dental Sciences*, pp. 109–114, 2019.

[19] B. Rezvan and H. Mahumoudhashemi, "Comparative survey on cardon dioxide laser and surgical scalpel removal of epulis fissuratum," *Journal of Oral Laser Applications*, vol. 7, pp. 187–190, 2007.

[20] M. Shapurik and F. Tozija, *Laser treatment for improvement of oral health in elderly*, 2019.

[21] A. Mersel and J. Israel, "Immediate or transitional complete dentures: gerodontic considerations," *International Dental Journal*, vol. 52, no. 4, pp. 298–303, 2002.

[22] A. Bouguezzi, J. Chagra, and A. Chokri, "Conventional surgery in the management of denture induced fibrous hyperplasia-a case report," *Journal of Dentistry and Dental Medicine*, vol. 3, no. 2, 2020.

[23] A. Sindel and A. M. Ali, "Evaluation of the efficacy of conventional surgery in the management of epulis fissuratum lesions rarely encountered on the lingual aspect of the alveolar crest," *Clinical Dentistry and Research*, vol. 41, no. 3, pp. 124–131, 2017.

10

Grafting with Bone Substitute Materials in Therapy-Resistant Periapical Actinomycosis

Saeed Asgary and Leyla Roghanizadeh

Iranian Center for Endodontic Research, Research Institute of Dental Sciences, Shahid Beheshti University of Medical Sciences, Tehran, Iran

Correspondence should be addressed to Leyla Roghanizadeh; leila_roghani@yahoo.com

Academic Editor: Giovanni Mergoni

Actinomycosis can be one of the causes of persistent periradicular lesions. This is the report of a patient who was first referred with complaint of pain in maxillary right incisors. A standard root canal therapy was carried out. Unluckily, the patient returned with recurrent symptoms; therefore, surgical endodontic retreatment was decided. While the large periradicular lesion was curetted, a whitish yellow granule-like material came out from the periapical area that was submitted for histopathological examination. The apices of both maxillary right incisors were resected. Root-end cavities were sealed with calcium-enriched mixture (CEM) cement. Finally, the remaining large defect was filled with natural bone substitutes. Since the histopathological diagnosis revealed actinomycotic infection, oral penicillin V was prescribed for four weeks. At two-year recall, the bone healing process was completed. Apical actinomycosis can cause therapy-resistant lesions. Root-end surgery employing CEM and bone substitutes might be an effective method to help bone healing in large periradicular lesions.

1. Introduction

Actinomycosis is a slowly progressive bacterial infection. The causative bacteria include facultative anaerobic, filamentous, gram-positive bacilli that belong to the *Actinomyces* genus [1]. They can be present as the microbial flora of tonsillar crypts, gingival crevices, periodontal pockets, and dental plaques [1]. Cervicofacial actinomycosis usually establishes following a disruption of the mucosal barrier, dental manipulations, or trauma to the mouth, such as a tooth extraction or a mandibular bone fracture, although it may arise spontaneously in patients with poor dental hygiene [2, 3].

Bone defects can be created by several etiologic factors such as infections, tumors, or genetic disorders. Those lesions do not simply heal, and assistance of bone substitute materials for bone regeneration is usually essential [4]. The applied biomaterials/grafts include "(i) barrier membranes used for guided tissue regeneration (GTR), (ii) bone replacement grafts (such as allografts, xenografts, and alloplastic materials), and (iii) wound modifiers (such as enamel matrix derivative)." Combinations of these types have been applied too [5].

This report presents a case of a large persistent endodontically induced periapical defect around the root of a maxillary lateral incisor that has undergone root canal therapy (RCT), although no healing resulted from the primary treatment. Thus, a surgical endodontic retreatment was planned.

2. Case Presentation

A 50-year-old woman was referred to the endodontic department of a private dental clinic. She had pain and discomfort upon mastication associated with her upper right incisors as the chief complaint. Her medical history was noncontributory. Intraoral examination of the region showed that teeth #11 and #12 had composite resin restorations; tooth #12 was tender to percussion and palpation. The probing depths of both teeth were within normal limits (i.e., ≤3 mm), and no abnormal mobility was found. No swelling or sinus tract was detected in the buccal or lingual mucosa. Both teeth did not respond to sensibility tests, including an electrical pulp tester (Parkell, Edgewood, NY, USA), and cold test with Endo-Frost (Coltène-Whaledent, Langenau, Germany). In the

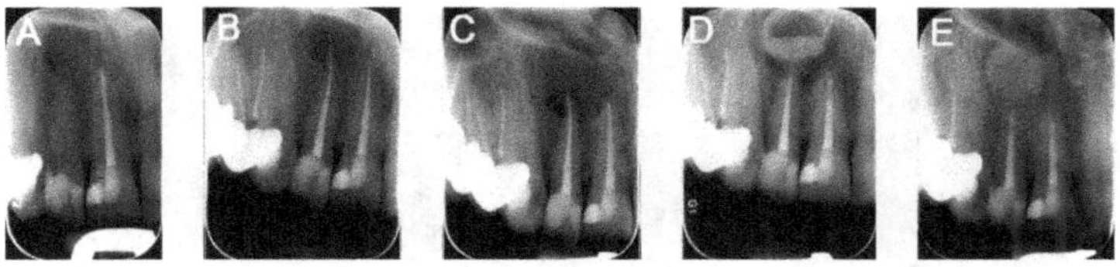

(a) (b) (c) (d) (e)

Figure 1: Periapical radiographs: (a) preoperative image of teeth #12, showing a large endodontic lesion; (b) immediate postendodontic radiograph; (c) at two-month follow-up, the patient returned with abscess formation and a larger periapical lesion; (d) applying bone substitute material during surgical retreatment; (e) at 6-month follow-up, bone healing can be observed.

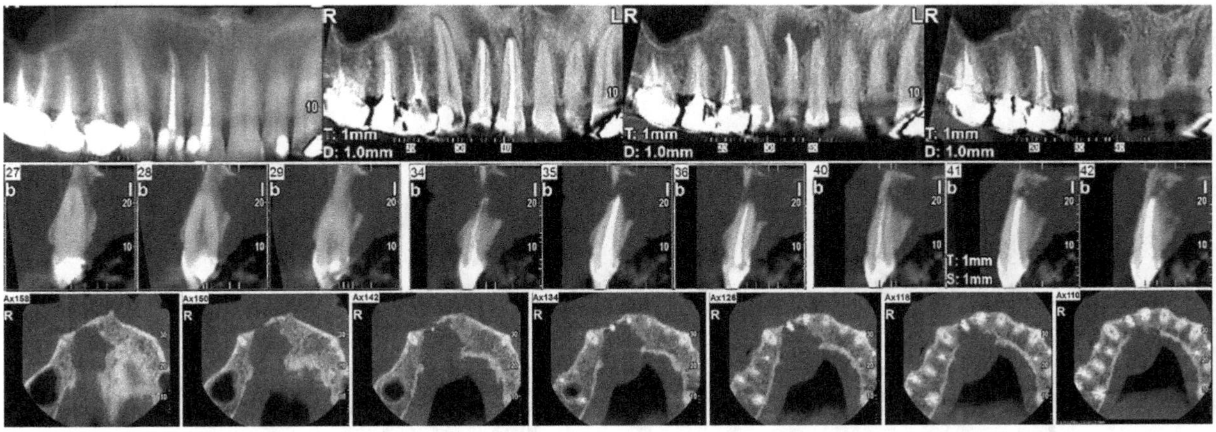

Figure 2: CBCT scan of the maxillary anterior region showing a large bony defect surrounding the periapex area of tooth #12, which extended from the distal aspect of the root of tooth #13 toward the mesial wall of the root of tooth #11.

radiographic evaluation (Figure 1(a)), tooth #11 had an adequate root canal filling and tooth #12 had a large well-defined radiolucent lesion.

Based on the clinical and radiographic findings, the diagnosis was asymptomatic apical periodontitis associated with a necrotic upper lateral incisor. Primary RCT was decided for tooth #12. The patient was informed about the diagnosis and the treatment plan. Informed consent was obtained.

On the treatment session, after local anesthesia with 2% lidocaine plus 1 : 80000 epinephrine (Darupakhsh, Tehran, Iran), access cavity was prepared, and treatment was continued with a rubber dam in place. There was no pus/exudate from the root canal. Cleaning and shaping by Flexofile (Dentsply, Maillefer, Switzerland) #15-40, accompanied by 5.25% sodium hypochlorite, were performed; then, the canal was obturated by a lateral condensation technique. Finally, the tooth was permanently restored with composite resin (Figure 1(b)).

After 2 months, the patient returned with no recovery from the signs/symptoms of tooth #12; clinically, a small localized abscess in the buccal vestibule and a large abscess in the palatal mucosa of the upper right incisors could be observed. Based on periapical radiograph (Figure 1(c)), with an adequate root canal filling, the size of the periapical lesion increased and the large bony defect extended toward the periapex of tooth #11. Cone-beam computed tomography (CBCT) was prescribed to scrutinize the associated region which showed a large radiolucent lesion in between the palatal aspect of teeth #13 and #11 (Figure 2). Considering all of the findings, the diagnosis was a therapy-resistant apical lesion, and surgical endodontic retreatment for both upper right incisors was judged to be favorable. The patient was thoroughly informed. She signed the informed consent form.

At the surgery appointment, the mouth was rinsed with 0.2% chlorhexidine and local anaesthesia via infiltration with 2% lidocaine plus 1 : 80000 epinephrine (Darupakhsh, Tehran, Iran) was administered. Then, a full mucoperiosteal flap was prepared and retracted. There was no buccal cortex over the root apex of tooth #11; after curettage of the granulation tissue, a through-and-through bony defect was appeared. During the procedure, a small whitish granule-like material was obtained. The specimen was stored in 10% formalin solution and submitted for histopathological examinations. Root-end resection/preparation for both incisors was carried out. Next, calcium-enriched mixture (CEM) cement (BioniqueDent, Tehran, Iran) was prepared according to the manufacturer's instructions and was delivered into the root-end cavities using a plastic instrument. After accomplishing the root-end fillings, the bony defect was filled with natural bovine bone grafting material (Cerabone, Botiss, Berlin, Germany). Following a confirmation radiography (Figure 1(d)), the flap was gently repositioned and sutured. Postsurgical recommendations were given to the patient.

Histopathological evaluations of sections of the specimen with conventional hematoxylin-eosin (H&E) staining (Figure 3) showed fragments of actinomycotic colony exhibiting club-shaped filaments arranged in a radiating rosette

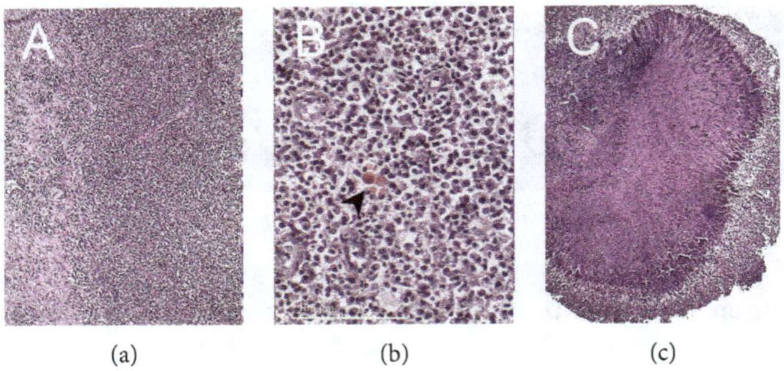

FIGURE 3: Pathological images: (a) granulation tissue (100× magnification); (b) showing in greater magnification (400×) collections of plasma cells, polymorphonuclear leukocytes, a few Russell bodies (which are marked with the arrow), and areas of erythrocyte extravasation; (c) club-shaped filaments in a radiating pattern demonstrating actinomycotic colonies (100× magnification).

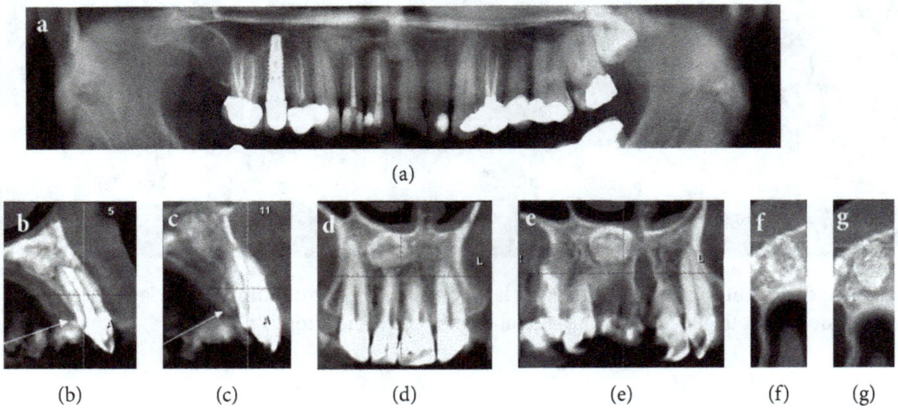

FIGURE 4: Two-year follow-up radiographic evaluation: (a) panoramic view: bone healing in the periapical areas of teeth #11 and #12; (b, c) axial views from teeth #11 and #12: bone augmentation in the palatal aspect of the maxilla; (d, e) frontal views of maxillary anterior teeth: there is no sign of radiolucent lesion around teeth #11 and #12 and bone substitute material can be observed; (f, g) transverse views of the area: successful bone augmentation.

pattern with a basophilic central core and eosinophilic peripheral portion. In addition, sections show granulation tissue with large collections of plasma cells, polymorphonuclear leukocytes, areas of erythrocyte extravasation, and a few Russel bodies. The diagnosis was periapical granuloma with actinomycotic infection.

After surgical intervention, the primary treatment outcome was satisfactory regarding symptom amelioration at the one-week follow-up. Based on the advice from her infectious disease specialist, the 500 mg tablets of penicillin V (one tablet per day for 4 weeks) was prescribed. At 6-month recall appointment, the tooth was in normal function, and there was no sensitivity to palpation or percussion. Radiographic examination (Figure 1(e)) demonstrated significant bone formation, and the periapical lesion was healed. After two years, the patient needed to take CBCT for implant surgery in posterior regions of both jaws. We made another study model for better assessment of periapical regions in right maxillary central and lateral incisors as two-year follow-up radiographic evaluation (Figure 4). The CBCT images show no radiolucent lesion in periapical areas of teeth #11 and #12. In addition, successful bone augmentation and healing can be observed (Figure 4).

3. Discussion

Actinomycosis in the oral cavity is an important disease to encounter. Sometimes, it is not timely diagnosed, due to general paucity of familiarity with the infection [1] and difficult culture of the causative bacteria, *Actinomyces* [6]. A precise and timely recognition of this infection requires a high degree of suspicion [1]. Furthermore, because of the resorptive potential of granulation tissue and extensive tissue destruction by actinomycotic infection, appropriate healing in apical actinomycosis is always demanding [1]. True diagnosis of this periapical infection can be reached only after surgical removal of the lesion and histopathological/microbiological examination. Definite diagnosis requires identification of the involved microorganisms such as *Actinomyces* species. However, commonly the infection has been diagnosed by the presence of sulfur granule, demonstrating actinomycotic colonies, obtained from endodontic surgery or through tooth extraction [7].

To treat and eliminate actinomycotic infection, combination of surgical removal of the involved tissue and suitable antibiotic therapy is necessary [6]. Penicillin is the traditional antibiotic of choice. The duration of antibiotic therapy can range from 4 weeks to 1 year based on the severity of the disease. Surgical management without antibiotic therapy might be associated with recurrence [1]. Recently, the concept that extraradicular infection may be established in the form of actinomycotic-like colonies and can cause treatment failure as an independent entity has been supported [8]. Endodontic surgery is an appropriate treatment plan for definitive removal of persistent extraradicular infections [9].

To decide eligibility for being a satisfactory root-end filling material, biocompatibility and sealing ability are crucial qualities. One of the biomaterials which has shown favorable characteristics in terms of sealability is CEM cement [10]. CEM not only can establish an effective bioseal but also has been able to stimulate osteogenesis and cementogenesis associated with regenerative periapical tissue responses [11]. CEM has high biostimulation potential for reproduction of dental hard tissues when it has been placed adjacent to live pulpal structure [12].

Another issue to discuss is that large bony defect secondary to endodontic surgeries may compromise the tooth function postoperatively. By application of GTR and/or bone graft approaches, the auxiliary materials can promote normal trabecular bone formation and also hinder migration of the proliferating oral epithelium into such lesions [13]. These techniques can improve the predictability of clinical, radiographic, and histological outcomes [14]. In this reported case, using bone substitute material resulted in successful healing. There are many studies in the literature in which large periradicular lesions with endodontic origin have been cured by the technique of GTR and bone grafting [13–15]. However, in some studies, just bone graft was applied and no membrane was used [16–18]. The outcome of endodontic surgeries in large lesions, especially in through-and-through defects, was more efficiently improved by the GTR technique [13]. In through-and-through defects, by this grafting approach, it would not be necessary to raise a flap on both sides of the alveolar process and would be technically easier to do than the application of membranes [18]. Finally, there is a need for more large-scale prospective clinical trials to assess added benefits of regenerative techniques for the outcomes of endodontic surgeries [15].

4. Conclusion

A therapy-resistant periapical lesion can be the result of an actinomycotic infection, which needs surgical intervention to promote the healing process. Using bone substitute material might facilitate healing and bone formation in large bone defects.

Consent

The authors certify that they have obtained an appropriate patient consent form.

Acknowledgments

The authors would like to acknowledge Dr. Mojgan Ghazi, DDS, MS, Oral and Maxillofacial Pathologist, for the histopathological examination of the sample. We also appreciate the patient for her permission to report the case.

References

[1] K. Moturi and V. Kaila, "Cervicofacial actinomycosis and its management," *Annals of Maxillofacial Surgery*, vol. 8, p. 361, 2018.

[2] W. Gomes-Silva, D. L. Pereira, E. R. Fregnani, O. P. Almeida, L. Armada, and F. R. Pires, "Clinicopathological and ultrastructural characterization of periapical actinomycosis," *Medicina Oral, Patología Oral y Cirugía Bucal*, vol. 25, pp. e131–e136, 2020.

[3] S. Asgary and L. Roghanizadeh, "Rapid bone healing after intentional replantation of a molar with apical actinomycosis," *Iranian Endodontic Journal*, vol. 13, p. 135, 2018.

[4] E. Garcia-Gareta, M. J. Coathup, and G. W. Blunn, "Osteoinduction of bone grafting materials for bone repair and regeneration," *Bone*, vol. 81, pp. 112–121, 2015.

[5] T. De Bruyckere, A. Eghbali, F. Younes et al., "A 5-year prospective study on regenerative periodontal therapy of infrabony defects using minimally invasive surgery and a collagen-enriched bovine-derived xenograft," *Clinical Oral Investigations*, vol. 22, no. 3, pp. 1235–1242, 2018.

[6] K. Gelada, R. Halli, H. Mograwala, and S. Sethi, "Actinomycosis which impersonates malignancy," *Annals of Maxillofacial Surgery*, vol. 8, no. 2, pp. 358–360, 2018.

[7] D. Ricucci and J. F. Siqueira Jr., "Apical actinomycosis as a continuum of intraradicular and extraradicular infection: case report and critical review on its involvement with treatment failure," *Journal of Endodontics*, vol. 34, no. 9, pp. 1124–1129, 2008.

[8] D. Ricucci, W. S. P. Lopes, S. Loghin, I. N. Rocas, and J. F. Siqueira Jr., "Large bacterial floc causing an independent extraradicular infection and posttreatment apical periodontitis: a case report," *Journal of Endodontics*, vol. 44, no. 8, pp. 1308–1316, 2018.

[9] J. F. Siqueira Jr., "Periapical actinomycosis and infection with Propionibacterium propionicum," *Endodontic Topics*, vol. 6, no. 1, pp. 78–95, 2003.

[10] S. Asgary and S. Ehsani, "Periradicular surgery of human permanent teeth with calcium-enriched mixture cement," *Iranian Endodontic Journal*, vol. 8, no. 3, pp. 140–144, 2013.

[11] S. Asgary, M. J. Eghbal, and S. Ehsani, "Periradicular regeneration after endodontic surgery with calcium-enriched mixture cement in dogs," *Journal of Endodontics*, vol. 36, no. 5, pp. 837–841, 2010.

[12] G. Ansari, S. P. Morovati, and S. Asgary, "Evaluation of four pulpotomy techniques in primary molars: a randomized controlled trial," *Iranian Endodontic Journal*, vol. 13, no. 1, pp. 7–12, 2018.

[13] G. Pecora, S. Kim, R. Celletti, and M. Davarpanah, "The guided tissue regeneration principle in endodontic surgery: one-year postoperative results of large periapical lesions," *International Endodontic Journal*, vol. 28, no. 1, pp. 41–46, 1995.

[14] S. Taschieri, S. Corbella, I. Tsesis, M. Bortolin, and M. Del Fabbro, "Effect of guided tissue regeneration on the outcome of surgical endodontic treatment of through-and-through lesions: a retrospective study at 4-year follow-up," *Oral and Maxillofacial Surgery*, vol. 15, no. 3, pp. 153–159, 2011.

[15] S. Corbella, S. Taschieri, A. Elkabbany, M. Del Fabbro, and T. von Arx, "Guided tissue regeneration using a barrier membrane in endodontic surgery," *Swiss Dental Journal*, vol. 126, no. 1, pp. 13–25, 2016.

[16] V. Chaturvedy and S. Chaturvedy, "Regenerative therapy as an adjunct to periapical surgery: a case report," *International Journal of Clinical Pediatric Dentistry*, vol. 5, no. 1, pp. 75–77, 2012.

[17] S. Asgary, L. Roghanizadeh, and A. Haeri, "Surgical endodontics vs regenerative periodontal surgery for management of a large periradicular lesion," *Iranian Endodontic Journal*, vol. 13, p. 271, 2018.

[18] G. Pecora, D. De Leonardis, N. Ibrahim, M. Bovi, and R. Cornelini, "The use of calcium sulphate in the surgical treatment of a 'through and through' periradicular lesion," *International Endodontic Journal*, vol. 34, no. 3, pp. 189–197, 2001.

11

Medication-Related Osteonecrosis of the Jaw Spontaneously Occurred in a Patient with Chronic Myelogenous Leukemia Only by Imatinib: A Report of a Rare Case

Makiko Okubo-Sato, Kenji Yamagata, Satoshi Fukuzawa, Kazuhiro Terada, Fumihiko Uchida, Naomi Ishibashi-Kanno, and Hiroki Bukawa

Department of Oral and Maxillofacial Surgery, Institute of Clinical Medicine, Faculty of Medicine, University of Tsukuba, 1-1-1 Tennodai, Tsukuba, Ibaraki 305-8575, Japan

Correspondence should be addressed to Kenji Yamagata; y-kenji@md.tsukuba.ac.jp

Academic Editor: Giuseppe Alessandro Scardina

The prevalence of medication-related osteonecrosis of the jaw (MRONJ) associated with molecular-targeted therapies such as bevacizumab and sunitinib has been constantly increasing in recent years. MRONJ frequently occurs after invasive dental procedures such as tooth extraction in patients currently or with a previous history of receiving antiresorptive agents including bisphosphonates and/or denosumab. Here, we report a rare case of spontaneously occurring MRONJ of the mandible in a 52-year-old Japanese woman with chronic myelogenous leukemia (CML) who was administered imatinib for 9 years. She had never been treated with antiresorptive agents, and her MRONJ developed spontaneously. Although there have been few reports of MRONJ related to imatinib, our case reported here indicates that imatinib may be capable of causing spontaneous MRONJ.

1. Introduction

Medication-related osteonecrosis of the jaw (MRONJ) is a severe adverse drug effect related to antiresorptive agents, and the number of reports of MRONJ cases associated with molecular-targeted therapies including antibody drugs and tyrosine kinase inhibitors (TKIs) has been increasing [1, 2]. Most cases are related to the administration of antiresorptive medications, such as bisphosphonates and receptor activator of nuclear factor κB ligand (RANKL) inhibitors, and precipitating events, such as tooth extraction, which may significantly increase the risk of developing MRONJ. Meanwhile, frequently reported agents among molecular-targeted therapies associated with MRONJ are bevacizumab [3, 4], sunitinib [5], sorafenib [6], everolimus [7], temsirolimus [3], and aflibercept [8].

Imatinib mesylate (Glivec®) is a TKI with specificity for the BCR–ABL protein resulting from the t(9, 22)-derived Philadelphia chromosome, platelet-derived growth factor receptors (PDGFRs), and c-kit. It is administered in patients with chronic myelogenous leukemia (CML), acute lymphocytic leukemia, and c-kit-positive gastrointestinal stromal tumor (GIST) [9]. The documented adverse effects of imatinib are nausea, vomiting, edema, tumor necrosis, muscle cramps, hematologic side effects, cardiovascular side effects, hepatic side effects, nephrotoxicity, and dermatologic side effects (such as skin rashes, pruritus, and petechiae); however, little is known about MRONJ [10]. The present report describes a very rare case of spontaneous MRONJ related to only imatinib in the absence of antiresorptive agents.

2. Case Report

A 52-year-old Japanese woman was referred to our department in July 2018. She complained of exposed bone with contact pain in the right mandible that had persisted for 6 months. She started using an oral antimicrobial mouthrinse, and the exposed bone was eliminated several times by her general practitioner, but her condition did not improve. She was diagnosed with CML in 2008 and administered only imatinib (400 mg daily) continuously with no apparent side effects. There was no other past medical history, and she had never received antiresorptive agents or undergone radiotherapy in the head and neck region. Clinical examination showed that the exposed bone measured approximately 5 mm on the lingual surface of the mandibular tori around the right premolars (Figure 1). Purulent discharge, swelling, tooth mobility, and percussion pain were not observed, and her oral hygiene was favorable. Although there were no significant findings on panoramic radiography (Figure 2(a)), computed tomography showed a separated sequestrum measuring approximately 25 mm, and magnetic resonance imaging indicated abnormal intramedullary signal intensity in the right mandible (Figures 2(b) and 2(c)). She was clinically diagnosed with MRONJ stage II. In November 2018, sequestrectomy and removal of the mandibular tori were performed under general anesthesia because of her vomiting reflex. Histopathological examination revealed necrotic lamellar bone with empty lacunae, bacterial aggregates, and an absence of neoplastic cells (Figure 3). Her postoperative course was uneventful, and at the 2-year follow-up, she was stable with no signs of MRONJ recurrence (Figures 4(a) and 4(b)).

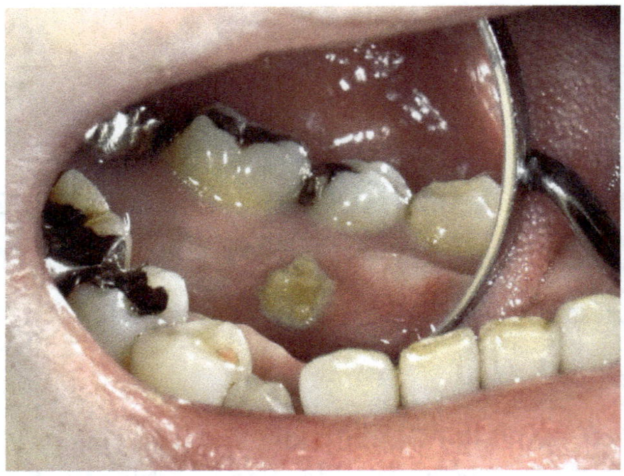

Figure 1: Examination of the oral cavity. Intraoral examination revealed bone exposure measuring approximately 5 mm on the lingual surface of the mandibular tori around the second premolar.

3. Discussion

In 2014, the American Association of Oral and Maxillofacial Surgeons (AAOMS) suggested that some cases of osteonecrosis of the jaw have been observed in patients with cancer following treatment with angiogenic inhibitors (bevacizumab), TKIs (sunitinib, sorafenib), and mammalian target of rapamycin (mTOR) inhibitors (sirolimus). The committee remains concerned about a similar potential risk associated with several other medications within the same drug class that have a similar mechanism of action [11]. Bevacizumab, sunitinib, and sorafenib inhibit vascular endothelial growth factor- (VEGF-) mediated angiogenesis and ultimately delay wound healing, which play relevant roles in the onset of MRONJ. Inhibition of mTOR, VEGF expression, and angiogenesis are also depressed [12].

Imatinib inhibits PDGFR and c-kit, which are both related to angiogenesis, and some reports have indicated that imatinib may partly reduce VEGF expression through the inhibition of these factors [13, 14]. Apart from its vascular effects, imatinib directly affects bone remodeling. The inhibition of c-fms and c-kit signaling by imatinib may decrease osteoclast number and activity. Imatinib also inhibits the proton-generating activity of carbonic anhydrase II and suppresses bone resorption [15]. In addition, the inhibition of PDGFR signaling in osteoblasts inhibits the production of macrophage colony-stimulating factor and RANKL, which are essential for osteoclast genesis, and decreases osteoblast proliferation [16]. Therefore, imatinib treatment should be included as a potential risk factor for developing MRONJ because of its inhibitory effects on angiogenesis and bone remodeling. Our patient had never received antiresorptive agents and spontaneously developed MRONJ, as suggested by the aforementioned mechanism.

There are only three reports describing MRONJ related to imatinib (Table 1). Nicolatou-Galitis et al. [17] reported a case of MRONJ that developed after tooth extraction in a woman with CML receiving imatinib for 19 months. Four years prior, she had received chemotherapy and rituximab for non-Hodgkin's lymphoma, as well as alendronate and one injection of zoledronate for osteoporosis. MRONJ was treated but recurred following an injection of denosumab. Mohamed et al. [18] reported a patient with chronic lymphocytic leukemia (CLL) treated with imatinib for 13 months. The patient was administered alendronate for 119 months, followed by denosumab for 5 months until 5 months before tooth extraction, which was a trigger for MRONJ. The last case reported by Viviano et al. [19] involved a patient with MRONJ after 22 months of receiving imatinib for a GIST. Although the patient had never received antiresorptive agents, a tooth was extracted prior to the patient developing MRONJ. Two of the three reported cases of MRONJ due to imatinib involved the administration of antiresorptive agents. Our case is the second case of MRONJ caused only by imatinib and is the first case of spontaneous development without any surgical invasion. Although the exposed bone was on the mandibular tori, which is usually considered an anatomical risk factor of mechanical stimulation, the patient had no clear history of trauma involved in the pathogenesis, such as wearing dentures and chewing hard foods. AAOMS (2014) recommended conservative treatments for patients

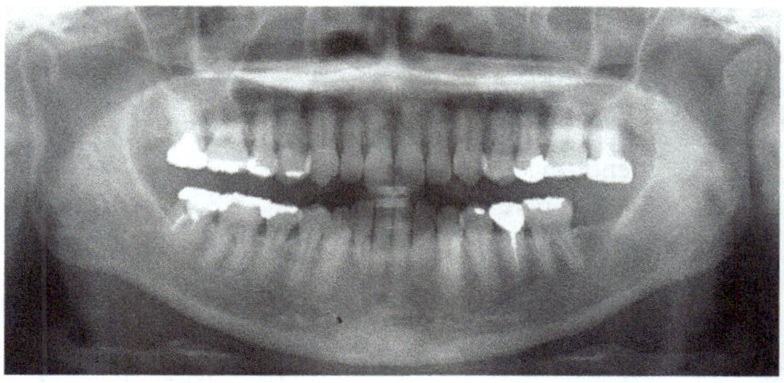

(a)

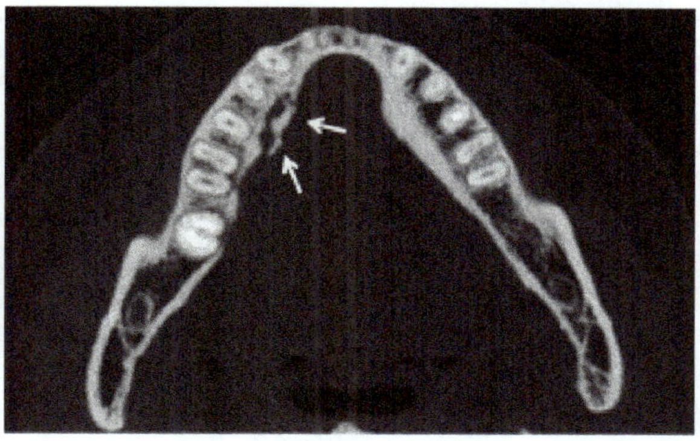

(b)

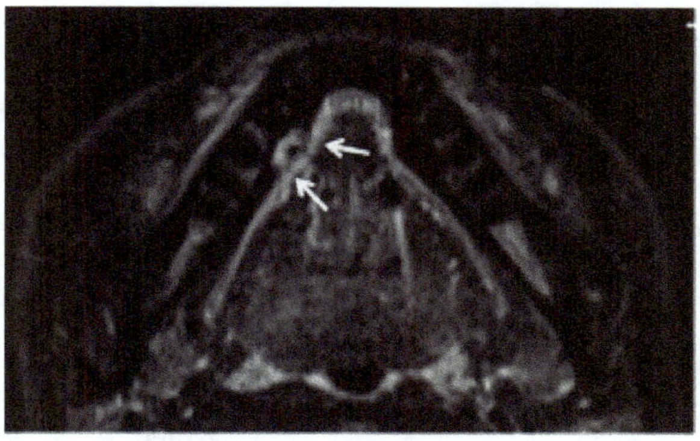

(c)

Figure 2: Imaging findings. (a) Panoramic radiography showed no obvious bone destruction or marginal and apical periodontitis. (b) Axial computed tomography depicted a sequestrum measuring approximately 25 mm (arrow). (c) Axial magnetic resonance short T1 inversion recovery imaging showed abnormal intramedullary signal intensity (arrow) on the lingual side of the right lower premolar.

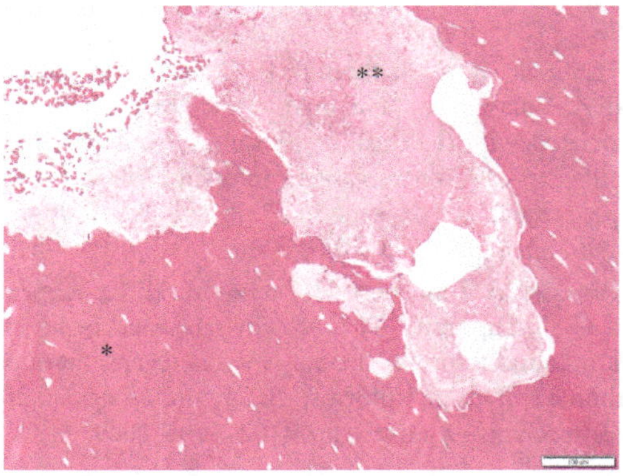

Figure 3: Microscopic findings. Histopathological examination revealed necrotic lamellar bone with empty lacunae (asterisk) and bacterial aggregates (double asterisk) (hematoxylin and eosin staining ×200 magnification).

with stage II MRONJ. However, the symptom of some patients with stage II and III do not respond to conservative treatments and reported that surgical management recently had a good prognosis [19]. The Position Paper 2017 of the Japanese Allied Committee on Osteonecrosis of the Jaw also recommended surgical treatments for stage II ONJ [20]. In our case, the patient continued to use antimicrobial mouthrinse but her condition did not improve. Therefore, we selected surgical treatment.

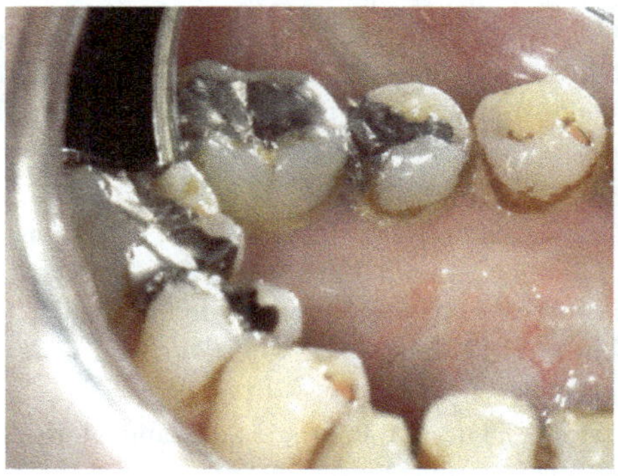

(a)

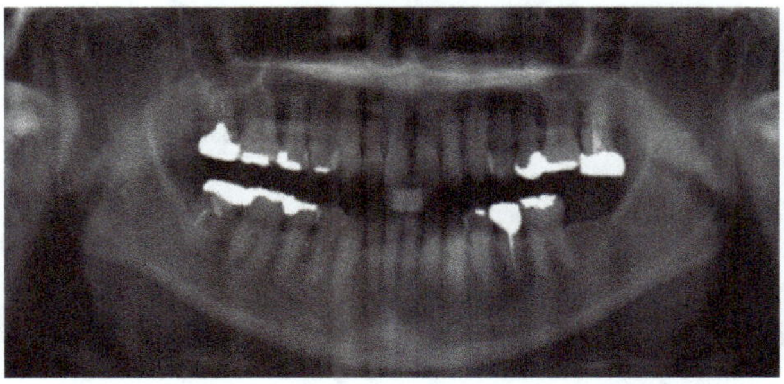

(b)

Figure 4: Follow-up oral examination 2 years after the surgery. (a) Follow-up observation revealed complete soft tissue healing with no signs of refractory osteonecrosis and exposed bone. (b) Panoramic radiography was also clear.

Table 1: Reported MRONJ cases related to imatinib [17–19].

No.	Study (yr)	Age (yr)/gender	Disease	Period of imatinib treatment (mo)	Antiresorptive agent	Trigger event	Stage	Treatment	Clinical outcome
1	Nicolatou-Galitis et al. (2013) [17]	71/M	CML	19	Alendronate Zoledoronate Denosumab	Tooth extraction	II	Antibiotic	Improved
2	Viviano et al. (2017) [19]	72/M	GIST	22	None	Tooth extraction	II	Antibiotic	Unknown
3	Mohamed et al. (2018) [18]	81/F	CLL	13	Alendronate Denosumab	Tooth extraction	II	Surgery	Healed
4	Present case (2020)	52/F	CML	111	None	None	II	Surgery	Healed

Abbreviations: MRONJ: medication-related osteonecrosis of the jaw; F: female; M: male; CML: chronic myelogenous leukemia; GIST: gastrointestinal stromal tumor; CLL: chronic lymphocytic leukemia.

To the best of our knowledge, we present the first case of spontaneous MRONJ attributed to the chronic use of imatinib with no history of receiving antiresorptive agents. The dental and medical communities must be aware that even if there are no apparent risk factors of MRONJ, the condition may develop in patients treated only with imatinib, and long-term monitoring and care are required.

References

[1] S. L. Ruggiero, T. B. Dodson, J. Fantasia et al., "American Association of Oral and Maxillofacial Surgeons position paper on medication-related osteonecrosis of the jaw–2014 update," *Journal of Oral and Maxillofacial Surgery*, vol. 72, no. 10, pp. 1938–1956, 2014.

[2] O. Nicolatou-Galitis, M. Kouri, E. Papadopoulou et al., "Osteonecrosis of the jaw related to non-antiresorptive medications: a systematic review," *Supportive Care in Cancer*, vol. 27, no. 2, pp. 383–394, 2019.

[3] A. R. Santos-Silva, G. A. Belizário Rosa, G. De Castro Júnior, R. B. Dias, A. C. Prado Ribeiro, and T. B. Brandão, "Osteonecrosis of the mandible associated with bevacizumab therapy," *Oral Surgery, Oral Medicine, Oral Pathology, Oral Radiology*, vol. 115, no. 6, pp. e32–e36, 2013.

[4] R. N. Hopp, J. Pucci, A. R. Santos-Silva, and J. Jorge, "Osteonecrosis after administration of intravitreous bevacizumab," *Journal of Oral and Maxillofacial Surgery*, vol. 70, no. 3, pp. 632–635, 2012.

[5] Y. Fleissig, E. Regev, and H. Lehman, "Sunitinib related osteonecrosis of jaw: a case report," *Oral Surgery, Oral Medicine, Oral Pathology, Oral Radiology*, vol. 113, no. 3, pp. e1–e3, 2012.

[6] F. Garuti, V. Camelli, L. Spinardi, L. Bucci, and F. Trevisani, "Osteonecrosis of the jaw during sorafenib therapy for hepatocellular carcinoma," *Tumori*, vol. 102, pp. S69–S70, 2016.

[7] D. Yamamoto, Y. Tsubota, T. Utsunomiya et al., "Osteonecrosis of the jaw associated with everolimus: a case report," *Molecular and Clinical Oncology*, vol. 6, no. 2, pp. 255–257, 2017.

[8] H. Mawardi, P. Enzinger, N. McCleary et al., "Osteonecrosis of the jaw associated with ziv-aflibercept," *Journal of gastrointestinal oncology*, vol. 7, no. 6, pp. E81–E87, 2016.

[9] S. Dulucq and M. Krajinovic, "The pharmacogenetics of imatinib," *Genome Medicine*, vol. 2, no. 11, pp. 1–8, 2010.

[10] H. Joensuu, J. C. Trent, and P. Reichardt, "Practical management of tyrosine kinase inhibitor-associated side effects in GIST," *Cancer Treatment Reviews*, vol. 37, no. 1, pp. 75–88, 2011.

[11] N. A. Valente, S. Chatelain, F. Alfonsi, C. Mortellaro, and A. Barone, "Medication-related osteonecrosis of the jaw," *The Journal of Craniofacial Surgery*, vol. 30, no. 4, pp. 1095–1101, 2019.

[12] H. A. Lane, J. M. Wood, P. M. J. McSheehy et al., "mTOR inhibitor RAD001 (everolimus) has antiangiogenic/vascular properties distinct from a VEGFR tyrosine kinase inhibitor," *Clinical Cancer Research*, vol. 15, no. 5, pp. 1612–1622, 2009.

[13] J. Litz and G. W. Krystal, "Imatinib inhibits c-kit-induced hypoxia-inducible factor-1α activity and vascular endothelial growth factor expression in small cell lung cancer cells," *Molecular Cancer Therapeutics*, vol. 5, no. 6, pp. 1415–1422, 2006.

[14] G. Vlahovic, Z. N. Rabbani, J. E. Herndon, M. W. Dewhirst, and Z. Vujaskovic, "Treatment with Imatinib in NSCLC is associated with decrease of phosphorylated PDGFR- β and VEGF expression, decrease in interstitial fluid pressure and improvement of oxygenation," *British Journal of Cancer*, vol. 95, no. 8, pp. 1013–1019, 2006.

[15] S. Parkkila, A. Innocenti, H. Kallio, M. Hilvo, A. Scozzafava, and C. T. Supuran, "The protein tyrosine kinase inhibitors imatinib and nilotinib strongly inhibit several mammalian α-carbonic anhydrase isoforms," *Bioorganic & medicinal chemistry letters*, vol. 19, no. 15, pp. 4102–4106, 2009.

[16] K. Vandyke, S. Fitter, A. L. Dewar, T. P. Hughes, and A. C. W. Zannettino, "Dysregulation of bone remodeling by imatinib mesylate," *Blood*, vol. 115, no. 4, pp. 766–774, 2010.

[17] O. Nicolatou-Galitis, E. Razis, D. Galiti, E. Vardas, F. Tzerbos, and S. Labropoulos, "Osteonecrosis of the jaw in a patient with chronic myelogenous leukemia receiving imatinib - a case report with clinical implications," *Forum of Clinical Oncology*, vol. 4, no. 4, pp. 29–33, 2013.

[18] H. A. M. Mohamed, C. E. N. Nielsen, and M. Schiodt, "Medication related osteonecrosis of the jaws associated with targeted therapy as monotherapy and in combination with antiresorptives. A report of 7 cases from the Copenhagen Cohort," *Oral Surgery, Oral Medicine, Oral Pathology, and Oral Radiology*, vol. 125, no. 2, pp. 157–163, 2018.

[19] M. Viviano, M. Rossi, and S. Cocca, "A rare case of osteonecrosis of the jaw related to imatinib," *Journal of the Korean Association of Oral and Maxillofacial Surgeons*, vol. 43, no. 2, pp. 120–124, 2017.

[20] Japanese Allied Committee On Osteonecrosis Of The Jaw, T. Yoneda, H. Hagino et al., "Antiresorptive agent-related osteonecrosis of the jaw: position paper 2017 of the Japanese Allied Committee on osteonecrosis of the jaw," *Journal of Bone and Mineral Metabolism*, vol. 35, no. 1, pp. 1–14, 2017.

Sialolipoma of the Floor of the Mouth with Immunohistological Analysis

Ahmed A. Zahrani[1] **Ahmed Qannam**[2] **Ra'ed Al Sadhan**[2] **and Ibrahim O. Bello**[2]

[1]*Department of Oral and Maxillofacial Surgery, King Saud University and University Dental Hospital, Riyadh, Saudi Arabia*
[2]*Department of Oral Medicine and Diagnostic Sciences, King Saud University and University Dental Hospital, Riyadh, Saudi Arabia*

Correspondence should be addressed to Ahmed A. Zahrani; azahran@ksu.edu.sa

Academic Editor: Sukumaran Anil

Lipomas are relatively rare in the head and neck, and sialolipoma was described as an entity about 20 years ago as lipoma that entraps salivary gland tissue. Less than 10 cases have been described in the floor of the mouth not related to the major salivary glands. Here, we report a case of sialolipoma affecting the floor of the mouth in a 47-year-old patient and reviewed the clinical, histologic, and immunohistochemical characteristics of the lesion.

1. Introduction

Lipomas of the oral cavity are relatively very rare lesions, unlike their counterparts in the trunk and extremities where they constitute the most common mesenchymal tumor. Based on many reports, lipomas constitute between 1% and 5% of all benign oral lesions [1]. They are traditionally classified as fibrolipoma, spindle cell lipoma, angiolipoma, chondroid lipoma, intramuscular lipoma, and pleomorphic lipoma [2, 3]. A less frequently reported variant characterized by entrapment of salivary gland tissue containing acini and ducts by neoplastic mature adipocytes is called sialolipoma, a term that was first described by Nagao et al. [4] in 2001. Here, we report a case of sialolipoma of the floor of the mouth unrelated to the sublingual salivary gland.

2. Case Report

A 47-year-old Saudi male presented at the Oral and Maxillofacial Surgery Clinic of the University Dental Hospital at King Saud University Medical City (KSUMC) for assessment of swelling of the floor of the mouth reportedly of more than 3-year duration. The swelling was noted as a slow-growing, painless mass which caused the patient minimal discomfort and slight interference with speech, mastication, and movement of the tongue. The patient reported neither a history of trauma to the floor of the mouth nor that of intense pain while eating. The medical and family histories were noncontributory, and the patient was generally in good health.

Oral examination revealed the presence of a circumscribed, soft mass located on the left side of the oral cavity that was beside the tongue. The overlying mucosa was intact and appeared normal (Figures 1(a) and 1(b)). In its vertical dimension, when felt with bimanual palpation, the mass extended into the submental region. It caused a slight elevation of the tongue but no restriction of its movement. The salivary flow of the submandibular (Wharton) duct was normal, and there was no sensory deficit in the area. Although the patient reported occasional globus pharyngeus, there were no symptoms of nausea, dysphagia, snoring, or strident breathing. Lymph node examination was carried out for all neck nodes with no lymphadenopathy detected.

Imaging studies by CT scan and MRI showed an irregular mass in the area of the genioglossus muscle extending from the base of the tongue to the skin overlying the mylohyoid muscle with a density similar to the adjacent subcutaneous fat (Figure 1(c)). A hypointense density mass was observed in fat suppression MRI section at the level of the first molar

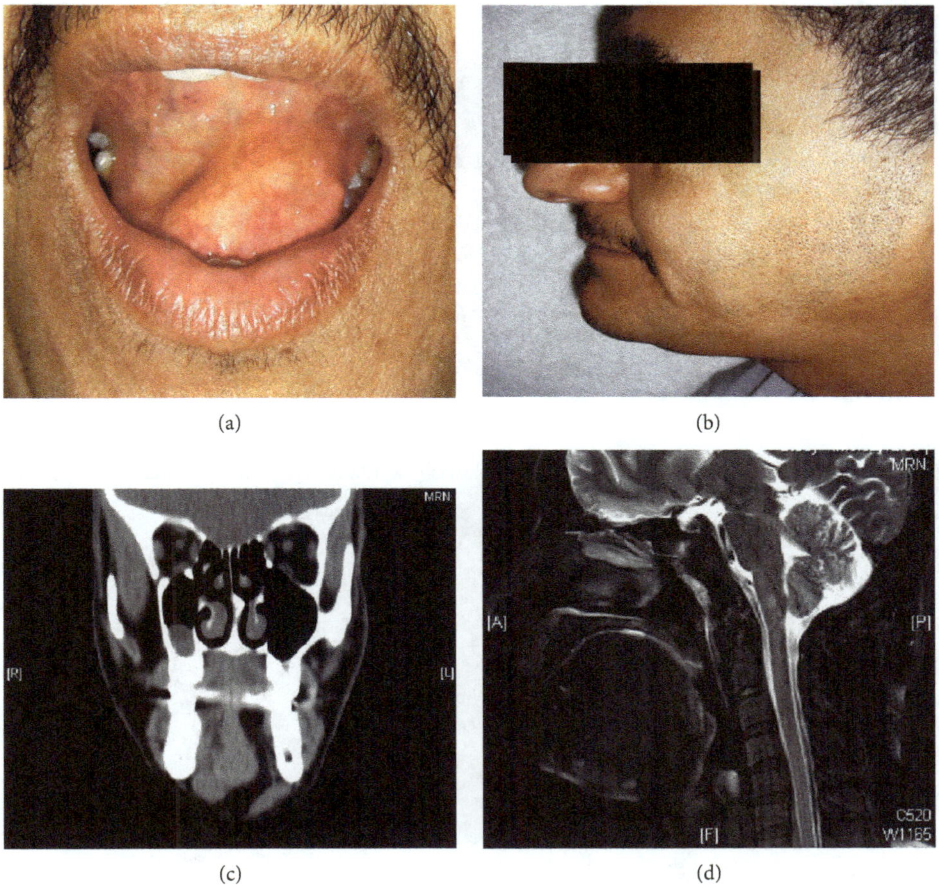

Figure 1: (a) Intraoral soft tissue mass in the floor of the mouth from the left ventral tongue surface extending beyond the midline to the right side. (b) Mild submental swelling as a result of an intraoral mass herniation beyond the mylohyoid muscle. (c) Coronal CT section at the level of the first molar in soft tissue window showing a markedly low density and clearly defined margin irregular mass within the left genioglossus muscle extending from ventral tongue to skin overlying the mylohyoid muscle. The density is homogenous and similar to adjacent subcutaneous fat. (d) Midsagittal MRI section in fat suppression showing the hypointense density mass.

suggesting an infiltrating intramuscular lipoma (Figure 1(d)). A tentative diagnosis of lipoma was made after clinical examination and radiographic examination, although the clinical differential diagnoses of the lesion included ranula, salivary gland neoplasm, and dermoid and epidermoid cyst.

The patient underwent surgical treatment under general anesthesia, and the lesion was excised through an intraoral approach. The specimen was formed of lobulated spherical masses, yellowish to pale pinkish in color, and measured $3.5 \times 4.7 \times 1.5$ cm in its greatest dimension (Figures 2(a) and 2(b)). The mass shelled out easily, with no adhesion to the sublingual gland or submandibular gland duct.

Histological examination showed an encapsulated lobulated tumor comprising mostly mature adipocytes. The lobules were separated by fibrovascular connective tissue septae in places. There were entrapped salivary gland acini and ducts scattered within the tumor mass (Figures 3(a) and 3(b)). The adipose tissue constituted about 90% of the tumor mass in comparison to the salivary gland tissue. A definitive diagnosis of sialolipoma was made. Immunohistochemical analysis of the tumor using pankeratin (AE1/AE3), epithelial membrane antigen (EMA), smooth muscle actin (SMA), S100, and Ki-67 immunostains was done. Acinar and ductal cells were strongly positive for AE1/AE3, luminal cells of ducts strongly expressed EMA alongside few acinar cells, and myoepithelial cells strongly stained by SMA and S100 with the latter also staining the fat cells. Proliferative activity as assessed by Ki-67 was less than 1% in both the adipose and salivary gland tissue (Table 1, Figures 3(c) and 3(d)).

The patient was followed up for more than 5 years, and there was no evidence of disease or recurrence.

3. Discussion

Sialolipoma was first described and reported as a series of 7 new cases in 2001 [4]. A subsequent review of 28 cases found in the literature as at 2009 showed that sialolipoma was seen in patients with a mean age of 52 years (range: 7 weeks to 84 years), occurred at relatively similar frequency in both males and females, and with most cases are seen in the parotid gland [5]. Sialolipoma of the minor salivary glands is very rare and is mostly found on the palate [4, 5]. Rare reports of cases occurring in the floor of the mouth have been reported mostly in females with all patients older than 60 years (Table 2) [6–9].

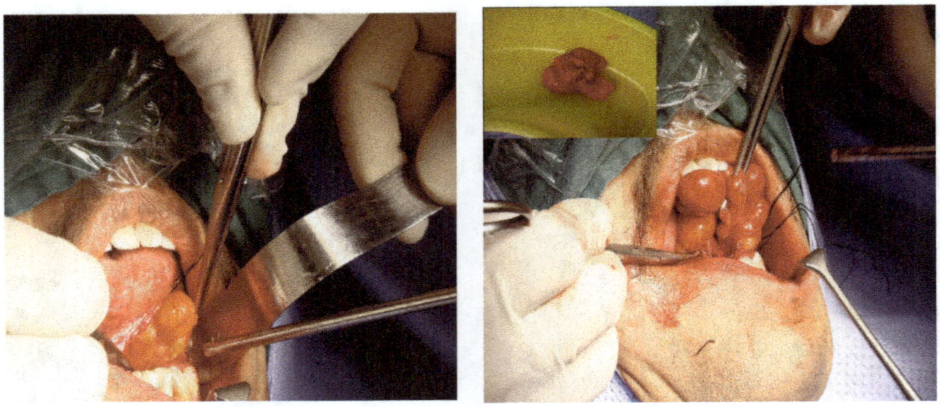

(a) (b)

Figure 2: (a, b) Surgical excision of the intraoral mass. Mass was yellowish, soft, and irregular in shape. Inset in (b) is the whole mass after excision.

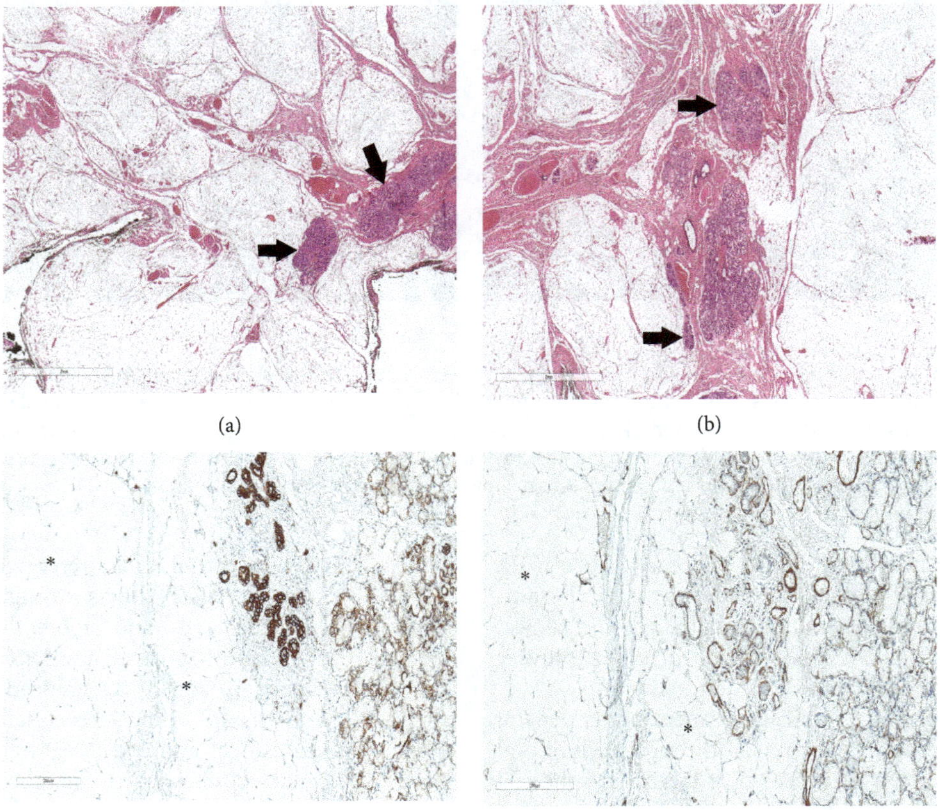

(a) (b)

(c) (d)

Figure 3: (a, b) Peripheral and inner areas of the tumor showing thin fibrous tissue capsule with numerous fat lobules and separated with fibrous tissue septae rich in vascular tissue with islands of salivary gland tissue (arrows) within the lipomatous proliferation. Scale bars: 2 mm. (c) Pancytokeratin (AE1/AE3) expression in the ductal and acinar cells in the entrapped salivary gland. The adipose tissue was negative (asterisk). Scale bar: 200 μm. (d) Smooth muscle actin highlighting the myoepithelial cells around the acini and ducts, and the smooth muscle in adjacent vascular structures. Lipomatous elements were negative (asterisk). Scale bar: 200 μm.

This report is that of a 47-year-old male patient with floor of the mouth sialolipoma, which coupled with its relatively large size is unusual for this specific entity. However, this is not a particularly rare finding in sialolipoma of other intraoral sites [9]. In general, this patient is younger than the mean age of presentation of sialolipomas [5]. Some reports have pointed to sialolipoma being more common in males [4, 10]. The lesion is generally characterized as being asymptomatic, slow-growing, soft, mobile, not associated with neurological deficits or mucosal or skin changes or other salivary gland lesions, or the presence of lipoma in other parts of the body [11]. All these features were seen in the present case. The occasional globus sensation reported by the patient could be attributed to the large size of the lesion

TABLE 1: Summary of immunohistochemical features of the floor of mouth sialolipoma.

Antibodies	Adipocytes	Acinar cells	Ductal cells	Antibody source
Epithelial membrane antigen (EMA)	—	+*	+	Roche (Ventana)
Ki-67	—	—	—	Roche (Ventana)
Pankeratin (AE1/AE3)	—	+	+	Roche (Ventana)
S-100	+	+	—	Roche (Ventana)
Smooth muscle actin	—	+	+	Roche (Ventana)

*Few acinar cell signals with bubbly positivity.

TABLE 2: Sialolipoma of the floor of the mouth.

Case	Author	Age	Sex	Duration	Size (cm)	Treatment	Follow-up
1	Lin et al. [6]	67	F	1 year	3 × 2	Excision	NED 2 years
2	Leyva Huerta et al. [7]	61	F	3 years	1.8 (diameter)	Excision	NA
3	Ponniah et al. [8]	60	M	NS	2 (diameter)	Excision	NED 2 years
4	Nonaka et al. [9]	73	F	NS	4 × 1	Excision	NA
5	Present case	47	M	3 years	4 × 5	Excision	NED 5 years

NA: not available; NED: no evidence of disease; NS: not specified.

and the elevation of the tongue as there was no pathology in the oropharynx, and this symptom was no longer present on follow-up after surgery.

Ultrasound examination would be the first choice among imaging investigations; however, lipomas may have a wide range of sonographic appearances [12]. The CT and MRI features are unique. On soft tissue window CT, it appears as a very low attenuation mass with minimal internal soft-tissue component [13]. MRI is the modality of choice for imaging lipomas, as it follows subcutaneous fat signal on all sequences appearing as high signal on T1 and saturates on fat-saturated sequences, with no or minimal contrast enhancement. On T2, it appears as a high signal on fast spin-echo sequences (FSE T2) and saturates on fat-saturated sequences [14].

Citing additional evidence from immunohistochemistry and ultrastructural studies, Nagao et al. [4] proposed that the salivary glandular elements seen in sialolipomas are non-neoplastic but rather became entrapped during the lipomatous proliferation. The glands are regularly organized and have normal phenotypes with little or no proliferative activity [4]. It is therefore assumed that the proliferative activity (which is relatively attenuated) resides in the adipocytes, although this is not demonstrable immunohistochemically. These features have been reaffirmed in other studies including a floor of mouth sialolipoma with some providing supportive immunohistochemical evidence for this hypothesis [6, 15], as in this present report. Microscopically, sialolipoma should be differentiated from salivary gland lipoadenoma (containing only dilated ducts along with fatty tissue but no salivary acini), lipomatous pleomorphic adenoma (containing chondromyxoid stroma), and salivary gland lipomatosis (unencapsulated proliferation of salivary acini, ducts, and mature adipocytes) [16, 17].

The treatment of choice is complete surgical removal as for all lipomas. In the present case in which the tumor arose in relation to minor salivary gland tissue in the floor of the mouth, there is no justification for removing the sublingual salivary gland as long as there is no proof that the tumor originates from the latter or found to be related to it during surgery. In the present case, the tumor shelled out without any adherence to the sublingual gland. Reported cases in the literature have shown no recurrence throughout the period of follow-up ranging from 7 to 91 months [5, 9, 10]. This patient was followed up for 62 months with no evidence of recurrence.

This report underlines that lipomas should be included in the differential diagnosis of asymptomatic, soft, mobile lesions of the floor of the mouth and that sialolipoma of the minor salivary glands could be the diagnosis found in microscopy after differentiation from relatively similar lesions such as lipoadenoma, lipomatosis, and pleomorphic adenoma with extensive lipomatosis. It may be more common than presently diagnosed as it is easy to overlook the presence of small scattered salivary gland elements. In addition, patients may be males younger than 60 years old.

References

[1] E. R. Fregnani, F. R. Pires, R. Falzoni, M. A. Lopes, and P. A. Vargas, "Lipomas of the oral cavity: clinical findings, histological classification and proliferative activity of 46 cases," *International Journal of Oral and Maxillofacial Surgery*, vol. 32, no. 1, pp. 49–53, 2003.

[2] M. A. Furlong, J. C. Fanburg-Smith, and E. L. B. Childers, "Lipoma of the oral and maxillofacial region: site and subclassification of 125 cases," *Oral Surgery, Oral Medicine, Oral Pathology, Oral Radiology, and Endodontics*, vol. 98, no. 4, pp. 441–450, 2004.

[3] T. Lombardi and E. W. Odell, "Spindle cell lipoma of the oral cavity: report of a case," *Journal of Oral Pathology & Medicine*, vol. 23, no. 5, pp. 237–239, 1994.

[4] T. Nagao, I. Sugano, Y. Ishida et al., "Sialolipoma: a report of seven cases of a new variant of salivary gland lipoma," *Histopathology*, vol. 38, no. 1, pp. 30–36, 2001.

[5] Y. W. Jang, S. G. Kim, H. Pai, J. W. Park, Y. C. Lee, and H. Rotaru, "Sialolipoma: case report and review of 27 cases," *Oral and Maxillofacial Surgery*, vol. 13, no. 2, pp. 109–113, 2009.

[6] Y. J. Lin, L. M. Lin, Y. K. Chen et al., "Sialolipoma of the floor of the mouth: a case report," *The Kaohsiung Journal of Medical Sciences*, vol. 20, no. 8, pp. 410–414, 2004.

[7] E. Leyva Huerta, D. Quezada Rivera, F. Tenorio Rocha, J. L. Tapia, J. Portilla Robertson, and L. A. Gaitán Cepeda, "Sialolipoma of minor salivary glands: presentation of five cases and review of the literature with an epidemiological analyze," *Indian Journal of Otolaryngology and Head & Neck Surgery*, vol. 67, Supplement 1, pp. 105–109, 2015.

[8] I. Ponniah, N. Lavanya, and P. SureshKumar, "Island of salivary gland in adipose tissue: a report of three cases," *Journal of Oral Pathology & Medicine*, vol. 36, no. 9, pp. 558-562, 2007.

[9] C. F. W. Nonaka, K. M. A. Pereira, P. P. de Andrade Santos, R. de Almeida Freitas, and M. C. da Costa Miguel, "Sialolipoma of minor salivary glands," *Annals of Diagnostic Pathology*, vol. 15, no. 1, pp. 6–11, 2011.

[10] N. Ramer, H. S. Lumerman, and Y. Ramer, "Sialolipoma: report of two cases and review of the literature," *Oral Surgery, Oral Medicine, Oral Pathology, Oral Radiology, and Endodontics*, vol. 104, no. 6, pp. 809–813, 2007.

[11] K. Sato, C. Gotoh, H. Uchida et al., "Sialolipoma of the submandibular gland in a child," *Journal of Pediatric Surgery*, vol. 46, no. 2, pp. 408–410, 2011.

[12] P. Inampudi, J. A. Jacobson, D. P. Fessell et al., "Soft-tissue lipomas: accuracy of sonography in diagnosis with pathologic correlation," *Radiology*, vol. 233, no. 3, pp. 763–767, 2004.

[13] M. D. Murphey, J. F. Carroll, D. J. Flemming, T. L. Pope, F. H. Gannon, and M. J. Kransdorf, "From the archives of the AFIP," *Radiographics*, vol. 24, no. 5, pp. 1433–1466, 2004.

[14] C. M. Gaskin and C. A. Helms, "Lipomas, lipoma variants, and well-differentiated liposarcomas (atypical lipomas): results of MRI evaluations of 126 consecutive fatty masses," *AJR. American Journal of Roentgenology*, vol. 182, no. 3, pp. 733–739, 2004.

[15] H. Okada, M. Yokoyama, M. Hara, Y. Akimoto, T. Kaneda, and H. Yamamoto, "Sialolipoma of the palate: a rare case and review of the literature," *Oral Surgery, Oral Medicine, Oral Pathology, Oral Radiology, and Endodontics*, vol. 108, no. 4, pp. 571–576, 2009.

[16] M. Hirokawa, Y. Bando, T. Tashiro, S. Kuma, I. Kawata, and T. Sano, "Parotid lipoadenoma with sclerotic and polycystic changes," *Virchows Archiv*, vol. 440, no. 5, pp. 549-550, 2002.

[17] H. A. Saleh, B. Ram, J. L. Harmse, B. A. Michie, and R. L. Blair, "Lipomatosis of the minor salivary glands," *The Journal of Laryngology and Otology*, vol. 112, no. 9, pp. 895–897, 1998.

13

BRIX3000® Papain Gel for Cavity Treatment in the Adult Patient

Leonardo Mancini,[1] **Alessia Pisaneschi**,[1] **Vincenzo Mancini**,[2] **Marino Ginoble**,[1] **Vincenzo Quinzi**,[1] **Enrico Marchetti**,[1] **and Giuseppe Marzo**[1]

[1]*Department of Life, Health and Environmental Sciences, University of L'Aquila, 67100 L'Aquila, Italy*
[2]*Private Practice in Via Degli Eroi n.4, 67051 Avezzano, Italy*

Correspondence should be addressed to Leonardo Mancini; mancinileonardo94@gmail.com

Academic Editor: Giuseppe Alessandro Scardina

Tooth decay is a multifactorial disease. Fermentable sugar, host factors, and cariogenic microbial flora are several agents that influence dental structure. In literature, alternative protocols for treating cavities are always of interest in terms of reducing pain and preserving tissue. In this case report, the use of a new gel-based on papain, which has a chemical effect on bacteria and allows the consistency of the altered tissue to be modified, leads to a less traumatic removal of the infected tissue. In this case report, BRIX3000, a gel with papain as its main ingredient, was used to treat an interproximal cavity on an upper premolar of a 35-year-old man frightened of the turbine. After a clinical check of all the systematic conditions and a first view of the oral cavity, the protocol was explained to the patient, and informed consent was obtained. The protocol involved applying the papain gel directly to the cavity, and after 2.5–3 minutes, it was removed. The complete removal of the infected tissue was achieved in three steps. The patient reported no discomfort, and the cavity was completely treated and ready to be restored. In conclusion, BRIX3000 seems to be a good alternative to the turbine in cavity treatment, particularly in patients who have discomfort during traditional treatments and are frightened of the turbine.

1. Introduction

Tooth decay is the most widespread disease in the world and has been defined by WHO as a major public health problem globally [1]. The Global Burden of Disease Study 2017 estimated that 2.3 billion people suffer from caries of permanent teeth, and more than 530 million children suffer from caries of primary teeth [2].

Dental caries is a noncommunicable disease (NCD), mediated by the interaction of various factors (physical, biological, environmental, behavioural, and lifestyle-related) that combine to create a degenerative process on the tooth surface with consequent loss of minerals in the hard tissue of the tooth [3]. Dental caries is a multifactorial pathology where all the participating factors increase the risk of developing the disease. There are several risk factors that contribute to the manifestation of tooth decay such as a high component of cariogenic bacteria, inadequate salivary flow, reduced exposure to fluoride, poor or incorrect oral hygiene, incorrect methods of feeding newborns, and poverty [4]. The carious lesion is caused by an imbalance between the continuous processes of demineralization and remineralization that occur naturally on the hard surface of the tooth. When demineralization processes prevail, they lead to a loss of the mineral component of enamel, dentin, or cement, reaching, if not arrested, a point of no return with the appearance of a severe cavitated lesion [5]. Tooth decay is a dynamic disease where several stages and symptoms follow one another. In early tooth decay (noncavitated), usually, there are no symptoms. When tooth decay advances, there is a progressive involvement of the dentine, and if not treated, there is an involvement of the dental pulp, and symptoms appear (tooth pain, infections, and abscesses, or even sepsis) [1]. When dental caries advances and arrives in dentine, the dentist has to remove the involved dentine: it is possible to do this through different methodologies, such as treatment with rotary instruments, manual excavator, air abrasion, sonic abrasion, ultrasonic methods, lasers, and chemo-mechanical methods. Conventional methods of caries removal (treatment with rotary instruments) are commonly associated with pain, discomfort, and fear [6]. Pain is a subjective experience and is a symptom that undermines the patient's physical and mental integrity; moreover, it is closely related to fear, which is the individual's response to a threatening event. Dental anxiety is regarded as a serious health issue worldwide [7]. A dental phobia is a persistent and excessive fear of dental stimuli and procedures that results in avoidance or significant distress with impact on individual's normal routine, social relationships, occupational or school functioning, and social relationships [8]. In DSM 5 (*Diagnostic and Statistical Manual of Mental Disorder, Fifth Edition*), dental phobia is classified as a specific-phobia and, more precisely, included in the blood-injection-injury (BII) phobia type [9]; furthermore, some studies suggest that patients with dental phobia often report more anxiety pertaining to other dental stimuli (e.g., the count of a drill and having a tooth extracted) than to blood and injections; indeed, anxiety regarding blood seems to be relatively uncommon or minor in individuals with dental anxiety [10, 11]. Dental anxiety is first and foremost an oral-health problem as it is associated with a lower frequency of dental visits and a higher prevalence of dental caries [12]. Dentists must diligently manage and care with patients who are anxious to receive dental care because this condition affects about one in seven people [13]. In one study, 67 potentially anxious stimuli were brought to the attention of participants, and the image of a "dentist drilling a tooth or molar" was the seventh most anxious stimulus. [14]. In recent years, research has moved towards the search for chemo-mechanical methods to remove dental caries in order to install a positive dental attitude [15]. Moreover, these methods belong to what is now identified as minimally invasive dentistry (MID). Such an approach adopts a philosophy that integrates prevention, remineralization, and minimal intervention for placement and replacement of restorations. The objective is tissue preservation, which means performing treatment with as little tissue loss as possible [16]. Chemo-mechanical cavity preparation is a new method of treatment that involves the chemical softening of carious dentine followed by its removal by gentle excavation [17]. Some studies in the literature have shown that the perceived pain was less when chemo-mechanical removal agents were used to remove caries compared to conventional rotary tools [18]. In other studies, it has emerged that chemo-mechanical caries removal agents have a very slow action compared to mechanical tools; moreover, it seems that they can be used together to completely remove the carious lesion tissue [7]. It has also emerged that the taste and odour of these used agents based on sodium hypochlorite were unpleasant [19]. Through the use of chemical-mechanical methods of caries removal, it is possible to bypass the use of the drill (reducing dental anxiety) but also to preserve a greater amount of healthy tooth tissue. In fact, these materials allow to create a further break in the collagen of the carious lesion to selectively remove the infected dentin while preserving the affected one that can remineralize. [20]. Chemical agents can be classified into two large families: on the one hand, there are those having sodium hypochlorite

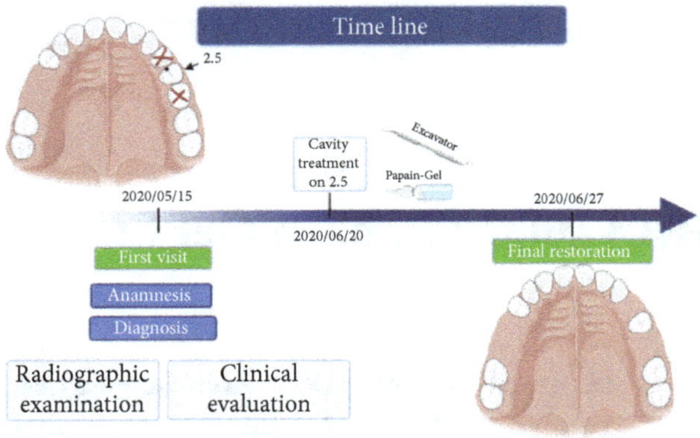

FIGURE 1: Timeline according to the CARE protocol.

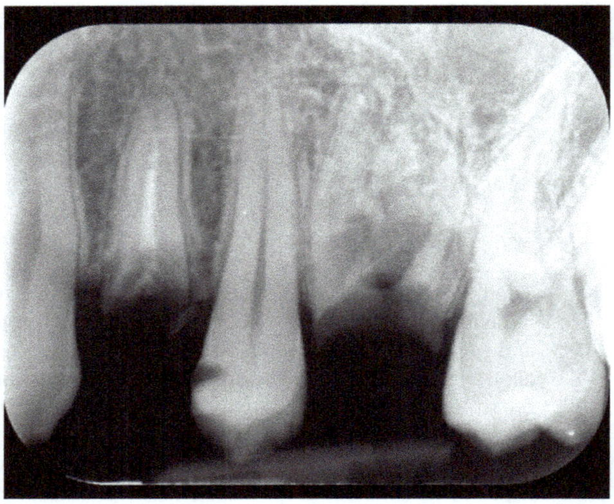

FIGURE 2: X-ray of the premolar with the presence of residual roots and the cavity on the crown.

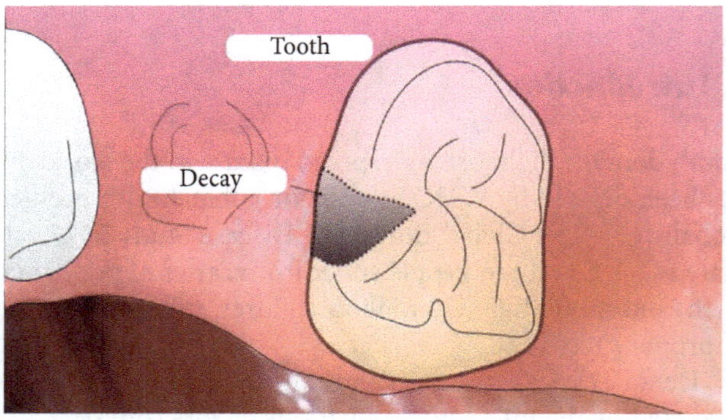

FIGURE 3: Iconographic representation of the tooth decay on the interproximal surface.

as main component, on the other those having enzymes. Over the years, there have been several chemical agents produced for the chemo-mechanical removal of dental caries (GK-101 ®/Nmonochloroglycerine, Caridex ®, and Carisolv ®, Papacarie). BRIX3000 was released in 2012 and is a chemical-mechanical agent based on a proteolytic enzyme and papain, which allows the chemical debridement of the collagen present in dentin. The amount of papain used

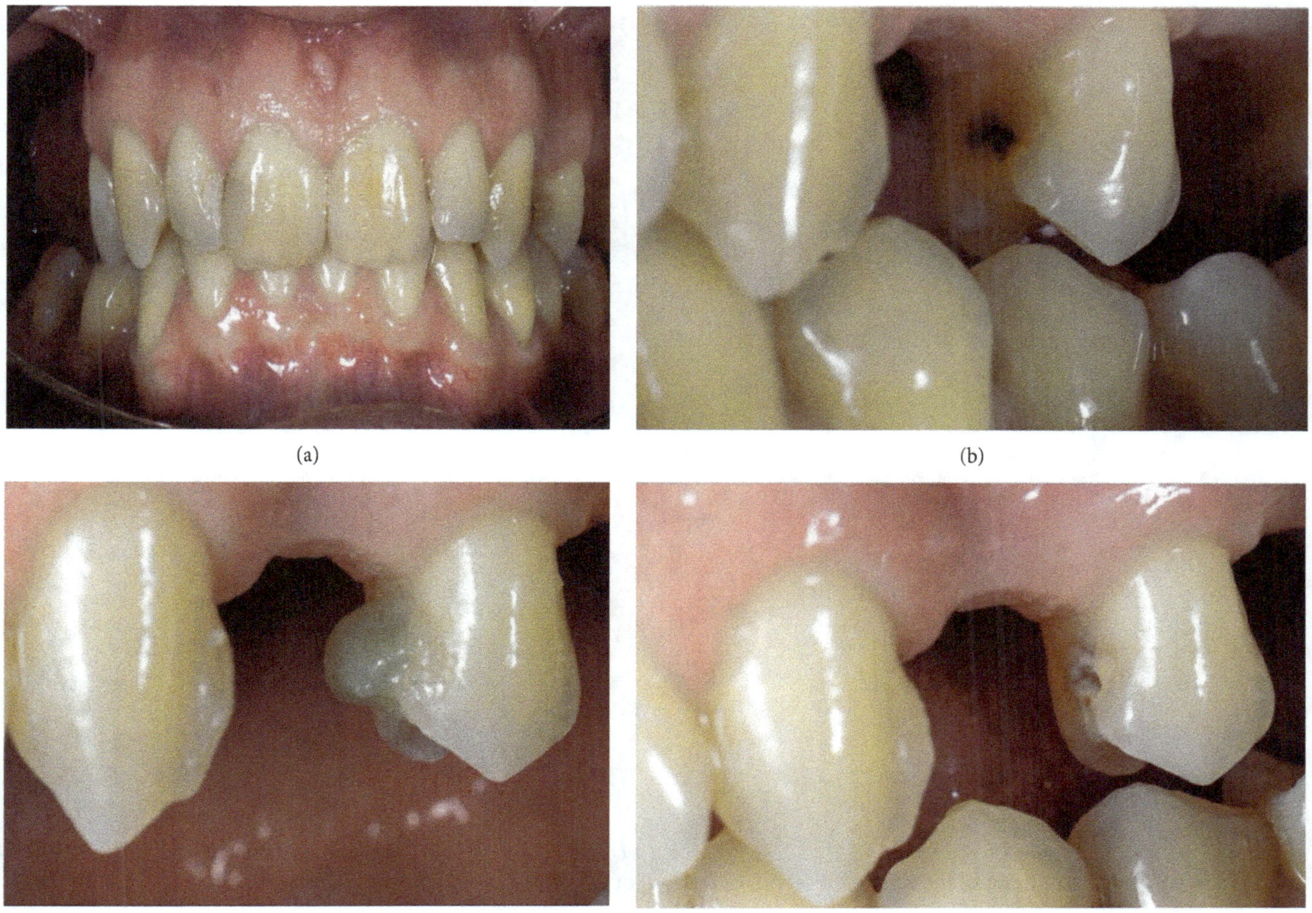

(a) (b) (c) (d)

Figure 4: (a) Initial photography. (b) High magnification of the cavity on the second premolar 2.5. (c) First application of BRIX3000. (d) After removing the altered tissue.

in the product, equal to 3,000 U/mg in a concentration of 10%, together with the capping by means of the Encapsulating Buffer Emulsion technology, would give the gel an ideal pH to ensure that the enzymes are able to perform a proteolysis, on the collagen of decayed dental tissue. The aim of the present study is to describe BRIX3000 as an alternative method to remove an interproximal cavity of an upper premolar tooth in a 35-year-old patient scared of the turbine.

2. Case Report

The present protocol was approved by the Ethics Committee of the University of L'Aquila (Document DR206/2013, 16 July 2013). This study follows the principles of Helsinki for human experimentation. This case report was assessed according to the CARE case report guidelines [21]. All the procedures were followed after the signs of the informed consent.

2.1. Patient Information. The patient was a 35-year-old nonsmoker who has not been followed by the dentist for some years. We found out through his medical history that he was in good general health and had no significant medical conditions or drug allergies. The man told us that he was afraid of the dentist and the turbine due to bad experiences in the past, and this fear was the cause of poor oral hygiene. He also reported having extracted the second premolar and first molar in the first sextant but could not remember the reason for the extraction. The patient came under our observation after suffering a crown fracture of 2.4 (endodontically treated tooth) and 2.6; he also suffered from dental sensitivity to hot, cold, and sweet stimuli in the days leading up to the visit.

2.2. Clinical Findings. During the intraoral visit, it has been found that the patient had poor oral hygiene with dental plaque, and he has been motivated to improve it. There were residual roots of the first premolar and first molar in the second sextant which have been extracted before the cavity's treatment. There was also a Class II interproximal cavity in the mesial tooth wall of the second upper left premolar; on the contrary, there were no fistula and endo-perio lesions.

2.3. Timeline. The general health and oral health status of the patient have been identified during the first visit. An intraoral radiography has been made in order to identify the residual roots and diagnose caries. After the extraction of the residual roots of 2.4 and 2.6, a mechanical-chemical removal of the

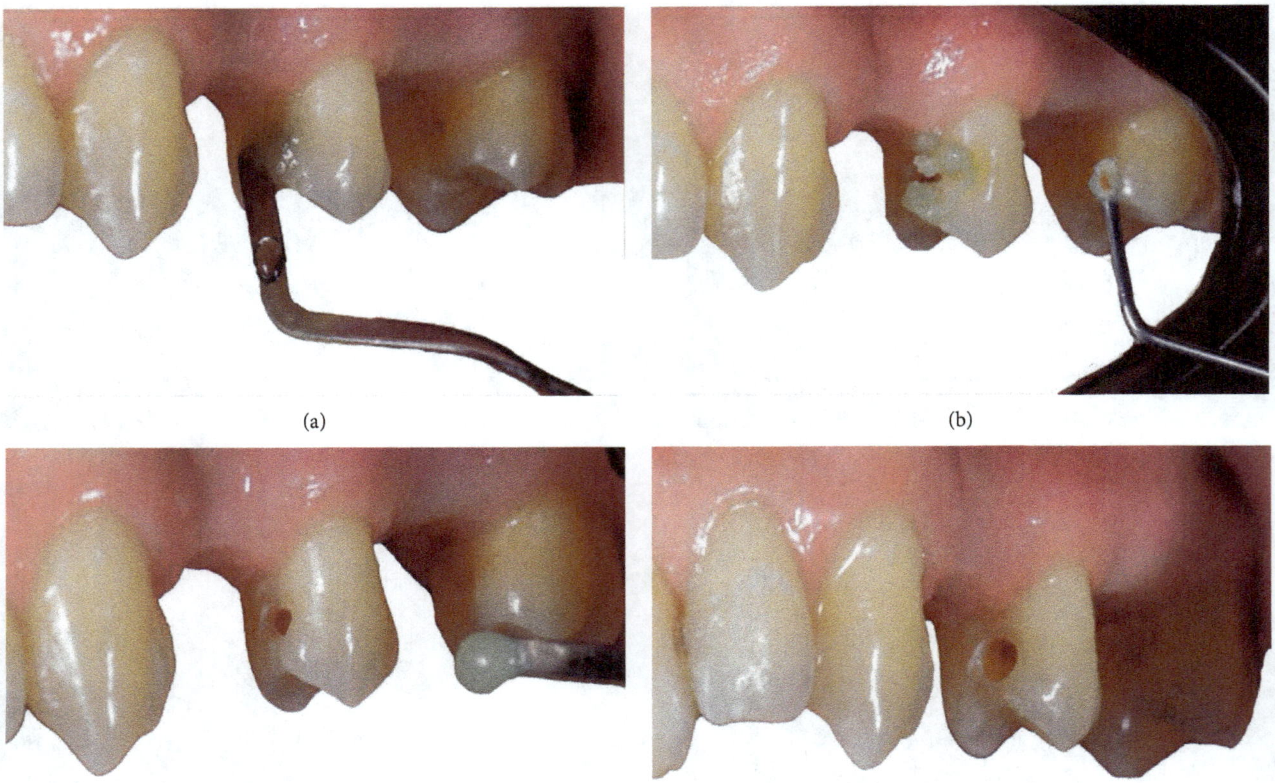

(a) (b) (c) (d)

FIGURE 5: (a) Second application of BRIX3000. (b) The cavity during a second application. (c) Tooth after removing the altered tissue in the second phase. (d) Cavity at the end of the third application. Correction of the profile was performed using the turbine.

dental cavity has been made allowing to control drill fear of the patient (Figure 1).

2.4. Diagnostic Assessment. The dental cavity in the interproximal level of the second premolar in the mesial wall has been diagnosed through an explorer (3A/6 Explorer, Hu-Friedy Mfg. Co., LLC 3232 N. Rockwell St.; Chicago) and a diagnostic X-ray. This diagnosis confirmed that caries reached the dentine by going beyond the amelo-dentinal junction (Figure 2).

2.5. Therapeutic Intervention. The clinical examination did not reveal the presence of a fistula or endo-perio lesion. Thus, a Class II stage DII according to the last classification from Anusavice et al. [22] interproximal cavity was diagnosed as represented in Figure 3.

The structure around the cavity was sufficient, and the tooth could be treated in a conservative mode, and the missing tissue restored. The man was afraid of dentists and the turbine due to negative experiences in the past. Therefore, a chemo-mechanical removal procedure was selected to reduce the discomfort. The product selected to remove the infected tissue was BRIX3000 papain gel (Brix Medical Science, Carcañá, Argentina). After the informed consent had been signed, the restorative procedure was initiated. The procedure was achieved without anesthesia, and for the first step of the treatment, the isolation was not obtained due to the use of the natural and nondangerous material papain gel. BRIX3000 was applied in the cavity of the 2.5 with a Heidemann spatula (ASA Dental, Bozzano, Italy), and after 2 minutes of activation, following the manufacturer's instructions, the gel started to modify its consistency, producing oxygen bubbles. Its color changed from translucent green to light grey, and at this phase, a dentine excavator (ASA Dental, Bozzano, Italy) was used to remove the altered tissue (Figure 4).

The complete removal of the decay was achieved with three applications of BRIX3000. The cavity was completely treated and ready to be restored with a treatment time of 10 minutes (Figure 5).

During the three steps, a visual analog scale was used (Figure 6). The patient consistently reported a Grade 0 except for the refinement phase, in which a rotary cutting instrument with a spherical cutting tip #014 (Komet Italia Srl, Milano, Italy) was used to modify the profile of the cavity, and Grade 2 was reported.

3. Patient Perspective

I received the treatment of the 2.5 premolar using a minimally invasive approach with a substance based on papain gel, and during the therapy, I did not feel disturbed by the treatment preferring the atraumatic remotion to the turbine.

4. Discussion

Conventional caries removal techniques are always associated with anxiety and discomfort in children and scared

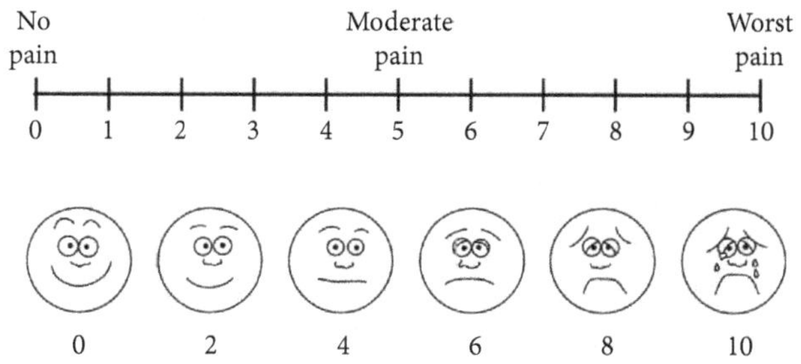

FIGURE 6: Visual analogue scale to assess pain perception and verify patient discomfort.

patients. This condition is related to the temperature increasing in the excavation phase which might cause irreversible pulp damage and tooth destruction reducing dentin structure and leading to an impairment of the tooth structure for future restorative therapy [23]. To overcome this condition, several alternative therapies were proposed as laser therapy [24], air abrasion [25], and chemo-mechanical caries removal [26]. Human dentin is composed of water and an organic matrix; the matrix is composed mainly of collagen, chondroitin sulphate, proteoglycans, and phosphoproteins. When carious start to impair the tooth, an acid releasing from several cariogenic bacteria leads to enamel dissolution and progressively in the dentinal tubules [27]. The pH reduction and the persistence presence of bacteria start to demineralize also the dentin which starts to differentiate in two layers, the first one which is the outer layer, and it is in intimate contact with bacteria without any possibilities to remineralized and a second layer where dentine could be remineralized after removing the outer layer [28]. The chemo-mechanical therapy might be more conservative and predictable concerning the traditional rotary instrumentation indeed the action of the papain enzyme is focused only on the outer infected layer where it starts to degrade the collagen of the infected tissue promoting the healthy dentine preservation [29]. The complete cavity treatment respect to the traditional method required more time but with a minimally invasive approach and in a more conservative way. The chemo-mechanical method is a promising alternative to traditional therapy and might be a possible alternative also during the recent issue for the presence of aerosol in the dental office during the COVID-19 outbreak [30, 31]. In this case report, Brix 3000 was used which is the last papain enzyme gel proposed to remove and treat tooth decay. This gel differs from the others for the papain preparation and concentration which might guarantee a better activity on the decay. During the application, the handling on the cavity was easy due to the dried surface which was achieved with a cotton roll. To reduce humidity and ensure a dry environment is possible to use rubber dam that is not tightly required because the gel is natural and in contact with the soft tissue does not arise adverse reactions. Moreover, to the best of our knowledge, the use of this alternative might facilitate, in the future, the approach to the turbine of several scared patients improving their confidence and collaboration for future dental therapies.

5. Conclusion

Minimally invasive dentistry is the future of dental practice and requires new materials to be conservative and produce less discomfort for patients. BRIX3000 papain gel seems to be a good alternative in the treatment of tooth decay, reducing the amount of removed tissue and making patients more confident and cooperative with their dentist.

Acknowledgments

This project could not have been accomplished without the support of One Flex technology Srl, Frosinone, Italy, and to the friendship demonstrated by Paolo Avveniri who donated all the materials for the work.

References

[1] X. Gao, S. B. Zhang, Y. Chang, F. Yang, and Y. Zhang, "Cryptanalysis of the Quantum Private Comparison Protocol Based on the Entanglement Swapping Between Three-Particle W-Class State and Bell State," *International Journal of Theoretical Physics*, vol. 57, no. 6, article 3697, pp. 1716–1722, 2018.

[2] GBD 2017 Oral Disorders Collaborators, E. Bernabe, W. Marcenes et al., "Global, regional, and national levels and trends in burden of oral conditions from 1990 to 2017: a systematic analysis for the Global Burden of Disease 2017 study," *Journal of Dental Research*, vol. 99, no. 4, pp. 362–373, 2020.

[3] V. Machiulskiene, G. Campus, J. C. Carvalho et al., "Terminology of dental caries and dental caries management: consensus report of a workshop organized by ORCA and Cariology Research Group of IADR," *Caries Research*, vol. 54, no. 1, pp. 7–14, 2020.

[4] R. H. Selwitz, A. I. Ismail, and N. B. Pitts, "Dental caries," *Lancet*, vol. 369, no. 9555, pp. 51–59, 2007.

[5] J. D. B. Featherstone, "Dental caries: a dynamic disease process," *Australian Dental Journal*, vol. 53, no. 3, pp. 286–291, 2008.

[6] W. H. O. Technical, I. Note, and K. E. Y. Facts, "Sugars and dental caries," *Journal of Public Health Dentistry*, vol. 4, no. 1, pp. 7–7, 1944.

[7] T. Yamada, S. Kuwano, S. Ebisu, and M. Hayashi, "Statistical analysis for subjective and objective evaluations of dental drill sounds," *PLoS One*, vol. 11, no. 7, article e0159926, 2016.

[8] C. M. Mak, H. M. Wong, and Y. F. Xu, "A four-part setting on examining the anxiety-provoking capacity of the sound of dental equipment," *Noise and Health*, vol. 13, no. 55, article 90291, pp. 385–391, 2011.

[9] L. D. Seligman, J. D. Hovey, K. Chacon, and T. H. Ollendick, "Dental anxiety: an understudied problem in youth," *Clinical Psychology Review*, vol. 55, pp. 25–40, 2017.

[10] "Oral Health in America: A report of the Surgeon General," *Journal of the California Dental Association*, vol. 28, no. 9, pp. 685–695, 2000.

[11] C. M. H. H. van Houtem, I. H. A. Aartman, D. I. Boomsma, L. Ligthart, C. M. Visscher, and A. de Jongh, "Is dental phobia a blood-injection-injury phobia?," *Depression and Anxiety*, vol. 31, no. 12, pp. 1026–1034, 2014.

[12] A. De Jongh, G. Bongaarts, I. Vermeule, K. Visser, P. De Vos, and P. Makkes, "Blood-injury-injection phobia and dental

phobia," *Behaviour Research and Therapy*, vol. 36, no. 10, pp. 971–982, 1998.

[13] G. Klingberg, U. Berggren, S. G. Carlsson, and J. G. Noren, "Child dental fear: cause-related factors and clinical effects," *European Journal of Oral Sciences*, vol. 103, no. 6, pp. 405–412, 1995.

[14] J. M. Armfield and L. J. Heaton, "Management of fear and anxiety in the dental clinic: a review," *Australian Dental Journal*, vol. 58, no. 4, pp. 390–407, 2013.

[15] F. M. D. Oosterink, A. De Jongh, and I. H. A. Aartman, "What are people afraid of during dental treatment? Anxiety-provoking capacity of 67 stimuli characteristic of the dental setting," *European Journal of Oral Sciences*, vol. 116, no. 1, pp. 44–51, 2008.

[16] P. A. Goyal, R. Kumari, V. P. Kannan, and S. Madhu, "Efficacy and tolerance of papain gel with conventional drilling method: a clinico-microbiological study," *Journal of Clinical Pediatric Dentistry*, vol. 39, no. 2, pp. 109–112, 2015.

[17] M. M. Jingarwar, N. K. Bajwa, and A. Pathak, "Minimal intervention dentistry - a new frontier in clinical dentistry," *Journal of clinical and diagnostic research: JCDR*, vol. 8, no. 7, pp. 4–8, 2014.

[18] J. A. Beeley, H. K. Yip, and A. G. Stevenson, "Chemochemical caries removal: a review of the techniques and latest developments," *Nederlands Tijdschrift voor Tandheelkunde*, vol. 188, no. 8, pp. 427–430, 2000.

[19] M. M. Alkhouli, S. F. Al Nesser, N. G. Bshara, A. N. AlMidani, and J. C. Comisi, "Comparing the efficacies of two chemomechanical caries removal agents (2.25% sodium hypochlorite gel and brix 3000), in caries removal and patient cooperation: a randomized controlled clinical trial," *Journal of dentistry*, vol. 93, article 103280, 2020.

[20] G. M. Maragakis, P. Hahn, and E. Hellwig, "Clinical evaluation of chemomechanical caries removal in primary molars and its acceptance by patients," *Caries Research*, vol. 35, no. 3, pp. 205–210, 2001.

[21] D. S. Riley, M. S. Barber, G. S. Kienle et al., "CARE guidelines for case reports: explanation and elaboration document," *Journal of clinical epidemiology*, vol. 89, no. 17, pp. 218–235, 2017.

[22] K. J. Anusavice, "Decision analysis in restorative dentistry," *Journal of Dental Education*, vol. 56, no. 12, pp. 812–822, 1992.

[23] M. Shabzendedar, H. Moosavi, M. Talbi, and M. Sharifi, "Permeability evaluation after decay removal in primary teeth with current caries-excavation techniques," *The Journal of Contemporary Dental Practice*, vol. 12, no. 6, pp. 441–446, 2011.

[24] Y. J. Wong, "Caries removal using lasers," *Evidence-Based Dentistry*, vol. 19, no. 2, p. 45, 2018.

[25] A. Banerjee, H. Pabari, G. Paolinelis, I. D. Thompson, and T. F Watson, "An in vitro evaluation of selective demineralised enamel removal using bio-active glass air abrasion," *Clinical Oral Investigations*, vol. 15, no. 6, pp. 895–900, 2011.

[26] F. Schwendicke, S. Paris, and Y. K. Tu, "Effects of using different criteria for caries removal: a systematic review and network meta-analysis," *Journal of Dentistry*, vol. 43, no. 1, pp. 1–15, 2015.

[27] N. B. Pitts, D. T. Zero, P. D. Marsh et al., "Dental caries," *Nature Reviews Disease Primers*, vol. 3, article 17030, 2017.

[28] D. Ricucci, S. Loghin, L. N. Niu, and F. R. Tay, "Changes in the radicular pulp-dentine complex in healthy intact teeth and in response to deep caries or restorations: a histological and histobacteriological study," *Journal of Dentistry*, vol. 73, pp. 76–90, 2018.

[29] Z. S. S. Júnior, S. B. Botta, P. A. Ana et al., "Effect of papain-based gel on type I collagen - spectroscopy applied for microstructural analysis," *Scientific Reports*, vol. 5, no. 1, article 11448, 2015.

[30] S. Saccomanno, V. Quinzi, S. Sarhan, D. Laganà, and G. Marzo, "Perspectives of tele-orthodontics in the COVID-19 emergency and as a future tool in daily practice," *European journal of paediatric dentistry*, vol. 21, no. 2, pp. 157–162, 2020.

[31] R. Izzetti, M. Nisi, M. Gabriele, and F. Graziani, "COVID-19 transmission in dental practice: brief review of preventive measures in Italy," *Journal of Dental Research*, vol. 99, no. 9, pp. 1030–1038, 2020.

14

Occurrence of Recurrent Aphthous Stomatitis (RAS) as a Rare Oral Manifestation in a Patient with Gilbert's Syndrome

Artak Heboyan,[1] **Anna Avetisyan**,[2] **Hans Erling Skallevold**,[3] **Dinesh Rokaya**,[4] **Vinay Marla**,[5] **and Anna Vardanyan**[1]

[1]*Department of Prosthodontics, Faculty of Stomatology, Yerevan State Medical University, Str. Koryun 2, Yerevan 0025, Armenia*
[2]*Department of Therapeutic Dentistry, Faculty of Stomatology, Yerevan State Medical University, Str. Koryun 2, Yerevan 0025, Armenia*
[3]*Christiania Tannlegesenter, Grønland 4, 0188 Oslo, Norway*
[4]*Department of Clinical Dentistry, Walailak University International College of Dentistry, Bangkok 10400, Thailand*
[5]*Department of Oral Pathology, Penang International Dental College, Penang 12000, Malaysia*

Correspondence should be addressed to Artak Heboyan; heboyan.artak@gmail.com

Academic Editor: Alberto Delbem

Recurrent aphthous stomatitis is an ulcerative disease of the oral cavity and can occur in isolation or as a manifestation of many systemic diseases. It is a quite common entity and may hence often be overlooked as an isolated lesion. Gilbert's syndrome is a genetic disorder where a deficiency of an enzyme associated with the conjugation of bilirubin results in unconjugated hyperbilirubinemia. The disease is generally asymptomatic and is aggravated by certain trigger factors. No associated oral manifestations are known. In this case report, we discuss the concomitant presence of recurrent aphthous stomatitis in a patient of Gilbert's syndrome. The presence of such recurrent stomatitis may represent as an oral manifestation of Gilbert's syndrome. Early identification of these entities may improve the overall quality of life of the patient.

1. Introduction

Recurrent aphthous stomatitis (RAS) is a chronic inflammatory ulcerative disease of the oral cavity, manifested with the formation of one or several aphthae in the oral mucosa [1]. The recurrence of the ulcers has no clear pattern, yet they are characterized by long-term course, lasting for several years. The disease affects 5% to 60% of the world population, affecting mostly females [2]. RAS manifests in several systemic diseases [3] and may be the initial symptoms in some. The presence of aphthae may contribute in the diagnosis of an underlying disease [1].

Recurrent aphthous stomatitis is further classified, based on lesion size and number, into three types, namely, recurrent aphthous stomatitis minor, recurrent aphthous stomatitis major, and herpetiform ulcers [4]. Minor RAS is the most common type and manifests as numerous ulcers measuring 8 to 10 mm in diameter which heal within 2 weeks without scarring [5]. Major RAS, on the other hand, are lesions larger than 1 cm in diameter, multiple, and require a longer duration to heal. These ulcers generally scar upon healing [1, 5]. Herpetiform ulcers presents as multiple crops (up to 100) of painful, small (2-3 mm in diameter) ulcers but later coalesce to form larger ones. This variant is more common in older women and predominantly affects the tongue and floor of the mouth [6].

Diagnosis of recurrent aphthous stomatitis is mainly made on the basis of history and clinical presentation. Histopathology may be prescribed to rule out any other chronic ulcerative pathology [7]. The presence of systemic disease is confirmed based on the findings related to that pathology. The common systemic diseases associated with recurrent aphthous stomatitis include Behcet's syndrome, Magic syndrome, Sweet's syndrome, cyclic neutropenia, and acquired

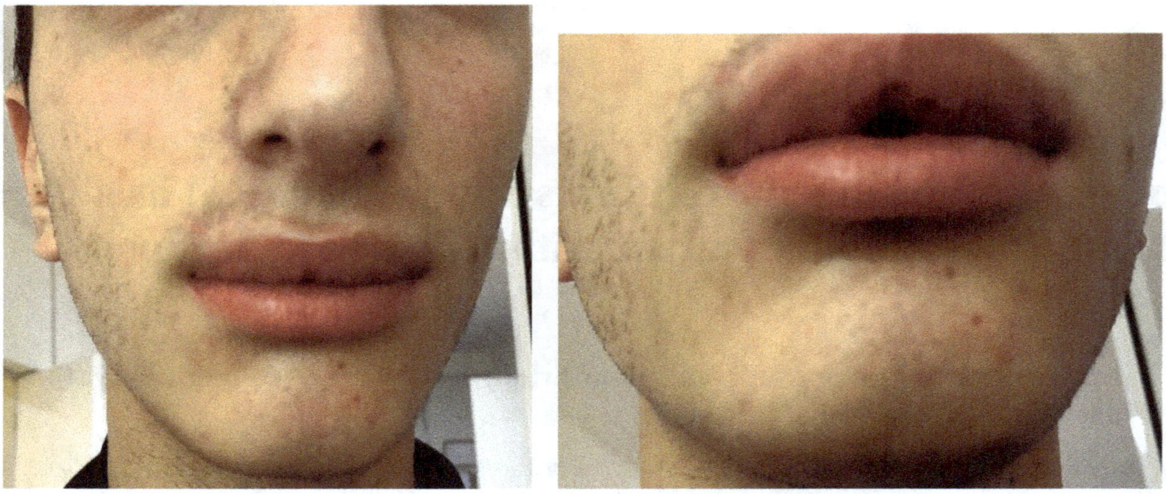

(a) (b)

FIGURE 1: (a, b) Significant swelling of the upper and lower lips.

immunodeficiency syndrome (AIDS) [8]. The association of RAS with Gilbert's syndrome has, to the authors' knowledge, not been reported so far in the literature.

Gilbert's syndrome is a genetic disorder which is caused due to the deficiency of the enzyme uridine diphosphoglucuronate-glucuronosyltransferase 1A1 (UGT1A1) which is involved in the process of conjugation of bilirubin, thereby resulting in unconjugated hyperbilirubinemia [9]. Gilbert's syndrome is generally asymptomatic and is aggravated in association with certain triggering factors [10]. Oral manifestations of Gilbert's syndrome have not been well documented. A metallic bitter taste sensation has been reported by some patients [11]. This case report presents an unusual case of RAS, highlighting its concurrence with Gilbert's syndrome. The objective of this case report is to highlight a possible association of RAS and Gilbert's syndrome which would aid in early identification of this condition.

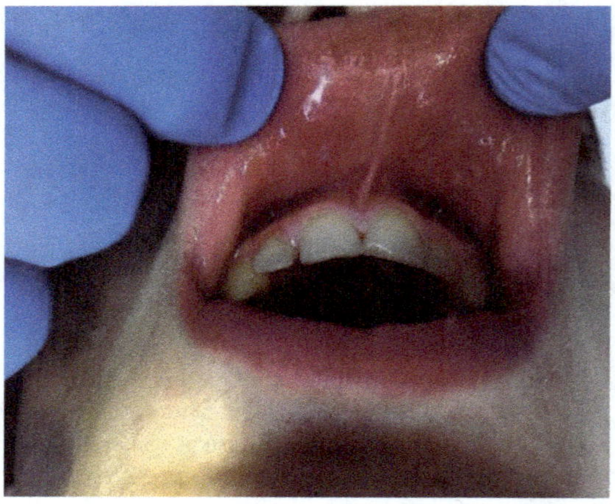

FIGURE 2: Aphthous ulcers on the mucous membrane of the lips.

2. Case Presentation

A 20-year-old male presented with general weakness, pain in the right hypochondrium, lip pain, difficulty of food intake, and speech. A thorough general physical, extraoral, and intraoral examination was performed. The patient was of normosthenic build. On external body examination, visible integuments/skin were yellowish. No enlarged lymph nodes were detected. Auscultation of the heart and lungs revealed, respectively, a regular heart rate with clear tones and bilateral vesicular breathing sound. Blood pressure measured 110/70 mm Hg, and pulse was 77 beats per minute. On palpation and percussion, the abdomen was painless and slightly inflated, the Pasternatsky sign was negative bilaterally, and urination was voluntary.

On extraoral examination, the upper and lower lips were swollen (Figure 1). Intraoral examination revealed several carious teeth and numerous painful aphthae in the mucous membrane of the lips (Figure 2).

Complete blood count revealed no deviations, and urine test showed leukocytes. Biochemical blood test values were within normal limits, apart from direct bilirubin level -10.6 μmol/L, 8.8 in dynamics, and indirect bilirubin counted 58.6 μmol/L, 40.1 in dynamics.

Abdominal ultrasound revealed that the spleen was 15.8 cm enlarged, the left kidney measured 11.2 cm, and the liver was enlarged and palpable under hypochondrium. There was moderate periportal infiltration and no portal hypertension. The gallbladder and pancreas showed no abnormal changes; all aforementioned organs were of homogenous structure.

Chest radiography did not reveal any abnormalities; echocardiography detected 0-1 mitral valve regurgitation. Antibodies to hepatitis and infections were negative. Specialists in hematology and infectious diseases were consulted and later examined for Gilbert's syndrome (GS) by molecular genetic testing. Homozygous UGT1A1*28 alleles were identified, confirming the diagnosis of Gilbert's syndrome.

Treatment was carried out in collaboration with different medical specialties. Initially, treatment started locally with oral prophylaxis and dental caries management. Aphthous ulcers were treated with DIPLEN-DENTA G and DIPLEN-DENTA X adhesive films. The first one or two applications

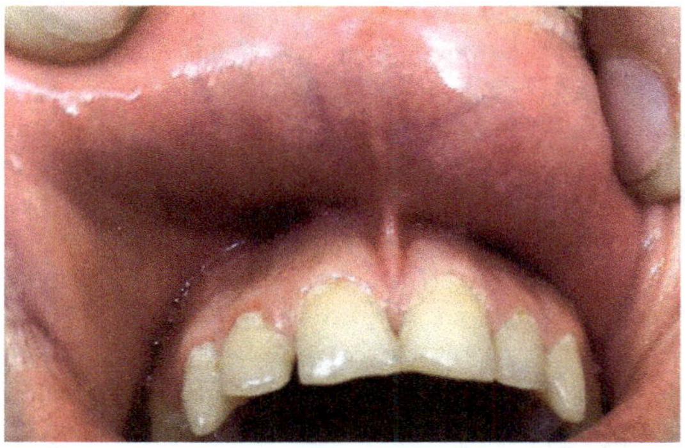

Figure 3: The mucous membrane of the lip with resolution of aphthous ulcers.

of adhesive films were performed in the clinic by the treating clinician, and later, it was applied by the patient at home. The patient was trained on how to use these films. The films were applied twice daily until the ulcers healed. In this reported case, aphthous ulcers in the mucous membrane cleared up within two weeks (Figure 3). The patient will be followed up by the general medical practitioner for monitoring any systemic conditions.

3. Discussion

Gilbert's syndrome, a benign hereditary hyperbilirubinemia, is caused by reduced UGT1A1 enzyme activity. Excretion of bilirubin is reduced following decreased glucuronidation, a prerequisite for bilirubin elimination. This results in an increase of indirect, or unconjugated, bilirubin (UCB). GS is inherited in an autosomal recessive manner, with a prevalence of 4-16% across varying populations [9]. Patients with GS are usually asymptomatic and require no treatment. Some patients may experience recurrent jaundice; about half of these may suffer from associated symptoms such as abdominal pain, fatigue, and bloating [12]. RAS has, to our knowledge, not been reported in association with GS in the literature.

Recurrent aphthous stomatitis is the most common encountered oral mucosal lesion [13]. Clinical characteristics include oval-shaped ulcers, with red hyperemic margins and a central fibrous coating, in nonkeratinized areas of oral mucosa, frequently affecting the vestibule, lips, and particularly areas subjected to trauma by teeth and solid food [1, 2]. Prodromal signs may include local intraoral burning sensation, fatigue, and mood swings. Relapses are sometimes accompanied by regional lymphadenitis and fever [3, 14]. Symptoms remain local but often change in frequency and severity with age and may include pain during speech and food intake. RAS may recur with certain regularity. Remissions can last for several days, months, or years [2, 3, 14].

The etiology of RAS is still not sufficiently clear [1]. However, several known factors contribute to RAS, including stress, viruses, bacteria, sensitivity to foods and drugs, gastrointestinal disease, vitamin deficiency, impaired immune system, autoimmune diseases, and trauma [1–3]. The commonly discussed etiological factors are genetic, nutritional, and immune-mediated. About 30%-40% of patients give a family history of RAS [2]. An increase in polymorphism of Toll-like receptor 4 has been observed in RAS patients, altering innate immunity and the cellular immune response [15].

Nutritional deficiencies of iron, folic acid, or vitamin B_{12} are implicated in up to 42% of cases [16]. Vitamin B_{12} deficiency has also been reported to cause unconjugated hyperbilirubinemia [17]. Histologically, RAS is characterized by a mucosal ulceration with inflammatory cell infiltrate dominated by T-cells [1]. This suggests that the immune system plays a vital part of RAS formation [2, 3]. RAS has also been found to be seen as oral manifestations of some systemic diseases like Behcet's disease, inflammatory bowel disease like Cohn's disease, and celiac disease [3]. There is no published literature currently which suggests an association between RAS and Gilbert's syndrome.

With regard to our case, the patient sought medical consultation for pain in the hypochondrium and oral cavity. The diagnosis of Gilbert's syndrome was based on the increased levels of direct and indirect bilirubin which was further confirmed by the identification of homozygous UGT1A1∗28 alleles in the individual. Gilbert's syndrome is a diagnosis of exclusion and is established by ruling out the other hepatic causes which result in hyperbilirubinemia [9]. The diagnosis of RAS was based on the clinical presentation of numerous small symmetrical ulcers surrounded by an erythematous halo and the presence of pain. It is possible that the aphthous stomatitis could be a manifestation of Gilbert's syndrome, but there is no evidence to prove this. As this is the first case report to document this concurrence, more such cases need to be documented before we can ascertain any association. Gilbert's syndrome is usually asymptomatic and is aggravated following a triggering factor such as stressful events such as surgery, rigorous exercise or sports activities, fasting, and alcohol intake [10]. There are reports of many cases of Gilbert's syndrome which has been reported during pregnancy [9] and as a postsurgical complication [18]. In our case, the symptoms would have been flared up due to stress considering his age and also the simultaneous occurrence of RAS which has also been associated with stress [3]. The patient experiencing difficulty in eating food could be a factor in further aggravation of Gilbert's syndrome. Hence, proper diet management should be considered while treating the patient. According to a study, the occurrence of jaundice during the aggravation of Gilbert's syndrome affects the quality of life of the individual, and therefore, the management of the patients should include avoidance of such episodes [12]. Knowledge of which medications that can be administered safely in patients with Gilbert's syndrome highlight's the importance of its early diagnosis [18].

Increased levels of Unconjugated Bilirubin (UCB) have been implicated in symptomatic improvements of rheumatoid arthritis, inflammatory bowel disease, and multiple sclerosis [19]. UCB levels are slightly elevated in patients with GS. Anti-inflammatory effects may occur at 2 and 12 mg/dL in adults, while proinflammatory effects, cytotoxicity, and oxidative stress may be evident at high concentrations of around 15–20 mg/dL. UCB is found to be toxic to a number of cell lines, in vitro, including platelets, fibroblasts, and leukocytes [20]. When UCB is unbound to albumin, it can easily enter plasma membranes [21]. This may explain the varying effects of UCB. The immune mediated effects implicated in RAS may therefore be modulated by UCB. Impaired lymphocyte proliferation can be observed at UCB levels as low as 6 mg/dL [19]. The proinflammatory process can additionally cause reduced neutrophil function in terms of impaired phagocytosis, production of oxidative species, and migration [22]. RAS is also associated with defective neutrophil function and reduced number of cells [23].

Research on UCB's impact on oral epithelium is scarce. However, bilirubin is known to accumulate in elastin and can be found in oral mucosa [24]. Considering this occurrence, it can be hypothesized that UCB may cause immune mediated changes inducing aphthous ulcers. The mouth is usually not an area investigated during diagnosis of GS, and RAS associated with GS may therefore go unnoticed. This calls for an interdisciplinary approach involving medical and dental practitioners for the effective diagnosis and management of a patient with Gilbert's syndrome. Addition of more such reports of the concurrent existence of GS and RAS will promote more future studies in this regard and lead to establishment of more diagnostic criteria for GS.

In our patient, DIPLEN-DENTA adhesive films were prescribed. The films consist of two layers. The self-adhesive lower layer, loaded with an active substance (gentamicin sulfate in DIPLEN-DENTA G, chlorhexidine digluconate in DIPLEN-DENTA X), was applied to the affected area. The top layer is a protective coating that protects aphthous ulcers from unfavorable external influence, allowing for less unpleasant oral intake. The films have strong wide spectrum antibacterial effects and are said to be effective [25].

4. Conclusion

In this case, we have attempted to present the existence of direct symptoms and clinical findings associated with Gilbert's syndrome and the presence of recurrent aphthous stomatitis in the patient. Since this a novel observation, it too early to directly establish an association between these two disease entities. However, at the same time, the simultaneous presentation of the two should not be taken as chance occurrences. Moving forward, it is recommended that all patients with Gilbert's syndrome should be thoroughly evaluated for any oral manifestations in order to effectively manage the patient. Early management of recurrent aphthous stomatitis may also be beneficial in reducing the trigger factors associated with Gilbert's disease.

References

[1] L. Preeti, K. T. Magesh, K. Rajkumar, and R. Karthik, "Recurrent aphthous stomatitis," *Journal of oral and maxillofacial pathology: JOMFP*, vol. 15, no. 3, pp. 252–256, 2011.

[2] S. I. M. L. Queiroz, M. V. A. D. Silva, A. M. C. Medeiros, P. T. Oliveira, B. C. V. Gurgel, and É. J. D. D. Silveira, "Recurrent aphthous ulceration: an epidemiological study of etiological factors, treatment and differential diagnosis," *Anais Brasileiros de Dermatologia*, vol. 93, no. 3, pp. 341–346, 2018.

[3] J. Sánchez, C. Conejero, and R. Conejero, "Aftosis oral recidivante," *Actas Dermo-Sifiliográficas (English Edition)*, vol. 111, no. 6, pp. 471–480, 2020.

[4] L. Cohen, "Etiology, pathogenesis and classification of aphthous stomatitis and Behcet's syndrome," *Journal of Oral Pathology*, vol. 7, no. 6, pp. 347–352, 1978.

[5] N. R. Edgar, D. Saleh, and R. A. Miller, "Recurrent aphthous stomatitis: a review," *The Journal of Clinical and Aesthetic Dermatology*, vol. 10, no. 3, pp. 26–36, 2017.

[6] B. Tarakji, G. Gazal, S. A. Al-Maweri, S. N. Azzeghaiby, and N. Alaizari, "Guideline for the diagnosis and treatment of recurrent aphthous stomatitis for dental practitioners," *Journal of International Oral Health*, vol. 7, no. 5, pp. 74–80, 2015.

[7] C. Rivera, "Essentials of recurrent aphthous stomatitis," *Biomedical Reports*, vol. 11, no. 2, pp. 47–50, 2019.

[8] S. R. Porter and J. C. Leao, "Review article: oral ulcers and its relevance to systemic disorders," *Alimentary Pharmacology & Therapeutics*, vol. 21, no. 4, pp. 295–306, 2005.

[9] S. Teoh, Y. L. Ng, N. Anuar, and R. Kamaludin, "A case of Gilbert's syndrome diagnosis during pregnancy," *Bangladesh Journal of Medical Science*, vol. 19, no. 2, pp. 333–335, 2020.

[10] D. Tzoneva, E. Aleksiev, K. Michova, and P. Stanimirov, "Perioperative management and anaesthetic considerations for adult patients with Gilbert's syndrome and oral cancer: review and case report," *Biotechnology & Biotechnological Equipment*, vol. 33, no. 1, pp. 1182–1186, 2019.

[11] A. R. Davidson, A. Rojas-Bueno, R. P. Thompson, and R. Williams, "Reduced caloric intake and nicontinic acid provocation tests in the diagnosis of Gilbert's syndrome," *British Medical Journal*, vol. 2, no. 5969, p. 480, 1975.

[12] S. Kamal, S. Abdelhakam, D. Ghoraba et al., "The frequency, clinical course, and health related quality of life in adults with Gilbert's syndrome: a longitudinal study," *BMC Gastroenterology*, vol. 19, no. 1, p. 22, 2019.

[13] J. A. Ship, E. M. Chavez, P. A. Doerr, B. S. Henson, and M. Sarmadi, "Recurrent aphthous stomatitis," *Quintessence International*, vol. 31, no. 2, pp. 95–112, 2000.

[14] S. O. Akintoye and M. S. Greenberg, "Recurrent aphthous stomatitis," *Dental Clinics of North America*, vol. 58, no. 2, pp. 281–297, 2014.

[15] J. Karasneh, M. Bani-Hani, A. Alkhateeb, A. Hassan, F. Alzoubi, and M. Thornhill, "TLR2, TLR4 and CD86 gene polymorphisms in recurrent aphthous stomatitis," *Journal of Oral Pathology & Medicine*, vol. 44, no. 10, pp. 857–863, 2015.

[16] L. Baccaglini, R. V. Lalla, A. J. Bruce et al., "Urban legends: recurrent aphthous stomatitis," *Oral Diseases*, vol. 17, no. 8, pp. 755–770, 2011.

[17] K. Naha, S. Dasari, G. Vivek, M. Hande, and V. Acharya, "Severe unconjugated hyperbilirubinaemia: one and one makes three?," *Case Reports*, vol. 2013, no. jun18 1, article bcr2013009962, 2013.

[18] D. S. Nag, N. Sinha, D. P. Samaddar, and P. R. Mahanty, "General anesthesia in a patient with Gilbert's syndrome," *Journal of Anaesthesiology Clinical Pharmacology*, vol. 27, no. 2, pp. 253–255, 2011.

[19] S. Jangi, L. Otterbein, and S. Robson, "The molecular basis for the immunomodulatory activities of unconjugated bilirubin," *The International Journal of Biochemistry & Cell Biology*, vol. 45, no. 12, pp. 2843–2851, 2013.

[20] V. Větvicka, P. Síma, I. Miler, and M. Bilej, "The immunosuppressive effects of bilirubin," *Folia Microbiologia (Praha)*, vol. 36, no. 2, pp. 112–119, 1991.

[21] S. D. Zucker, W. Goessling, and A. G. Hoppin, "Unconjugated bilirubin exhibits spontaneous diffusion through model lipid bilayers and native hepatocyte membranes∗," *The Journal of Biological Chemistry*, vol. 274, no. 16, pp. 10852–10862, 1999.

[22] E. Mortaz, S. D. Alipoor, I. M. Adcock, S. Mumby, and L. Koenderman, "Update on neutrophil function in severe inflammation," *Frontiers in Immunology*, vol. 9, p. 2171, 2018.

[23] A. Broides, B. Yerushalmi, R. Levy et al., "Imerslund-Grasbeck syndrome associated with recurrent aphthous stomatitis and defective neutrophil function," *Journal of Pediatric Hematology/Oncology*, vol. 28, no. 11, pp. 715–719, 2006.

[24] D. R. Schafer and S. H. Glass, "A guide to yellow oral mucosal entities: etiology and pathology," *Head and Neck Pathology*, vol. 13, no. 1, pp. 33–46, 2019.

[25] D. S. Abakarova, "Two-layer adhesive film Diplen-denta C–a new compound containing polymer base and active component Solcoseryl," *Stomatologiia (Mosk)*, vol. 86, no. 1, pp. 70-71, 2007.

15

Maxillary Sinus Natural Killer/T-Cell Extranodal Lymphoma Mimicking a Dentoalveolar Abscess

Erika Antonia dos Anjos Ramos,[1] Luciana Munhoz,[1] Basílio Almeida Milani,[2] Tomás Zecchini Barrese,[3] Stephanie Kenig Viveiros,[1] and Emiko Saito Arita[1]

[1]*Department of Stomatology, School of Dentistry, University of São Paulo, 2227 Lineu Prestes Avenue, 05508-000 São Paulo, SP, Brazil*
[2]*Department of Maxillofacial Surgery, Hospital Municipal do Campo Limpo, 1661 Estrada da Itapecerica, 05835-005 São Paulo, Brazil*
[3]*Department of Pathological Sciences, School of Medicine, Santa Casa de Sao Paulo School of Medical Sciences, 61 Dr. Cesário Motta Junior Street, 01221-020 São Paulo, SP, Brazil*

Correspondence should be addressed to Erika Antonia dos Anjos Ramos; erika.antonia.ramos@usp.br

Academic Editor: Ricardo Alves Mesquita

Extranodal natural killer/T-cell lymphoma (ENKL) is an aggressive and infrequent malignant neoplasm. Early sinonasal ENKL clinical symptomatology is often not specific which can mimic several clinical odontogenic processes such as dentoalveolar abscesses. A 41-year-old female was referred to our institution due to facial pain with skin rash, fever, and intraoral swelling in the left side of the maxillary region. Computed tomography (CT) revealed a soft tissue hypodense area in the left side with bone discontinuity in anterior and lateral maxillary sinuses. Initial laboratorial tests showed no alterations on hemogram, coagulation profile, and immune phenotype ($CD3^+/CD4^+$). However, the lesion progressed fastly showing an evident growth, so it was decided that an intraoral biopsy should be performed. The diagnosis was sinonasal ENKLs. This case is an example that the rare T-cell lymphoma can mimic an odontogenic lesion, thus puzzling the clinician. Fortunately, the rapid growth of the lesion prompted the correct diagnosis and early treatment.

1. Introduction

Extranodal natural killer/T-cell lymphoma (ENKL) is an infrequent malignant neoplasm [1] that arises primarily from the natural killer cell [2] and accounts for 15% of all non-Hodgkin lymphomas located in the nasal fossae and maxillary sinuses [3]. The sinonasal ENKL location is unusual [4]. Formerly, the lesion was not recognized as a neoplastic process, and it was named "malignant centrofacial granuloma," [4] "lethal midline granuloma," or angiocentric lymphoma, due to its necrotizing and invasive evolution features [2].

Sinonasal ENKL presents as a highly aggressive neoplasm [2], which is characterized by the progressive destruction of the midline facial and/or nasal structures [3, 5] and eventually also may affect the orbit by contiguity [3]. Early sinonasal ENKL clinical symptomatology is often not specific and may include headache, facial pain, nasal congestion, and fever [1]. Although most of the sinonasal ENKL patients exhibit locoregional disease, systemic involvement may be present [5].

Due to the anatomical proximity with oral cavity and paranasal sinuses, ENKL can affect intraoral elements, which can mimic several clinical odontogenic origin entities, including inflammatory and infectious diseases, such as dentoalveolar abscesses [6].

Accordingly, the objective of this report is to describe the main clinical, radiographic, and histologic characteristics of a

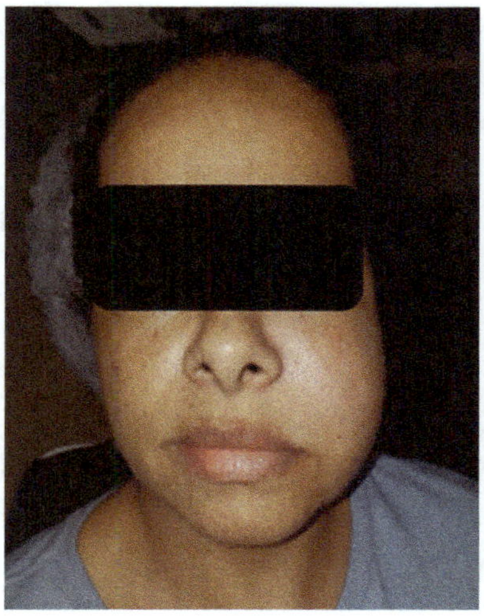

(a)

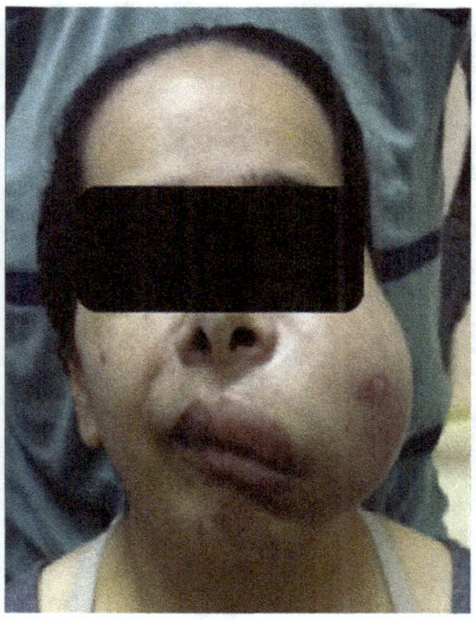

(b)

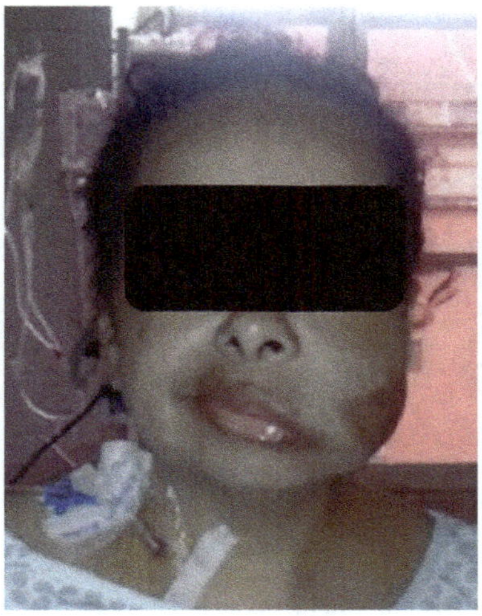

(c)

FIGURE 1: From left to right: (a) exhibits patient facial aspect at the first consultation, note the slight bulging in the left side of the face; (b) demonstrates the lesion fast progress by showing the evident lesion growth in 3 weeks; (c) shows lesion shrink after 4 weeks of chemotherapy.

sinonasal ENKL case in the maxillary sinuses, first diagnosed as an odontogenic abscess due to its early clinical features. Furthermore, the aggressive lesion development is also illustrated in tomographic examinations performed in different short time interval moments.

2. Case Report

A 41-year-old Caucasian woman noticed left cheek swelling and pain in corresponding upper premolars and molars and attended to a consultation in the Oral and Maxillofacial service at Hospital Municipal do Campo Limpo (São Paulo, Brazil). Her medical history revealed a previously ischemic cerebrovascular accident and continuous use of anticoagulants but no other past disease.

Extraoral examination showed no lymphadenopathy or paresthesia but an evident swelling in the left cheek (Figure 1(a)) with a hardened consistency. The patient mentioned she noticed the symptoms for a period of time higher than a week. Intraorally, she showed severe periodontal disease and pain during vertical/horizontal percussion tests. Pulp vitality could not be determined at this point, due to the severity of pain presented during teeth percussion tests. Buccoalveolar sulcus bulging and a floating tumefaction in the left upper molar root region were observed. Although the first diagnostic hypothesis was dental abscess, due to the unusual duration of the tumefaction, the patient was then referred to imaging examinations (multislice computed tomography—MCT). However, due to the presence of an intraoral floating tumefaction and dental origin symptomatology, drainage was performed, and antibiotic treatment was prescribed.

Despite of accomplishing imaging examinations as requested in the first consultation, the patient only came back to the Oral and Maxillofacial service after three weeks, when she felt paresthesia and severe pain in her left face. Figure 1(b) exhibits the patient left face swelling aspect at this moment. Due to the increase in painful symptomatology and evident speedy lesion development, the patient was immediately hospitalized, and a new CT examination was

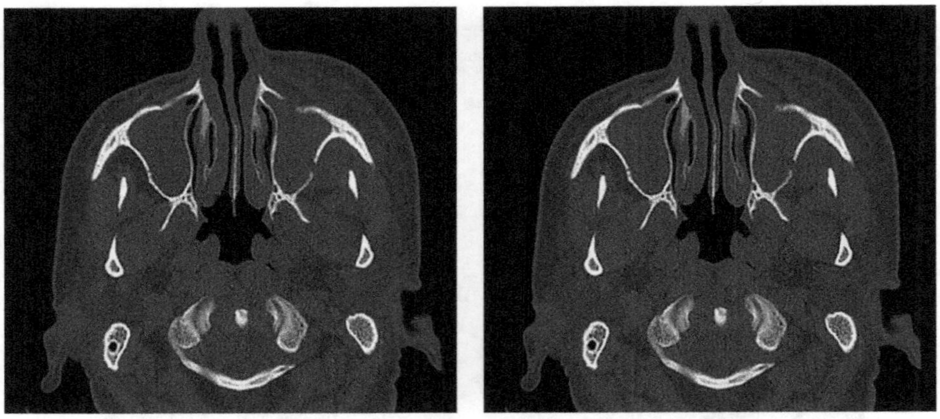

(a) (b)

FIGURE 2: First consultation examination. (a) The axial MCT scan shows a soft-tissue mass anterior to the maxillary sinus, left side, and sinus anterior and lateral wall bone erosion. (b) Coronal MCT scan exhibits nasal cavity involvement by soft-tissue mass, as well as sinus lateral wall bone destruction.

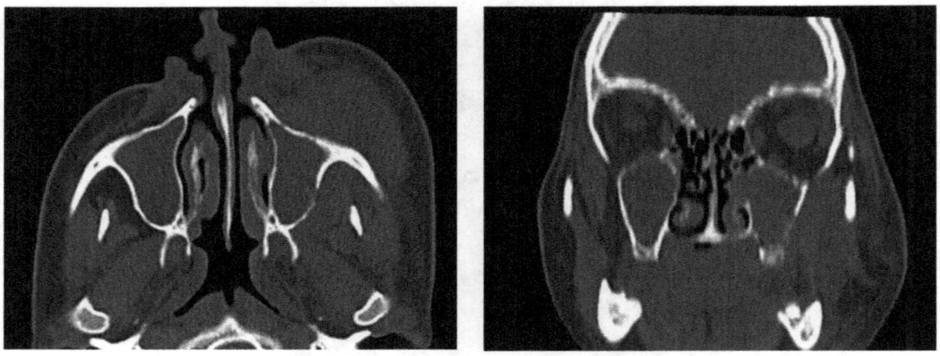

(a) (b)

FIGURE 3: MCT examination 3 weeks after the first consultation. (a) Axial MCT scan, note the prominent increasing of extensive soft tissue. In (b), the nasal cavity involvement is even more evident when compared to the first consultation imaging examination.

performed, as well as routine and biochemical blood test examinations. Intraoral floating was now absented.

No alterations were verified in the patient hemogram, coagulation tests, and immune phenotype ($CD3^{+}$/$CD4^{+}$) examinations, as well as blood tests for hormones, especially the parathyroid hormone.

2.1. Imaging Evaluations. Noncontrast-enhanced, high resolution MCT with 16 slices (Toshiba Activion, Medical Systems Corporation, Japan) was used for MCT imaging. Acquisition imaging parameters were 0.5 mm slice thickness, 1.0 mm *Spacing* Between Slices, 250 mm field of view, 120 kV peak, and 250 mA. The first consultation MCT axial slices revealed a soft tissue hypodense area in the left side, comprising the maxillary sinus area and bone discontinuity in the anterior and lateral maxillary sinus wall (Figure 2(a)) orbital cavity floor. Frontal slices showed discrete nasal cavity involvement (Figure 2(b)).

The second consultation MCT axial slices revealed that the soft tissue hypodense area in the left side increased in size, with greater nasal cavity involvement and bone destruction than Figure 2.

At this point, the main diagnostic hypothesis was osteosarcoma, sinonasal diffuse large B-cell lymphoma, parathyroid brown tumor, and extranodal malignant lymphoma, particularly maxillary ENKL. The hypothesis of dentoalveolar abscess was disregarded: floating tumefaction might be coincidentally previously present due to the periodontal disease severe status.

2.2. Histopathological Results/Histopathology. A biopsy was taken from the lesion (oral cavity) and sent to the hospital's pathology department. The histopathological examination with hematoxylin and eosin (H&E) showed a diffuse proliferation of small to medium-sized atypical lymphocytes with areas showing an angiocentric pattern effacing the normal architecture of the oral mucosa. Mild epithelium tropism and espongiosis were observed (Figures 4(a) and 4(b)). Focal areas of ulceration and necrosis were also seen. Trial immunohistochemical and in situ hybridization reactions were made (Figures 4(c)–4(i)). The findings were consistent with ENKL. As part of staging, a bone marrow biopsy was done, and no abnormalities were found.

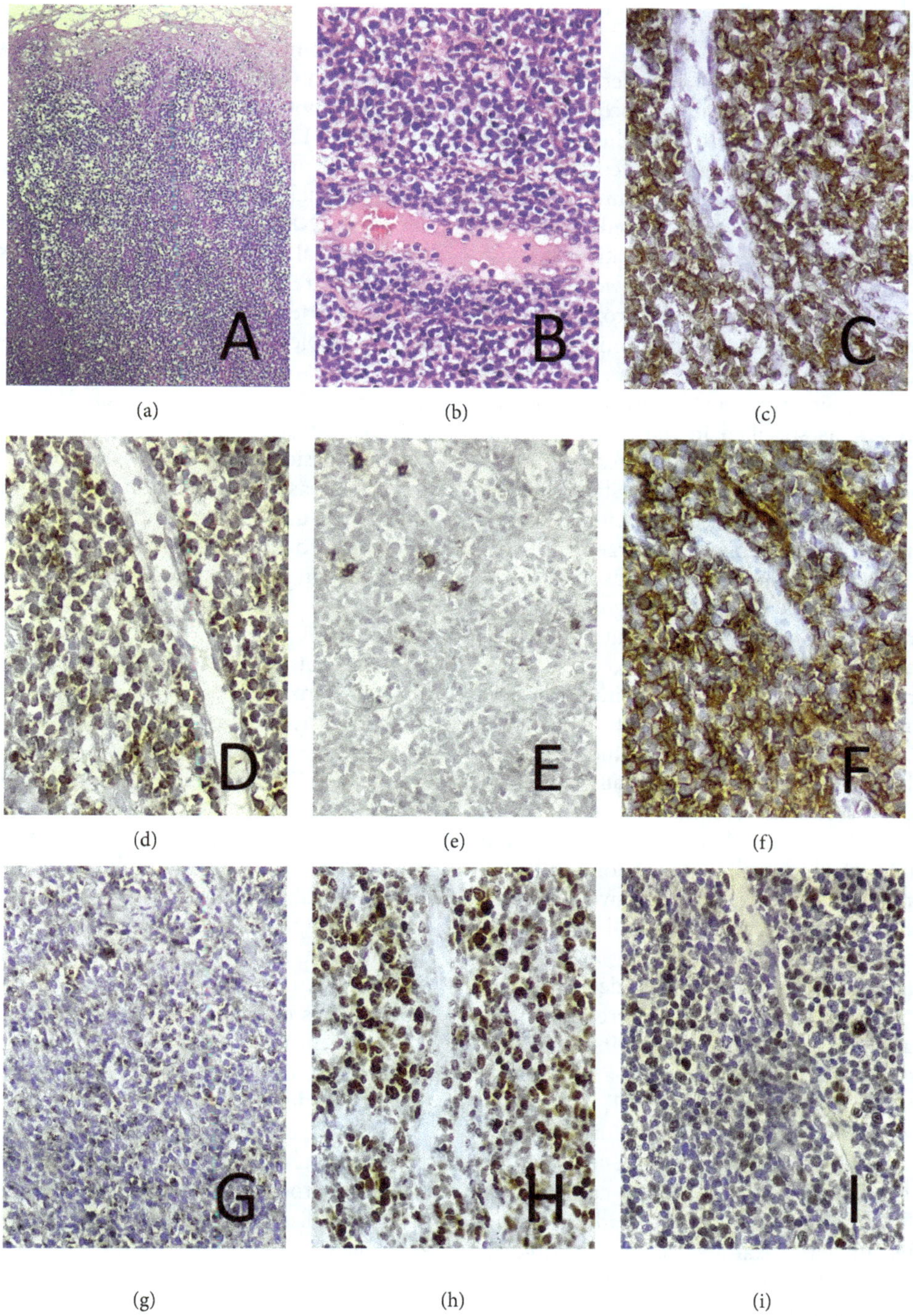

FIGURE 4: Histopathological features: in (a), the histologic section from the lesion biopsy sample shows a diffuse and permeative infiltrate of small to medium-sized atypical lymphocytes (H&E, ×100); in (b), an evident angiocentric and angiodestructive growth pattern is represented (H&E, ×400). Immunohistochemical and in situ hybridization reactions: in (c), the neoplastic cells show immunopositivity for CD45 (×400); in (d), immunopositivity (partial/weak) for CD3 (×400); in (e), immunonegativity for CD20 (×400); in (f), immunopositivity for CD56 (×400); in (g), immunopositivity (cytoplasmic granules) for TIA1 (×400); in (h), Ki67 index (×400); and in (i), positive nuclear labeling for in situ hybridization for EBV (×400).

2.3. Treatment. Before the diagnostic definition, the patient was treated with one cycle of CHOP (cyclophosphamide, doxorubicin, vincristine, and prednisolone). Once the diagnosis was established, the AspaMetDex (L-asparaginase, methotrexate, and dexamethasone) regimen was started, but no response was observed after two cycles of chemotherapy; on the contrary, the lesion became larger, and the acute inflammatory signs turned more evident. Facing this, the DICE (dexamethasone, isofosfamide, cisplatin, and etoposide) regimen and local radiotherapy (30 Gy) were started. After two cycles, the lesion presented a significant reduction, but her general condition deteriorated and was associated with mucositis and persistent neutropenia. Before even starting another cycle, five months after the diagnosis, the patient passed away.

3. Discussion

Although malignant lymphomas are also considered opportunistic neoplasms as they usually affect immunocompromised patients [7], in the present case, there were no history, blood laboratory results, or signs that suggested compromised immunity, as previously described in the literature [1].

Sinonasal ENKL is an aggressive and speedy evolution lesion [1]. Our case confirms this, demonstrating the fast disease progress clinically observed in three weeks and at MCT. Furthermore, due to the anatomical proximity with the oral cavity, sinonasal ENKL may compromise intraoral structures and, eventually, in the presence of a concomitant odontogenic disease, mimic infectious diseases [6], such as dentoalveolar abscesses, as specified in the case described. Lymphomas and infectious diseases may present similar MCT images, mainly during the early disease stage, such as the slight bone destruction [6]. Furthermore, clinical symptoms such as mobile teeth, gingival enlargement, oral masses, and swelling next to the oral cavity as chief complaints may lead clinicians to misdiagnose lymphomas as dentoalveolar abscesses [8] in an initial consultation which may delay the final diagnosis.

Imaging features in MCT often shows infiltrative or permeative bony discontinuity, with different destruction degrees [9]; in our case, evident destruction of sinonasal walls was also observed. The presence of the partially preserved sinus wall for the most extensive tumor involvement, as noticed in Figure 3, is also a usual characteristic of sinonasal lymphomas [9], although sinus wall bone erosion can be the result of other aggressive neoplasm [10]. Extensive soft-tissue mass can be observed in sinonasal ENKLs [10] particularly with lesion progression.

The differential diagnosis should include malignant maxillary tumors, such as sinonanasal undifferentiated and nasopharyngeal carcinoma [1], or other midline ulcerative destructive lesions [3], squamous cell carcinoma [9, 10], oral manifestations of Wegner's granulomatosis [1, 4, 10], primary orbit tumors [3], malignant melanoma, adenoid cystic carcinoma [10], and sinonasal diffuse large B-cell lymphomas, which have similar characteristics when compared to sinonasal ENKLs [2]. In the present case, the leading diagnosis hypothesis after imaging examination evaluation was sinonasal ENKL mainly due to the bony wall destruction noticed and concomitant right and left maxillary sinus opacification, resembling to another case previously described, in which sinonasal ENKL has also mimicked an odontogenic origin infection, delaying the final diagnosis [6].

Outcomes for sinonasal malignancies, enclosing ENKL, have improved recently [2]; nonetheless, prognosis is still relatively poor [2, 4], particularly to patients who have systemic disease [5, 6], and even worse in the case of recurrence [5]. Early precise disease diagnosis for any maxillofacial malignant lymphoma is crucial to achieve better treatment results [1, 11, 12].

Overall, paranasal sinus malignant lymphomas usually present nonspecific early clinical symptomatology [2, 12]. The dental professional can play a valuable role in the diagnosis of patients with sinonasal malignancies which warrants immediate referral to an appropriate specialist when the combination of patient clinical signs arouses suspicion, mainly due to the fact that the mucosa of paranasal sinuses is not accessible as the oral mucosa for further inspection [12].

Notwithstanding, considering the aforementioned nonspecific signals and symptoms, the final diagnosis of the sinonasal ENKLs is achieved by histological and immunohistochemical evaluations [1, 6]. The histological features of ENKLs are usually the same no matter the site affected. The lesions tend to have a diffuse and permeative infiltration of atypical lymphocytes that can be small, medium-sized, large, or anaplastic. The neoplastic cells can be accompanied by a mixture of inflammatory cells. An angiocentric and angiodestructive growth pattern is often present. Besides, this entity frequently shows extensive necrotic areas and ulceration, and multiple biopsies may be required until representative material is acquired. Fortunately, and due to the dimensions of the tumor described here, one single biopsy was enough to the diagnosis. Typically, the immunophenotype of ENKT is CD45 positive, surface CD3 negative, CD2 positive, CD5 negative, and, although not specific, CD56 positive. Cytotoxic molecules such as granzyme B, TIA1, and perforin are positive. The diagnosis virtually requires the presence of EBV, and the most reliable way to demonstrate it is the *in situ* hybridization for EBER, since immunostaining for LMP1 is frequently negative [13].

Treatment for ENKL is mainly dependent on the disease stage at the diagnosis and, although controversial [13], the histologic subtype [2] and is not as yet well codified [4]. Radiotherapy and chemotherapy may be applied [4], but it has often unsatisfactory results [5, 6]. Unfortunately, in our case, the patient have not had a satisfactory response by the moment this manuscript was written.

In conclusion, sinonasal ENKL is an infrequent aggressive disease that can resemble to odontogenic origin diseases, which can delay the diagnosis. Imaging examinations are essential to guide diagnostic hypotheses; however, histological and immunohistochemical examinations are essential in the diagnosis process. The speedy neoplasm progress of this malignant disease was illustrated in this report by the CT examinations performed in distinct moments, with short time interval.

References

[1] N. Nikolaos, P. Grigorios, K. Konstantinos et al., "Extranodal nasal-type NK/T-cell lymphoma of the palate and paranasal sinuses," *American Journal of Case Reports*, vol. 13, pp. 79–85, 2012.

[2] P. M. Dubal, R. Dutta, A. Vazquez, T. D. Patel, S. Baredes, and J. A. Eloy, "A comparative population-based analysis of sinonasal diffuse large B-cell and extranodal NK/T-cell lymphomas," *Laryngoscope*, vol. 125, no. 5, pp. 1077–1083, 2015.

[3] A. Hervás-Ontiveros, E. España-Gregori, P. Hernández-Martínez, F. J. Vera-Sempere, and M. Díaz-Llopis, "Orbital involvement by non-Hodgkin lymphoma NK T cells," *Archivos de la Sociedad Española de Oftalmología*, vol. 89, no. 11, pp. 450–453, 2014.

[4] M. Hmidi, M. Kettani, A. Elboukhari, N. Touiheme, and A. Messary, "Sinonasal NK/T-cell lymphoma," *European Annals of Otorhinolaryngology, Head and Neck Diseases*, vol. 130, no. 3, pp. 145–147, 2013.

[5] C. C. Li, H. F. Tien, J. L. Tang et al., "Treatment outcome and pattern of failure in 77 patients with sinonasal natural killer/T-cell or T-cell lymphoma," *Cancer*, vol. 100, no. 2, pp. 366–375, 2004.

[6] T. Yamada, K. Mishima, A. Ota et al., "A case of ATLL (adult T-cell leukemia/lymphoma) mimicking odontogenic infection," *Oral Surgery, Oral Medicine, Oral Pathology, Oral Radiology, and Endodontology*, vol. 109, no. 6, pp. e51–e55, 2010.

[7] E. Zapater, J. V. Bagán, F. Carbonell, and J. Basterra, "Malignant lymphoma of the head and neck," *Oral Diseases*, vol. 16, no. 2, pp. 119–128, 2010.

[8] L. Ardekian, A. Rachmiel, D. Rosen, I. Abu-El-Naaj, M. Peled, and D. Laufer, "Burkitt's lymphoma of the oral cavity in Israel," *Journal of Cranio-Maxillofacial Surgery*, vol. 27, no. 5, pp. 294–297, 1999.

[9] H. Kato, M. Kanematsu, H. Watanabe, S. Kawaguchi, K. Mizuta, and M. Aoki, "Differentiation of extranodal non-Hodgkins lymphoma from squamous cell carcinoma of the maxillary sinus: a multimodality imaging approach," *SpringerPlus*, vol. 4, no. 1, p. 228, 2015.

[10] G. C. Ooi, C. S. Chim, R. Liang, K. W. T. Tsang, and Y. L. Kwong, "Nasal T-cell/natural killer cell lymphoma: CT and MR imaging features of a new clinicopathologic entity," *AJR American Journal of Roentgenology*, vol. 174, no. 4, pp. 1141–1145, 2000.

[11] L. Munhoz, F. P. M. Marsan, and E. S. Arita, "Radiographic enlargement of mandibular canal as an extranodal primary non-Hodgkin's lymphoma early sign in an asymptomatic patient," *Case Reports in Dentistry*, vol. 2017, Article ID 9193165, 4 pages, 2017.

[12] G. W. Bell, B. B. Joshi, and R. I. Macleod, "Maxillary sinus disease: diagnosis and treatment," *British Dental Journal*, vol. 210, no. 3, pp. 113–118, 2011.

[13] S. H. Swerdlow, E. Campo, N. L. Harris et al., *World Health Organization Classification of Tumors of Haematopoietic and Lymphoid Tissues*, IARC Press, Lyon, 5th edition, 2017.

16

Chairside Restorations of Maxillary Anterior Teeth with CAD/CAM Porcelain Laminate Veneers Produced by Digital Workflow: A Case Report with a Step to Facilitate Restoration Design

Elif Öztürk Bayazıt[1] **and Murat Karabıyık**[2]

[1]*Hacettepe University, Faculty of Dentistry, Department of Restorative Dentistry, 06100 Sıhhiye, Ankara, Turkey*
[2]*32 Diş Dünyası Ağız ve Diş Sağlığı Polikliniği, 34940 Tuzla, İstanbul, Turkey*

Correspondence should be addressed to Elif Öztürk Bayazıt; dtelifoz@gmail.com

Academic Editor: Mine Dündar

Since the introduction of porcelain laminate veneers in the early 1980s, the anterior esthetic rehabilitation with PLVs has been provided with a conventional restorative technique for many years. Recently, a new concept named digital workflow has been raised that will lead to the abandonment of conventional procedures during the fabrication of PLVs. Digital workflow is a new concept facilitating applications by adapting digital systems to clinical applications, including intra- and extraoral photographs, diagnostic wax-up, mock-up, intraoral camera, and use of the CAD/CAM device. The aim of this case report is to describe the clinical procedures of porcelain laminate veneers using digital workflow with a facilitating step in a single session and to evaluate the PLVs after one year of clinical service.

1. Introduction

During the last few decades, the demand for the computer-aided design and manufacturing systems in dentistry has dramatically increased because of the rapid developments in computer technology and science [1]. The idea of CAD/-CAM was emerged with the aim of creating excellent restorations with the least possible error by the computer, as opposed to the conventional manufacturing techniques by free hand, which is prone to numerous subjective failures [2]. CAD/CAM systems can be categorized as either chairside or laboratory systems [3]. Chairside CAD/CAM systems allow the clinicians in private offices to independently design and also machine dental ceramic restorations within a few hours during a single visit [1, 4]. Inlay, onlay, porcelain laminate veneer, crown, and bridge can be produced with today's CAD/CAM systems.

The clinical technique for porcelain laminate veneers includes bonding very thin restorations to tooth adhesively in order to correct an unesthetic appearance of the anterior teeth [5]. The main reason why PLVs are so demanded restorations is that they are very minimally invasive restorations and very good esthetic results can be achieved with them [6]. With the improvements in CAD/CAM systems, such thin restorations with a thickness of 0.3 - 0.7 mm could be created almost perfectly with the help of computer design [7, 8]. Excellent esthetic results can be provided by these restorations especially with the use of digital workflow in recent years [9].

Several medium-to-long-term clinical studies have evaluated the clinical performance of PLVs produced by conventional techniques. The success of conventional PLVs in these clinical trials ranges from 100% to 67% [6, 10]. However, to the authors' knowledge, only limited clinical data about the porcelain laminate veneers (PLVs) produced by CEREC CAD/CAM chairside systems have been reported and no long-term clinical results have existed. Therefore, the aim of this case report is to explain the clinical procedures

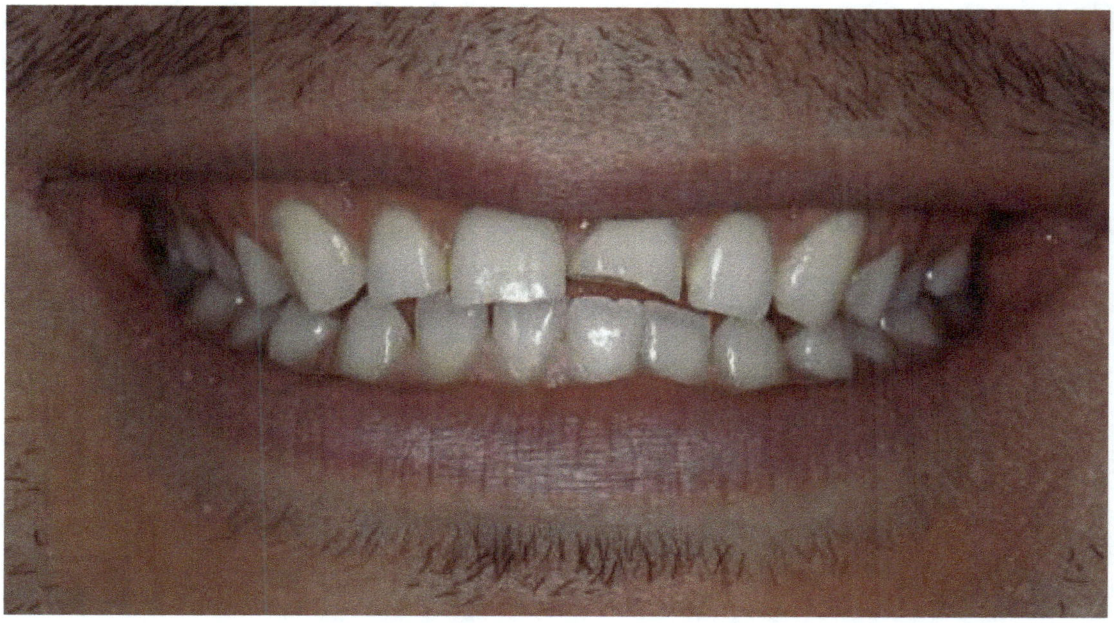

Figure 1: Initial smile of the patient.

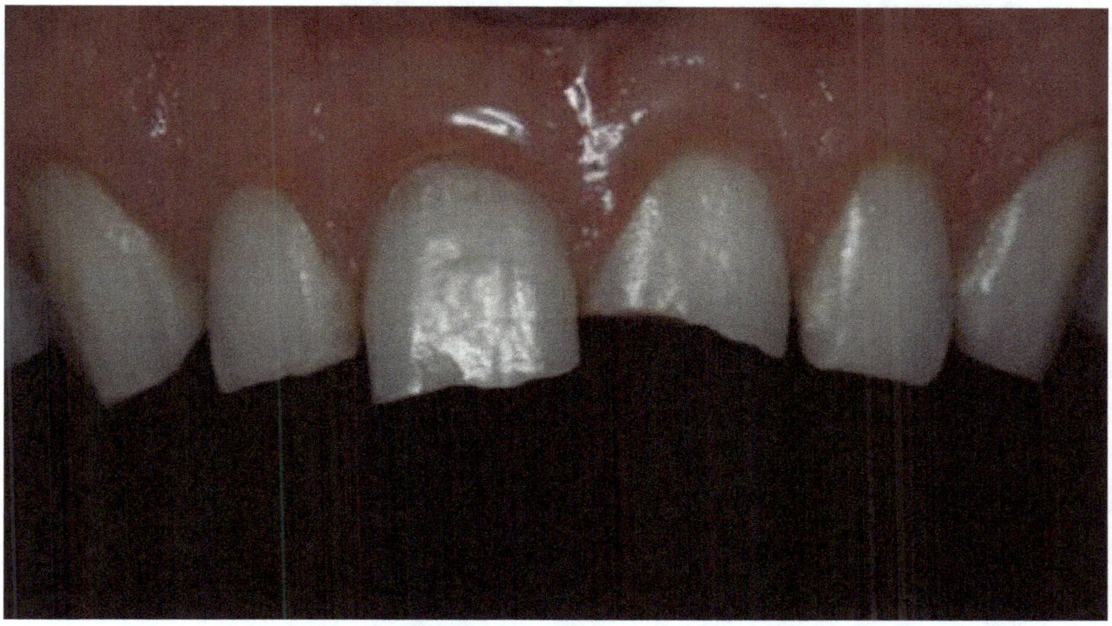

Figure 2: Intraoral view of the fractured anterior teeth.

for fabricating PLVs with CAD/CAM in a single session using digital workflow with a facilitating step and to report a year of clinical results.

2. Case Report

A healthy 19-year-old male patient attended to our clinic with a chief complaint of maxillary anterior teeth because of the fractures (Figures 1 and 2). All the documents related to the patient including dental anamnesis, intra- and extra-oral photographs, and bite registration with impressions from the maxilla and mandible were collected at the first visit. In the dental anamnesis obtained from the patient, it was found that his upper anterior teeth were broken as a result of the fall in childhood. The patient has used his teeth until this age, and he has not had any complaints from his teeth except for the aesthetic appearance. In the intraoral examination, fractured maxillary 12-11-21-22 teeth were found vital and noncarious. In addition, the patient's oral hygiene was good, and the periodontal tissues were healthy. Immediately after the examination in the first visit, the impressions of the maxilla and mandible were taken using alginate. In addition, bite registration was prepared with heated dental wax.

Cast models were provided from the impressions and a wax-up model was prepared by free-hand technique. The wax-up model was duplicated, and vacuum sheet

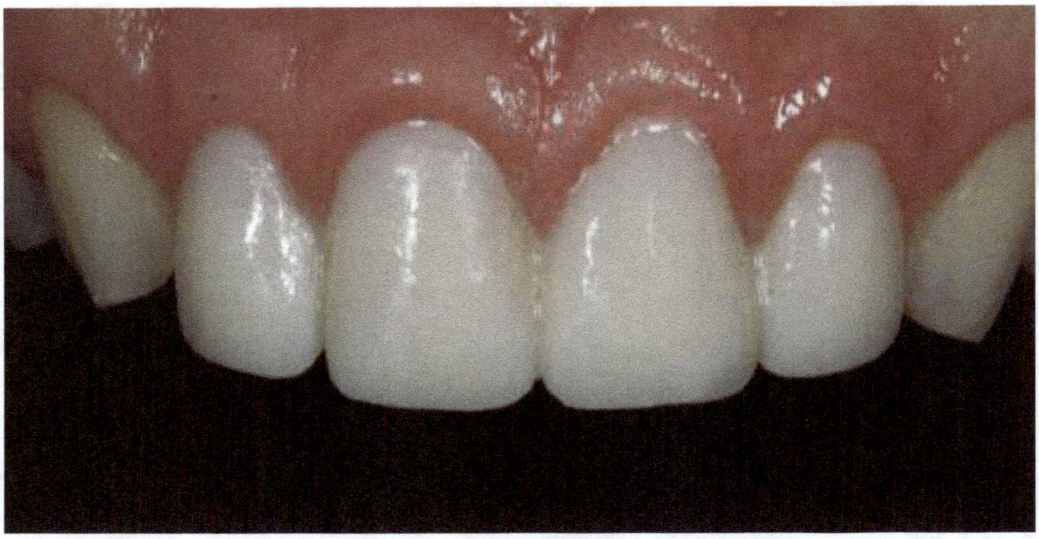

Figure 3: Mock-up made in the mouth through the wax-up prepared in laboratory by free-hand technique.

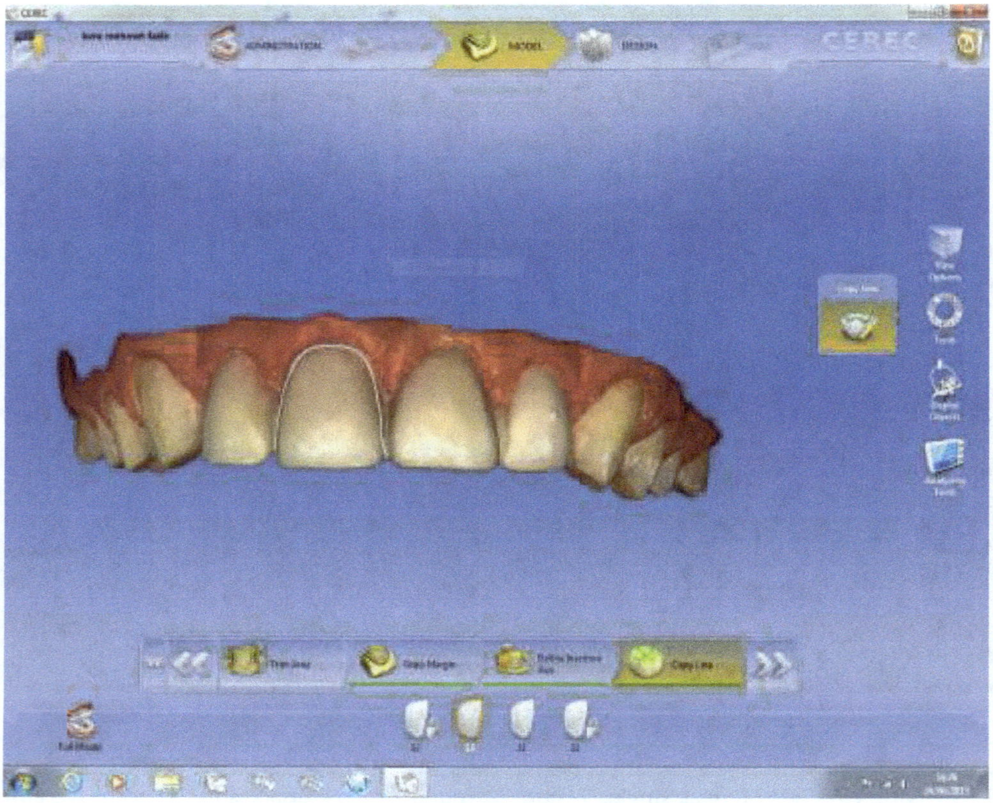

Figure 4: Digital impression via mock-up.

was prepared on the stone cast model for mock-up. At the second appointment, the final volume of the provisional restorations was made with temporary flowable composite resin (Systemp.link, Ivoclar Vivadent) using transparent, rigid, and vacuum-shaped sheets (VacuFormer System, Cavex, Haarlem, Netherlands). The patient was able to preview the estimated finished restoration from the provisional restorations. After patient approval of the mock-up (Figure 3), the first digital impression (Figure 4) was taken on the mock-up from the maxilla with CEREC Omnicam (CAD/CAM, Sirona Dental, Istanbul, Turkey) using the biocopy design mode on the CAD/CAM software. In addition, the patient's photo and digital impression were uploaded to the system, and digital smile design was done on the computer (Figures 5 and 6). The smile design was shown to the patient, and reapproval was obtained (Figure 6). Afterward, preparations were performed over the provisional composite restorations using an operation microscope with

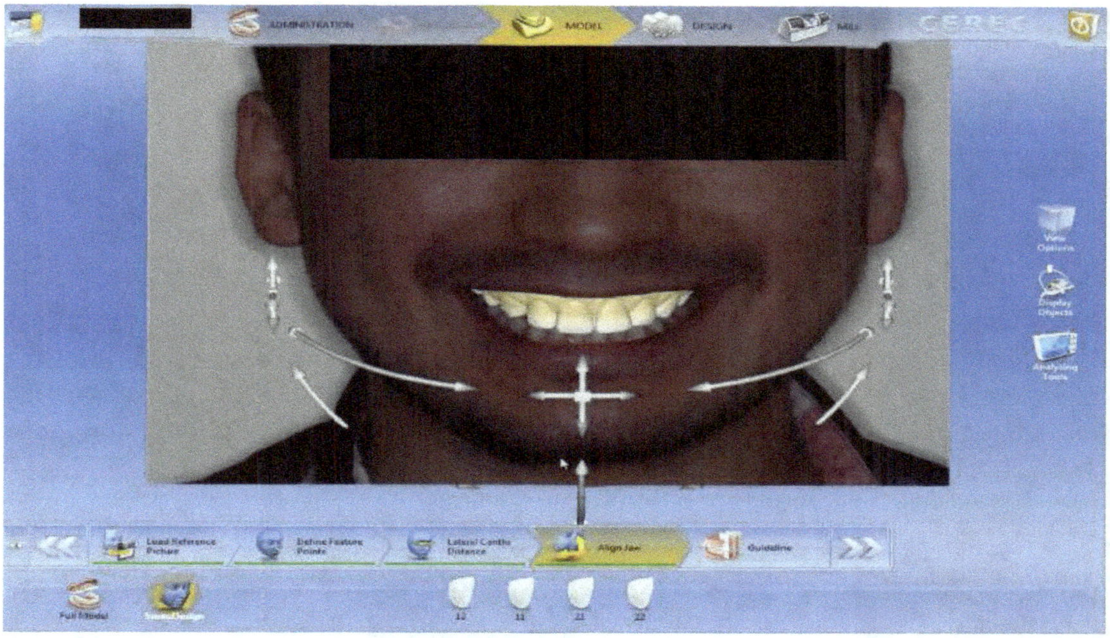

FIGURE 5: Adaptation of the digital impression with smile design on the patient's photo converted from 2D to 3D by the program.

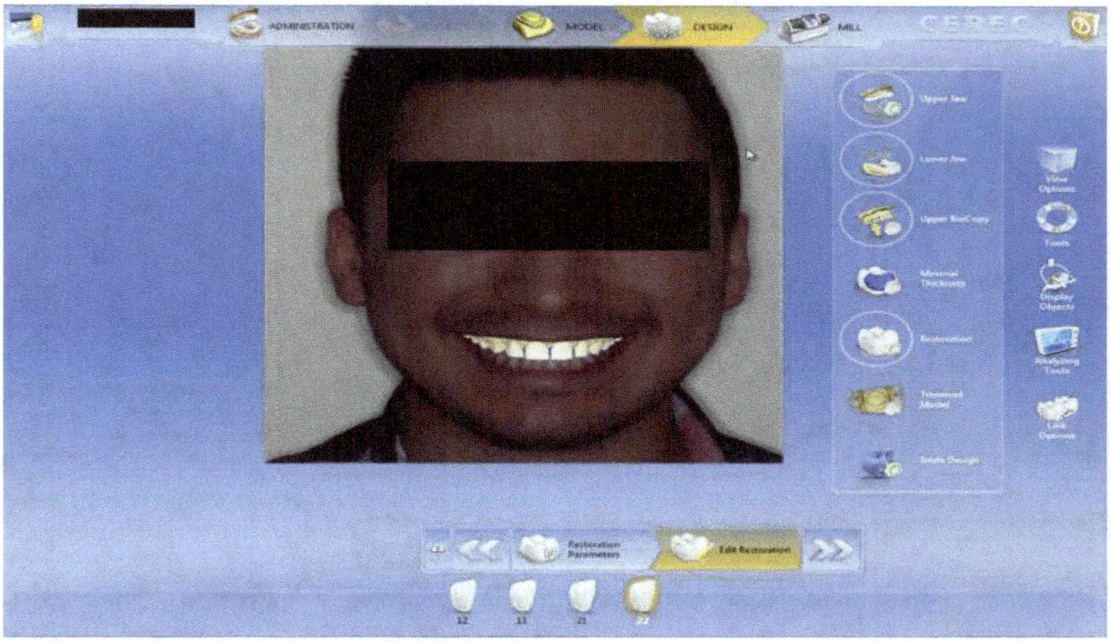

FIGURE 6: The final appearance of the smile design with the corrected version of the restorations on the digital impression taken with mock-up.

a magnification of 40x (Carl Zeiss; Oberkochen, Germany) (Figure 7(a)). Facial surfaces of the teeth were prepared by making depth-orientation grooves (0.3 mm in depth) with a depth preparation diamond bur (Diatech, Coltène Whaledent, Altstätten, Switzerland). The facial reduction was continued with a tapered rounded-end diamond bur (Diatech) until a flat surface was provided under the microscope (Figure 7(b)). All sharp edges and corners were smoothened with an extra-coarse aluminum-oxide polishing disk (Opti-Disc, Kerr, Orange, CA, USA) to reduce stress concentrations. Minimal invasive preparations with incisal bevel were provided within the enamel for each tooth. When the teeth were prepared the final shape, the teeth were almost uncut (Figure 8).

After finishing the preparations of the teeth, the second digital impression of the maxilla, as well as the first digital impression of the mandible and occlusal bite registration, were taken with the CEREC Omnicam. The mock-up model was copied to the computer, errors on the copy were corrected manually on the computer, and designs of the restorations were completed (Figure 9). The mesiodistal and insicogingival dimensions of the restorations were measured

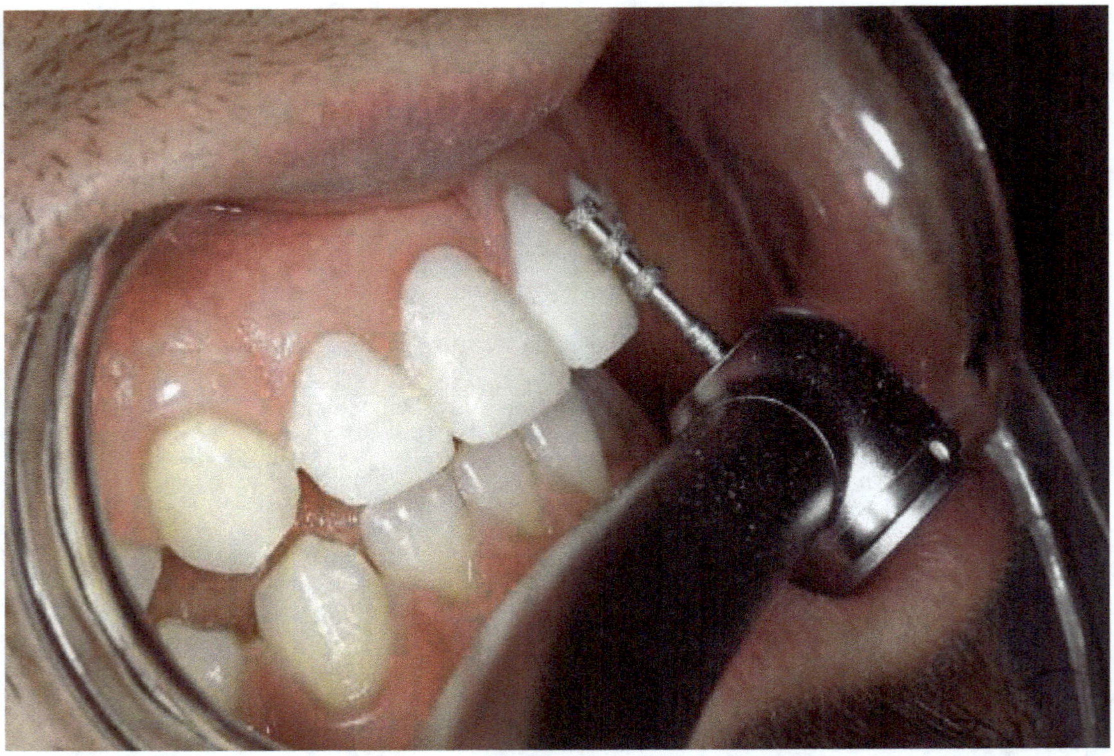

(a)

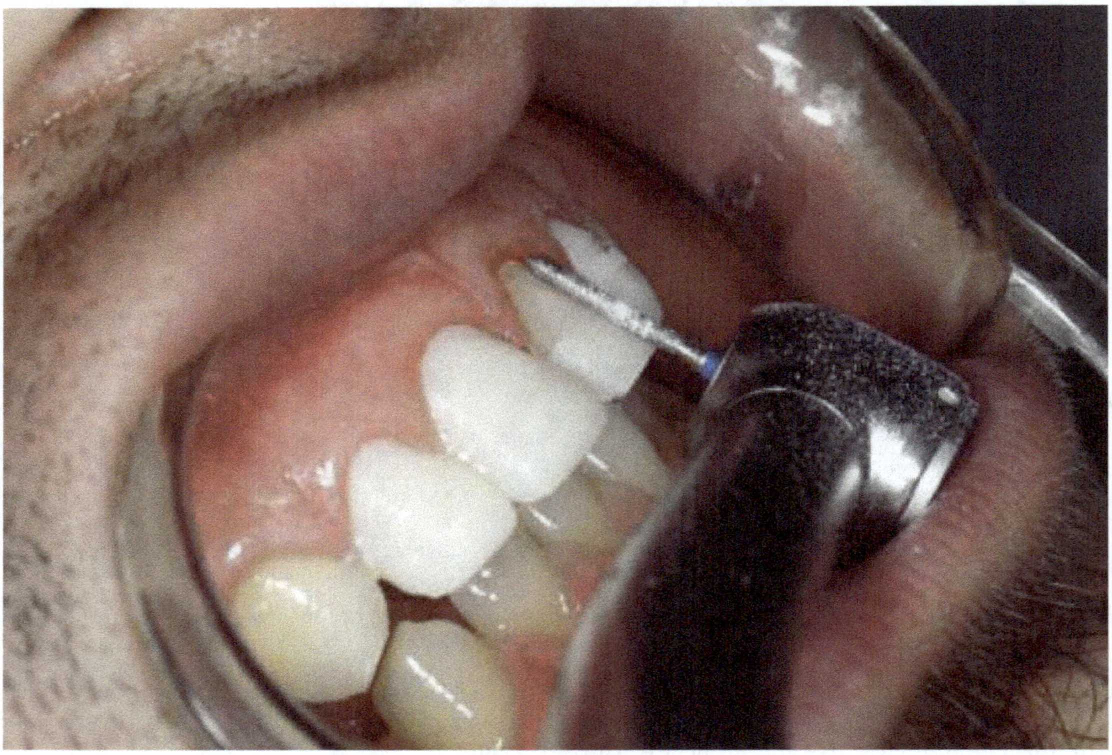

(b)

Figure 7: (a, b) Preparation steps on the mock-up after the first digital impression.

on the computer and were corrected. Symmetry between the teeth was achieved. After completing the restoration design, restorations were milled by CEREC Blocs (Sirona Dental). After the intraoral controls, the restorations were glazed (Figure 10).

A light-curing adhesive resin cement (Variolink Veneer, Ivoclar Vivadent, Schaan, Liechtenstein) was used for the adhesive cementation of the PLVs according to the manufacturers' instructions. The adhesion surfaces of all the veneers were etched with hydrofluoric acid (Vita Ceramics Etch,

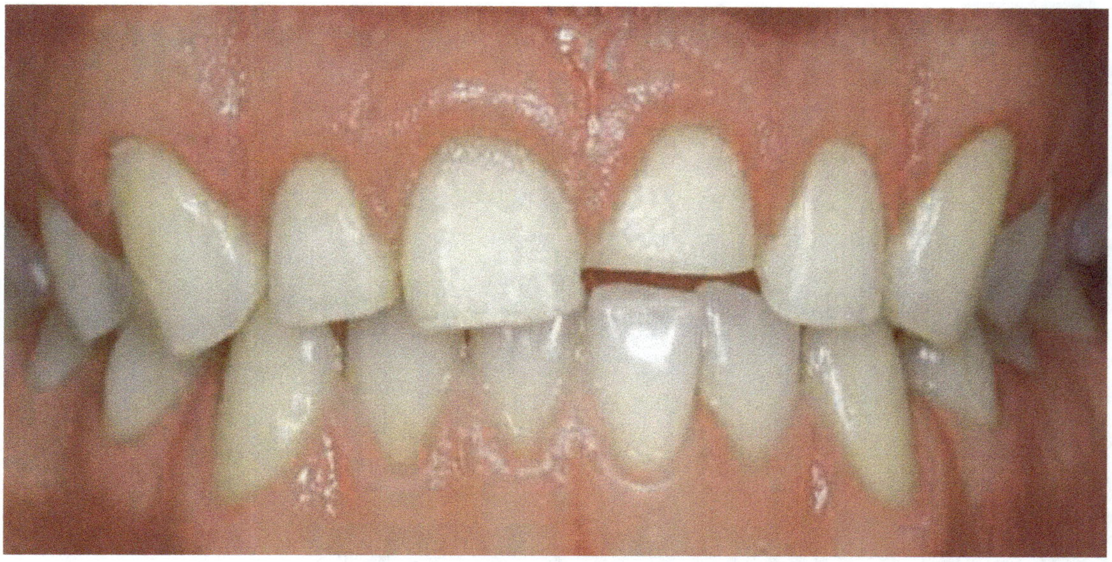

FIGURE 8: Final view of the almost uncut preparation.

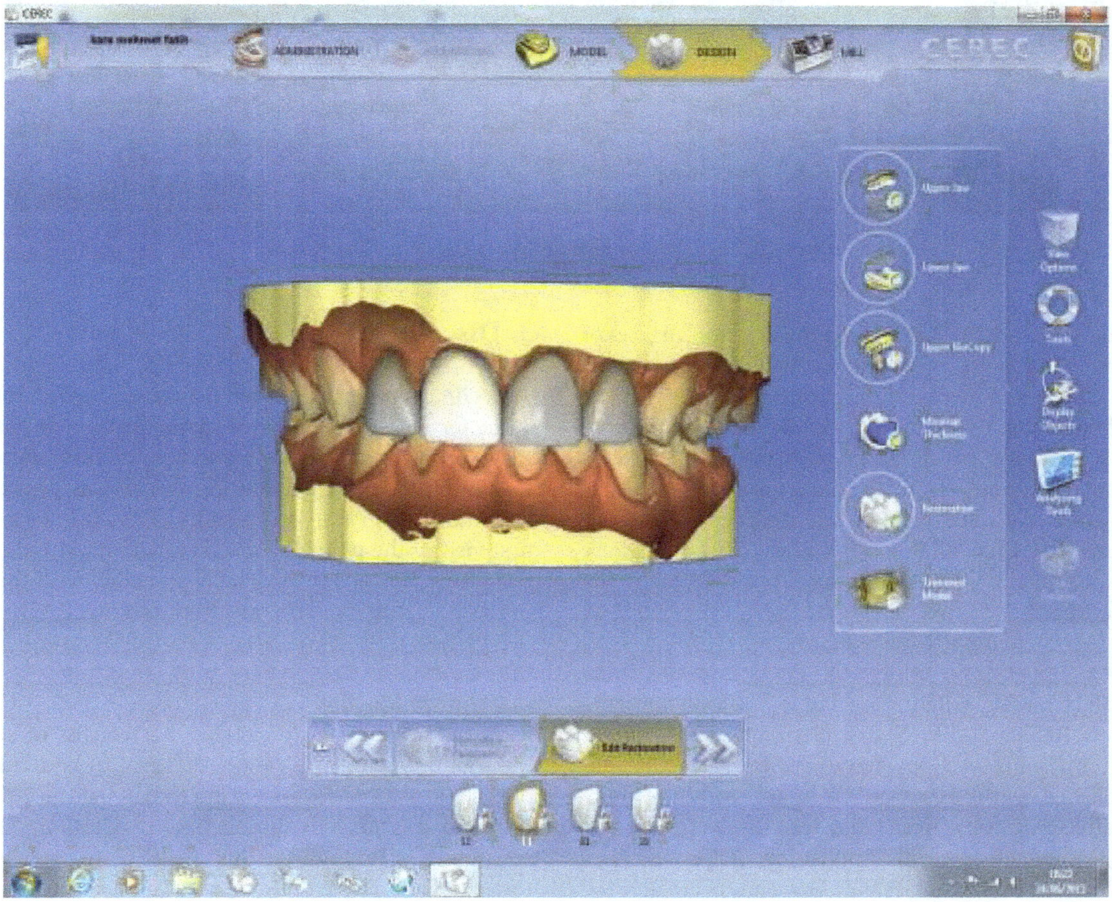

FIGURE 9: Final view of the restoration design with the corrected restorations on digital impressions completed after the preparation.

VITA Zahnfabrik, Bad Säckingen, Germany) for 60 s and subsequently rinsed with water and dried. Monobond S (Ivoclar Vivadent) was applied as a silane for 60 s to the inner surfaces of the veneers. Phosphoric acid (37% Total Etch, Ivoclar Vivadent) was applied to the prepared tooth surfaces including enamel for 30 s and dentine (incisal edge of the left upper central tooth) for 15 s. Adhesive bonding agent (Heliobond, Ivoclar Vivadent) was applied to both the adhesion surfaces of the teeth and the PLVs for 10 s. Resin cement in the selected translucent value (Medium Value 0, Variolink

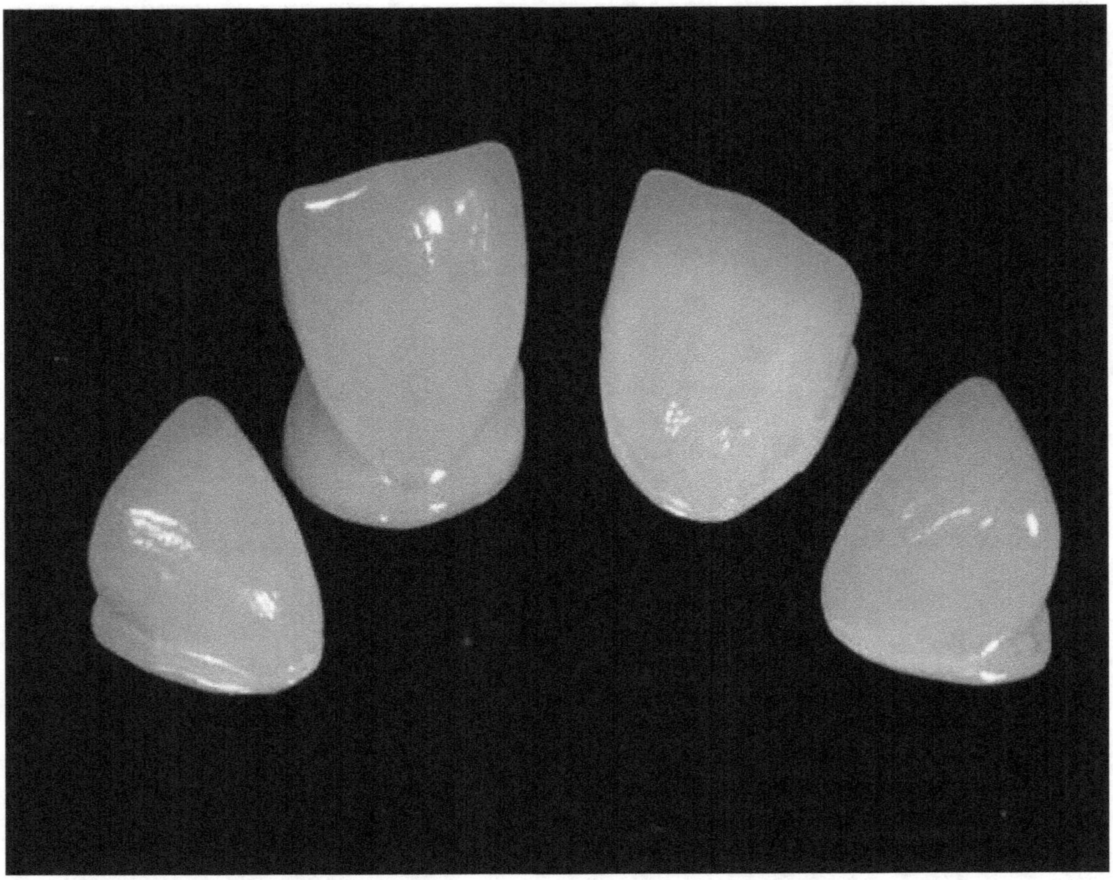

Figure 10: Final view of restorations milled with CAD/CAM.

Veneer, Ivoclar Vivadent) was applied to the inner surfaces of the veneers. After these procedures, the PLV restorations were positioned, and excess luting cement was removed with hand instruments and a brush. Before final curing, PLVs were cervically precured for 5 s to remove excess resin cement completely from the cervical and interproximal areas using hand instruments and dental floss without any pressure. For each of the PLVs, these processes were separately made and the PLVs were cemented one by one before the final cure. Final curing was performed according to the manufacturer's instructions for 40 s on each surface (upper- and midbuccal, cervical, mesial, distal, and palatal) with a light-emitting diode polymerizing unit (Elipar S10, 3M ESPE; Neuss, Germany; light output: 1200 mW/cm^2). Restoration margins were finished and further polished with extrafine diamond finishing burs (Diatech), polishing cups (Kerr HiLuster Plus, Kerr, Orange, CA, USA), and interproximal polishing strips (Sof-Lex Finishing Strips, 3M ESPE, Seefeld, Germany). Finally, the occlusion was checked in protrusive and lateral movements of the mandible.

PLV restorations produced in a single session with CAD/CAM provided the patient's aesthetic rehabilitation and satisfaction quickly (Figures 11 and 12). The patient was recalled after one year, and the restorations were evaluated. PLV restorations were observed to be very good after one year (Figure 13).

3. Discussion

This clinical report described how to achieve an esthetic outcome for anterior teeth as minimal invasive as possible with PLVs produced by digital workflow. In addition, to facilitate the computer design, a wax-up model was prepared in the laboratory from the impressions taken immediately in the first visit of the patient. Esthetic rehabilitation of the 4 maxillary anterior teeth was quickly provided with the chairside porcelain laminate veneers produced by CAD/CAM, and the patient satisfaction was provided. Even after one year, the restorations were in very good condition.

The production of a restoration with CAD/CAM includes step by step processes that consist of selection of the tooth, type of restoration, material to be used, selection of the restoration design, taking the digital impressions with intraoral camera, designing the restoration, and finally sending the data to the milling machine to print out the restoration [11]. Three options are available in the software for designing of the restoration: bioreference, biocopy, or biogeneric [12]. In the bioreference project, the design of the restoration incorporates the anatomical features of the corresponding contralateral tooth, if it is present. The biocopy project reproduces the anatomy of the tooth before the preparation, the temporary restoration or a prepared mock-up on the patient, in order to keep as well as to achieve the esthetics and function. In the biogeneric project, the

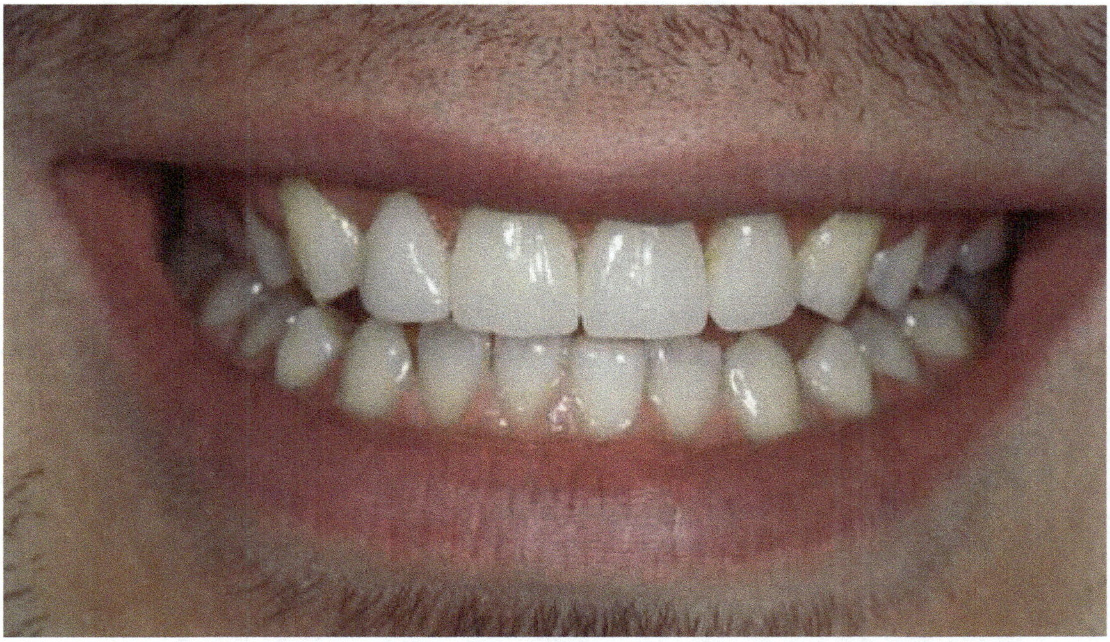

FIGURE 11: The patient's smile immediately after cementation of the restorations.

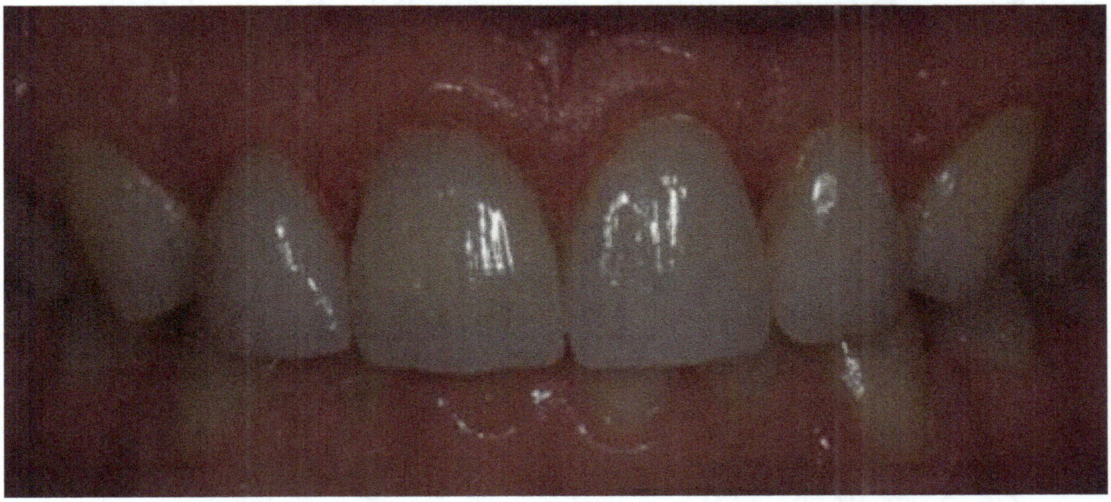

FIGURE 12: Intraoral appearance of restorations immediately after cementation.

software reads the morphology of the patient's dentition to predict the right form and function. Within the clinical experience of the authors', it can be very difficult to achieve the ideal restoration design with the computer automatically when biogeneric and bioreference are selected, especially in cases where several anterior teeth are needed to be restored with such as PLVs because of inappropriate and/or incomplete anatomic crowns. For this reason, we preferred the biocopy method in this case. In addition, we achieved the perfect restoration design by making corrections on the first digital impression received through the mock-up. Thus, we used mock-up as a step to facilitate the final restoration design.

Different clinical methods can be found in the dental literature to produce porcelain laminate veneers with CAD/CAM. Zandinejad et al. [9] prepared a mock-up in the laboratory before PLVs produced with CAD/CAM and carried out the preparation via this mock-up. After preparation, they sent the digital impressions to the laboratory and produced the PLVs in the laboratory on these impressions. On the other hand, Cattoni et al. [13] used a totally digital process with CAD/CAM from the initial photo shoot to CAD/CAM-milling mock-up. However, the authors did not give any detailed information about the restoration design. Within the knowledge of the authors, there is no published protocol to facilitate computer design in the restoration of anterior unesthetic teeth with PLVs. For this reason, as in this case, time-consuming steps like restoration design can be reduced by the clinical techniques modified according to the patient.

A recent clinical study was published and reported the survival of chairside CAD/CAM porcelain laminate veneers [14]. The authors found that chairside computer-aided

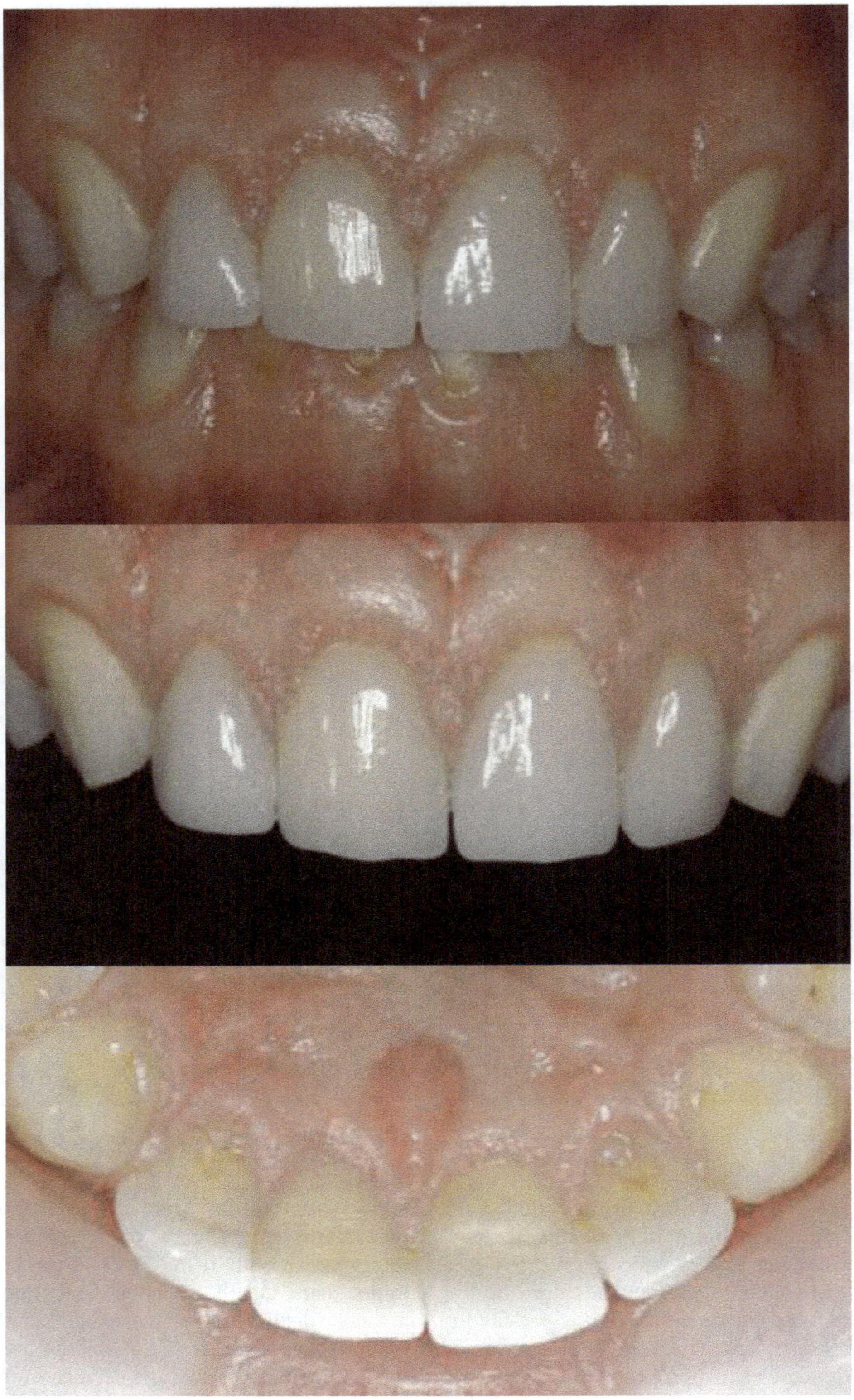

FIGURE 13: One year follow-up of the restorations.

design/computer-aided manufacturing porcelain laminate veneers were clinically successful restorations with the mean survival rate of 99.0% after 5 years. Another study evaluating the 2-year clinical success of PLVs produced by the CEREC inLab system in the laboratory reported the success rate of these restorations as 100% and found no significant difference between the porcelain laminate veneers fabricated with CAD/CAM and heat-pressed techniques in terms of marginal and internal adaptation [15]. In both studies, the old software of the CEREC system and BlueCam were used for the restoration design. Therefore, further long-term clinical studies are needed to report the clinical success of chairside PLV restorations produced by new digital techniques. In addition, the introduction of different and/or new clinical techniques into the literature as in this case report would be useful in promoting the applicability of these methods with digital systems.

4. Conclusions

PLVs can be produced with CAD/CAM systems in perfect harmony to the teeth with minimal error. The digital workflow facilitates the relationship between dentist and patient. The mock-up model to be prepared can be created and applied by the computer first and can also be implemented by the free-hand technique with heated wax-up before computer design. The clinician can perform whatever technique is more feasible for him or her. A differently modified technique, as here, can help the clinician in designing the restorations with CAD/CAM, especially for the multiple anterior teeth.

Acknowledgments

The authors kindly appreciate Sirona Turkey for their contribution and support.

References

[1] G. Sannino, F. Germano, L. Arcuri, E. Bigelli, C. Arcuri, and A. Barlattani, "CEREC CAD/CAM chairside system," *ORAL & Implantology*, vol. 7, no. 3, pp. 57–70, 2014.

[2] T. Miyazaki, Y. Hotta, J. Kunii, S. Kuriyama, and Y. Tamaki, "A review of dental CAD/CAM: current status and future perspectives from 20 years of experience," *Dental Materials Journal*, vol. 28, no. 1, pp. 44–56, 2009.

[3] V. Alt, M. Hannig, B. Wostmann, and M. Balkenhol, "Fracture strength of temporary fixed partial dentures: CAD/CAM versus directly fabricated restorations," *Dental Materials*, vol. 27, no. 4, pp. 339–347, 2011.

[4] W. Mormann and I. Krejci, "Computer-designed inlays after 5 years in situ: clinical performance and scanning electron microscopic evaluation," *Quintessence International*, vol. 23, no. 2, pp. 109–115, 1992.

[5] M. Peumans, B. Van Meerbeek, P. Lambrechts, and G. Vanherle, "Porcelain veneers: a review of the literature," *Journal of Dentistry*, vol. 28, no. 3, pp. 163–177, 2000.

[6] E. Ozturk and S. Bolay, "Survival of porcelain laminate veneers with different degrees of dentin exposure: 2-year clinical results," *The Journal of Adhesive Dentistry*, vol. 16, no. 5, pp. 481–489, 2014.

[7] D. Edelhoff, F. Beuer, J. Schweiger, O. Brix, M. Stimmelmayr, and J. F. Guth, "CAD/CAM-generated high-density polymer restorations for the pretreatment of complex cases: a case report," *Quintessence International*, vol. 43, no. 6, pp. 457–467, 2012.

[8] B. Stawarczyk, A. Krawczuk, and N. Ilie, "Tensile bond strength of resin composite repair in vitro using different surface preparation conditionings to an aged CAD/CAM resin nanoceramic," *Clinical Oral Investigations*, vol. 19, no. 2, pp. 299–308, 2015.

[9] A. Zandinejad, W. S. Lin, M. Atarodi, T. Abdel-Azim, M. J. Metz, and D. Morton, "Digital workflow for virtually designing and milling ceramic lithium disilicate veneers: a clinical report," *Operative Dentistry*, vol. 40, no. 3, pp. 241–246, 2015.

[10] A. Aykor and E. Ozel, "Five-year clinical evaluation of 300 teeth restored with porcelain laminate veneers using total-etch and a modified self-etch adhesive system," *Operative Dentistry*, vol. 34, no. 5, pp. 516–523, 2009.

[11] V. Marsango, R. Bollero, N. D'Ovidio, M. Miranda, P. Bollero, and A. Barlattani Jr., "Digital workflow," *ORAL & Implantology*, vol. 7, no. 1, pp. 20–24, 2014.

[12] Y. Arslan, S. Karakoca Nemli, M. Bankoglu Gungor, E. Tamam, and H. Yilmaz, "Evaluation of biogeneric design techniques with CEREC CAD/CAM system," *The Journal of Advanced Prosthodontics*, vol. 7, no. 6, pp. 431–436, 2015.

[13] F. Cattoni, F. Mastrangelo, E. F. Gherlone, and G. Gastaldi, "A new total digital smile planning technique (3D-DSP) to fabricate CAD-CAM mockups for esthetic crowns and veneers," *International Journal of Dentistry*, vol. 2016, Article ID 6282587, 5 pages, 2016.

[14] F. Nejatidanesh, G. Savabi, M. Amjadi, M. Abbasi, and O. Savabi, "Five year clinical outcomes and survival of chair-side CAD/CAM ceramic laminate veneers - a retrospective study," *Journal of Prosthodontic Research*, vol. 62, no. 4, pp. 462–467, 2018.

[15] M. Yuce, M. Ulusoy, and A. G. Turk, "Comparison of marginal and internal adaptation of heat-pressed and CAD/CAM porcelain laminate veneers and a 2-year follow-up," *Journal of Prosthodontics*, 2017.

17

Long-Term Follow-Up following Condylotomy in a Case of Traumatic Unilateral Anterosuperior Mandibular Condyle Dislocation

Syed Nabil, Elavarasi Kuppusamy, Rifqah Nordin, Abdul Jabar Nazimi, and Roszalina Ramli

Oral and Maxillofacial Surgery, Faculty of Dentistry, The National University of Malaysia, Jalan Raja Muda Abdul Aziz, 50300 Kuala Lumpur, Malaysia

Correspondence should be addressed to Syed Nabil; dr_syednabil@yahoo.com.my

Academic Editor: Wen Lin Chai

Anterosuperior temporomandibular joint dislocation is rare. Manual reduction of such dislocation is difficult especially when treatment is delayed. Therefore, it has an increased likelihood of needing surgical intervention to achieve reduction. The authors report a case of an anterosuperior temporomandibular dislocation in a 19-year-old male following a motor vehicle accident. Difficulties were encountered in reducing the dislocation necessitating surgically assisted reduction. The long-term outcome following management by condylotomy is reported. This present report also reviews the literature regarding the classification and management of this uncommon dislocation.

1. Introduction

Temporomandibular joint dislocation (TMJD) is an abnormal condition in which the head of the condyle displaces from its usual position in the glenoid fossa in the squamotemporal portion of the cranial base [1]. TMJD can involve only one or bilateral joints, and it can be dislocated either anteriorly, laterally, medially, posteriorly, or superiorly [1]. The cause of TMJD can either be traumatic or nontraumatic [2]. Nontraumatic dislocations are more common and precipitated by events such as forceful or excessive opening of the mouth during laughing, yawning, and dental or endoscopy treatment, during anesthetic intubation, and during eating or as consequences of seizures [1]. The nontraumatic TMJD is caused by the laxity of the surrounding connective tissue and generally can be managed by conservative reduction [2]. Traumatic TMJD meanwhile has been reported to occur following a fall, road traffic accident, domestic accident, or interpersonal violence [1]. TMJD can also be classified as acute, recurrent/habitual, or long-standing/chronic based on the dislocation duration [3]. Acute dislocation is the most frequent. When acute dislocations are not reduced for more than 72 hours, it can be defined as long-standing dislocations [4]. Recurrent or habitual dislocation occurs in repeated episodes and may become more frequent if left untreated [3].

A subtype of TMJD that is notoriously difficult to reduce is the anterosuperior dislocation (ASD) [5, 6]. ASD is described as a condition where the condyle is displaced anteriorly beyond the articular eminence then superiorly medial to the zygomatic arch to enter into the temporal fossa [6]. This type of dislocation is uncommon with only a handful of cases reported. The authors report a case of ASD in an intact condyle following a motor vehicle accident. Additionally, this article would describe the long-term outcome of such case following management with intraoral condylotomy.

2. Case Report

A 19-year-old man was brought to the emergency department following a road traffic accident after his motorcycle skidded and hit the road divider. His Glasgow Coma Scale (GSC) on initial examination was 12/15. He sustained laceration of his upper lip and tongue, comminuted fracture of the right mandible parasymphysis, and avulsed teeth 11, 12, 41, 42, 43, and 44 (Figure 1). He was intubated immediately for airway protection. An emergency head CT scan showed that he also sustained depressed fracture of the frontal bone with subdural and epidural hemorrhage. CT scan also showed right parasymphysis mandible fracture and dislocated left condyle (Figure 2(a)). The left condyle was dislocated anteriorly and superiorly into the infratemporal fossa medial to the zygomatic arch. There were no fractures of the condyle and zygomatic arch.

He underwent emergency craniotomy with evacuation of blood clot by the neurosurgical team. In the same setting, the facial laceration injury was sutured and an arch bar with intraosseous wiring was placed to stabilize the fractured mandible. Condyle dislocation reduction was also attempted. Due to the orotracheal intubation tube, the occlusion was not assessed following reduction. The patient was then transferred to the intensive care unit (ICU) subsequently with the orotracheal intubation kept in place. Following extubation 5 days later, it was noted that the patient kept his mouth open without any closure movement. There was also excessive drooling of saliva due to the inability to close his mouth. On examination, his mandible movement appeared restricted and the mandible was unable to move in any direction. He was not obeying instruction well. Multiple manual reduction attempts at bedside were unsuccessful.

An open reduction and internal fixation was planned for the right parasymphysis of mandible fracture, and it was planned to perform reduction of the dislocated condyle on the left side. Owing to the patient's neurological injury, the surgery could only be done 2 weeks after the injuries were sustained. In view of the ASD condyle and the prolonged period of dislocation, we anticipated difficult reduction. This was discussed with the patient and his family, and it was decided if the need for open or surgical reduction arises, they prefer surgical approach to be done intraorally. During the surgery under general anesthesia with muscle relaxation, initial attempts were made to reduce the left condylar dislocation by using manual traction by Hippocratic method and then with the assistance of a mouth gag but proved to be unsuccessful. Our next attempt was to release the intraosseous wiring at the parasymphysis fracture site effectively rendering the mandible in two separate pieces to simulate mandibulotomy-assisted reduction as described by previous clinicians [7, 8]. Once this was not successful, we went ahead with an intraoral condylotomy on the left side by piezoelectric surgery. First, a coronoidectomy was done to get access to the condyle. Then, the condylar neck was osteotomized using the piezosurgery, and the mandible was then able to be pushed back into occlusion. Finally, open reduction and fixation of the right parasymphysis fracture was performed and stable occlusion was achieved.

Postoperative CT scan confirmed the reduction of the dislocation (Figure 2(b)). There was a slight deviation of the jaw to the left and mouth opening was 19 mm. Occlusion was acceptable and elastics were placed for 6 weeks. Jaw exercises were encouraged, and review after 2 months postoperatively showed improvement in mouth opening

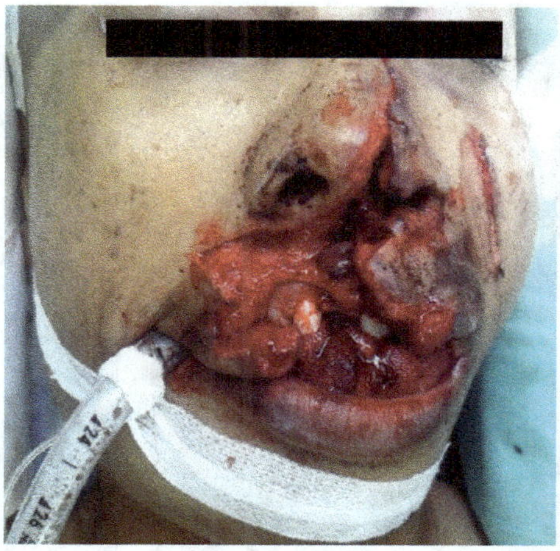

FIGURE 1: Facial injury sustained.

at 40 mm with stable occlusion. The patient was then referred to a prosthodontist for further rehabilitation and treatment of the missing teeth.

On 1-year follow-up, the patient presented with no complaint. Clinically, there was no tenderness at the joint or muscle of mastication on palpation or during movement. However, there was mild asymmetry of the jaw with the chin deviated 2 mm to the left (Figure 3). Mouth opening was maintained at 40 mm with deviation to the left on opening (Figure 4). Occlusion was good with upper and lower dentures in place. CT scan shows union between the condyle head and the condylar process stump (Figure 2(c)). Its position remains as seen immediately after surgery. The stump of the condylar process meanwhile has remodeled to form a neocondyle.

3. Discussion

The description of ASD can be rather confusing. Several previous authors used different terms for dislocation of the condyle medial to the zygomatic arch similar to this reported case including superolateral dislocation (SLD) [9], anteromedial dislocation (AMD) [2], and ASD [6]. We describe our case as ASD as the condyle is anterior and superior to its original position in the glenoid fossa. Technically, the terms SLD and AMD for such dislocation are inaccurate as the condyle is not located medial/lateral to the glenoid fossa but instead is medial/lateral to the zygomatic arch. To add further confusion, ASD has been suggested to be included under lateral dislocation classification. Allen and Young first attempted to classify cases of lateral TMJD to types I and II for lateral subluxation and lateral complete dislocation, respectively [10]. Later, Satoh et al. suggested further refinement of lateral TMJD by dividing type II to subtypes IIA, IIB, and IIC [11]. They described unhooked condyle in lateral TMJD (type IIA), laterally hooked condyle above the zygomatic arch (type IIB), and lodgment of the condyle under a fractured zygomatic arch (type IIC) [11]. The next revision of this classification was made by Prabhakar and Singla who described the condyle of an intact mandible being medial to unfractured zygoma [6]. Type III as defined by Prabhakar and

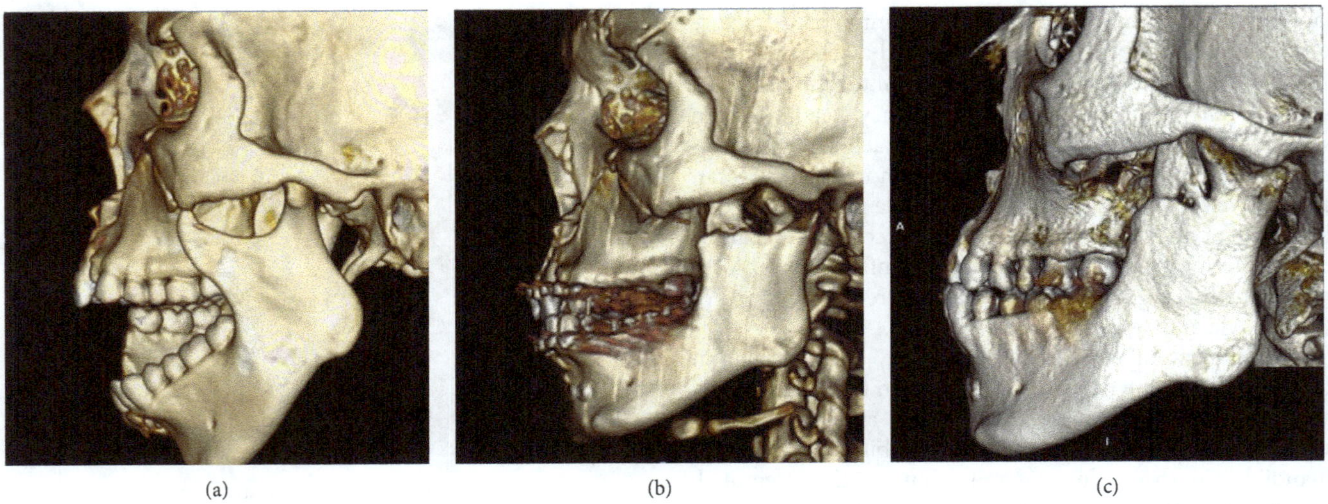

FIGURE 2: CT scan image of the left temporomandibular joint at (a) day 1 of trauma, (b) two days postsurgery, and (c) one year postsurgery.

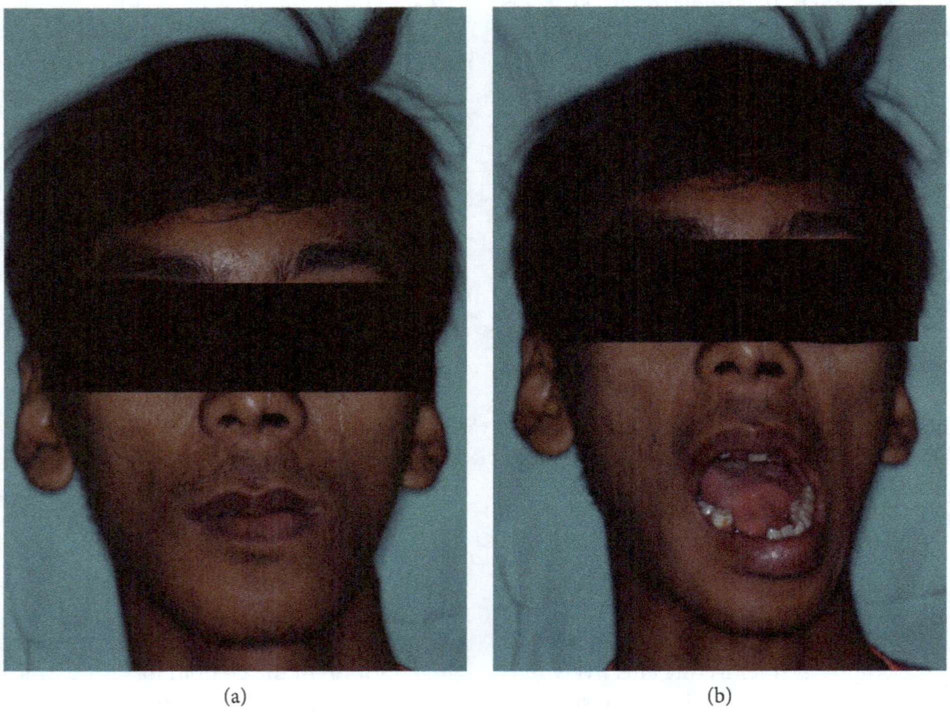

FIGURE 3: Extraoral presentation on closing and opening of the mouth one year postsurgery.

Singla is more precisely an anterior-superior dislocation (as described by the authors themselves); thus, together with type IIC from Satoh et al. has deviated from the "lateral" TMJD classification as described initially by Allen and Young [6, 10, 11]. Further refinement was made to complete the type III classification to type IIIA or type IIIB based on the presence or absence of mandibular fracture [5]. Most recently, Rahman et al. analyzed previous classification and suggested a complete classification for lateral TMJD [12]. While the classification is comprehensive, it technically lumps together an anterior vector dislocation (anterosuperior) with a lateral vector dislocation (lateral and superolateral).

Untreated or persistent acute condyle displacement due to failure to diagnose or inadequate treatment rendered for the patient can lead to "long standing" TMJD [3]. Once the condyle becomes abnormally positioned for a period of time, it causes muscle spasm, soft tissue fibrosis, and soft tissue ingrowth into the glenoid fossa [2–4]. Thus, prolonged dislocations will be more difficult to be repositioned [2–4]. Several authors agree with this and further suggest the use of the duration of the dislocation as a guide in managing long-standing TMJD cases [2, 4]. Huang et al. suggested closed reduction in a dislocation of less than 3 weeks, open reduction using wire traction at the angle of mandible for a

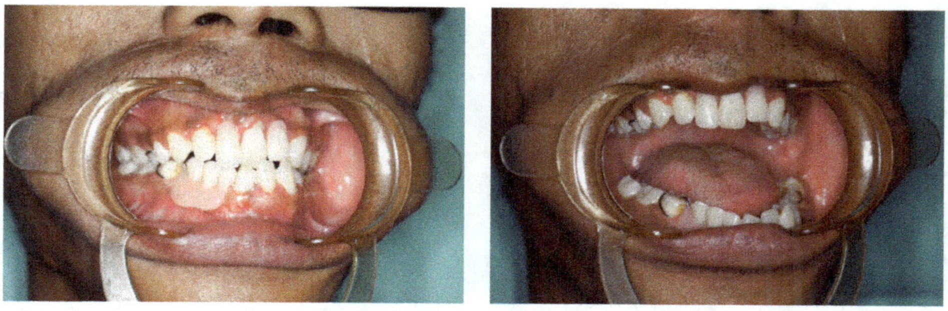

(a) (b)

FIGURE 4: Occlusion on biting and opening of the mouth with dentures one year postsurgery.

dislocation persisting more than 4-12 weeks, and more complicated surgical procedures such as condylectomy, condylotomy, myotomy, and TMJ prosthesis for dislocations persisting for more than 6 months [4]. Rattan and Rai meanwhile proposed trial of manual reduction and anterior traction using elastics before proceeding with indirect open reduction with the use of transosseous wires or hooks, direct open reduction via preauricular approach in TMJD that persist for more than one month, and orthognathic surgical procedure in cases of more than 6 months [2]. There is no consensus yet on when should an acute dislocation phase ends and the long-standing starts [3]. Huang et al. define a dislocation which has been left untreated or inadequately treated for more than 72 hours while Rattan et al. suggest a longer period of 1 month [2, 4]. In the presented case, the dislocation was attempted to be reduced at 14 days. The difficulty in manual reduction clearly shows the extent of spasm, fibrosis, and tissue ingrowth to be well advanced. There is also a possibility of a mechanical obstruction with the condyle under the zygomatic arch. Hence, an invasive procedure was eventually needed involving condylotomy and coronoidectomy on the left side as described by Pappachan et al. [13].

In ASD, the need for surgical reduction should be anticipated. From the literature, it is noted that in the nine previously reported cases, 56% (5/9) of the cases with this type of dislocation need open surgery reduction [5]. The remaining 33% (3/9) had assisted manual reduction such as the use of mouth gags [9] and zygomatic bone hook traction [5, 14]. Furthermore, the period of time before reduction in cases of ASD further contributes to the failures in manual reduction [5]. Several surgical modalities have been reported in the management of difficult cases of TMJ dislocation. These include direct reduction via preauricular incision [2], condylectomy [15], condylotomy [13], inverted L-shaped ramus osteotomy [16], bilateral vertical-oblique osteotomy of ramus [17], and midline mandibulotomy [7]. In the reported case, after conservative attempts and using of the right parasymphysis fracture to simulate midline mandibulotomy reduction failed, we proceed to perform condylotomy. Due to the expected shortening of the ramus height, long-term undesirable changes that could possibly develop include the presence of malocclusion, the deviation to the operated side when opening the mouth, loss of lateral excursion, TMJ dysfunction symptoms, and open bite [18, 19]. Clinical examination at 1-year postsurgery showed deviation of the mandible to the left side on jaw opening and the chin was noted to be shifted 2 mm to the left when resting. The patient however gained an excellent range in mouth opening with good occlusion, and normal function of the jaw was restored. Radiographically, although the left condyle head was still at its dislocated position, the stump of the condylar process has remodeled to form a neocondyle allowing satisfactory functioning of the jaw. While this shows acceptable outcome, a long-term effect of a unilateral shortening of the ramus height is still not clear. Previous reported case of condylotomy for anteriorly displaced condyles also reported similar favorable outcome [13, 20].

Condylotomy can be performed transorally, which avoids the cutaneous scar and risk for facial nerve injury. Risks to the other surrounding structures such as maxillary artery meanwhile differ among the different devices used to perform the osteotomy. Osteotomy around the condyle can be performed using piezosurgery, drill, saw, osteotome, and even gigli saw. The use of piezosurgical instruments has the advantage of not damaging the soft tissue and at the same time allowing and improving precision in osteotomy. This allows access to this limited area with minimal damage to the surrounding tissue. The fact that the joint was dislocated anteriorly provides an advantage for the surgeon to access the condyle in the reported case.

In summary, ASD is a rare occurrence of condyle dislocation anterior to the glenoid fossa and should not be classified together with lateral vector dislocations. When ASD is identified, surgical management should be anticipated and planned due to the low likelihood of success for manual reduction especially when treatment provision is delayed. There is no proper evidence to suggest or guide which surgical intervention would provide the best long-term outcome for the management of ASD. Condylotomy especially with piezoelectric surgery is a viable and safe option especially when intraoral approach is preferred.

References

[1] B. O. Akinbami, "Evaluation of the mechanism and principles of management of temporomandibular joint dislocation. Systematic review of literature and a proposed new classification

of temporomandibular joint dislocation," *Head & Face Medicine*, vol. 7, no. 1, 2011.

[2] V. Rattan and S. Rai, "Management of long-standing anteromedial temporomandibular joint dislocation," *Asian Journal of Oral and Maxillofacial Surgery*, vol. 19, no. 3, pp. 155–159, 2007.

[3] D. A. Baur, J. R. Jannuzzi, U. Mercan, and F. A. Quereshy, "Treatment of long term anterior dislocation of the TMJ," *International Journal of Oral and Maxillofacial Surgery*, vol. 42, no. 8, pp. 1030–1033, 2013.

[4] I. Y. Huang, C. M. Chen, Y. H. Kao, and C. W. Wu, "Management of long-standing mandibular dislocation," *International Journal of Oral and Maxillofacial Surgery*, vol. 40, no. 8, pp. 810–814, 2011.

[5] R. L. Silveira, I. Ranuzia, M. F. S. Melo, R. A. de Oliveira, A. A. de Brito, and V. L. Vidigal, "Traumatic anterosuperior dislocation of the intact mandibular condyle into the temporal fossa," *Craniomaxillofacial Trauma & Reconstruction*, vol. 11, no. 4, pp. 296–301, 2018.

[6] V. Prabhakar and S. Singla, "Bilateral anterosuperior dislocation of intact mandibular condyles in the temporal fossa," *International Journal of Oral and Maxillofacial Surgery*, vol. 40, no. 6, pp. 640–643, 2011.

[7] S. H. Lee, S. I. Son, J. H. Park, I. S. Park, and J. H. Nam, "Reduction of prolonged bilateral temporomandibular joint dislocation by midline mandibulotomy," *International Journal of Oral and Maxillofacial Surgery*, vol. 35, no. 11, pp. 1054–1056, 2006.

[8] V. Rattan, S. Rai, and A. Sethi, "Midline mandibulotomy for reduction of long-standing temporomandibular joint dislocation," *Craniomaxillofacial Trauma and Reconstruction*, vol. 6, no. 2, pp. 127–132, 2013.

[9] S. S. Bu, S. L. Jin, and L. Yin, "Superolateral dislocation of the intact mandibular condyle into the temporal fossa: review of the literature and report of a case," *Oral Surgery, Oral Medicine, Oral Pathology, Oral Radiology, and Endodontology*, vol. 103, no. 2, pp. 185–189, 2007.

[10] F. J. Allen and A. H. Young, "Lateral displacement of the intact mandibular condyle. A report of five cases," *British Journal of Oral Surgery*, vol. 7, no. 1, pp. 24–30, 1969.

[11] K. Satoh, H. Suzuki, and S. Matsuzaki, "A type II lateral dislocation of bilateral intact mandibular condyles with a proposed new classification," *Plastic and Reconstructive Surgery*, vol. 93, no. 3, pp. 598–602, 1994.

[12] T. Rahman, G. S. Hashmi, S. S. Ahmed, and S. A. Rahman, "Posttraumatic lateral dislocation of mandibular condyle: a proposed new classification with report of 14 dislocated condyles," *Craniomaxillofacial Trauma & Reconstruction*, 2019, In press.

[13] B. Pappachan, M. Alexander, and B. Snehal, "Intraoral high condylotomy for a case of chronic mandibular dislocation," *British Journal of Oral and Maxillofacial Surgery*, vol. 50, no. 3, pp. e38–e40, 2012.

[14] M. F. S. Melo, R. B. de Oliveira, R. L. Silveira, and M. B. F. Amaral, "Anterosuperior dislocation of the intact condyles into the temporal fossa," *Journal of Craniofacial Surgery*, vol. 26, no. 3, pp. 990-991, 2015.

[15] K. Chul-Hwan and K. Dae-Hyun, "Chronic dislocation of temporomandibular joint persisting for 6 months: a case report," *Journal of the Korean Association of Oral and Maxillofacial Surgeons*, vol. 38, no. 5, pp. 305–309, 2012.

[16] E. O. Adekeye, R. I. Shamia, and P. Cove, "Inverted L-shaped ramus osteotomy for prolonged bilateral dislocation of the temporomandibular joint," *Oral Surgery, Oral Medicine, Oral Pathology*, vol. 41, no. 5, pp. 568–577, 1976.

[17] S. C. Debnath, S. M. Kotrashetti, R. Halli, and S. Baliga, "Bilateral vertical-oblique osteotomy of ramus (external approach) for treatment of a long-standing dislocation of the temporomandibular joint: a case report," *Oral Surgery, Oral Medicine, Oral Pathology, Oral Radiology, and Endodontology*, vol. 101, no. 6, pp. e79–e82, 2006.

[18] U. Silvennoinen, T. Iizuka, K. Oikarinen, and C. Lindqvist, "Analysis of possible factors leading to problems after nonsurgical treatment of condylar fractures," *Journal of Oral and Maxillofacial Surgery*, vol. 52, no. 8, pp. 793–799, 1994.

[19] L. M. H. Smets, P. A. van Damme, and P. J. W. Stoelinga, "Non-surgical treatment of condylar fractures in adults: a retrospective analysis," *Journal of Cranio-Maxillofacial Surgery*, vol. 31, no. 3, pp. 162–167, 2003.

[20] K. Matsushita, E. Nakamura, I. Kobayashi et al., "Traumatic dislocation of the mandibular condyle into the temporal fossa," *Asian Journal of Oral and Maxillofacial Surgery*, vol. 14, no. 4, pp. 250–254, 2002.

18

A Case of Oral Histoplasmosis Concomitant with Pulmonary Tuberculosis

Silas Antonio Juvencio de Freitas Filho ,[1] Natália Galvão Garcia ,[1] Mário César de Souza,[2] and Denise Tostes Oliveira [1]

[1]*Department of Surgery, Stomatology, Pathology and Radiology (Area of Pathology), Bauru School of Dentistry, University of São Paulo, Bauru, São Paulo, Brazil*
[2]*Department of Dentistry, Northern State University of Paraná, Jacarezinho Unit, Paraná, Brazil*

Correspondence should be addressed to Denise Tostes Oliveira; denisetostes@usp.br

Academic Editor: Evanthia Chrysomali

The superficial intraoral lesions of histoplasmosis occurring concomitant to tuberculosis, in a 46-year-old man, are reported. The human immunodeficiency virus (HIV) infection test was negative. The immunosuppression caused by tuberculosis in our patient probably had an important role in the development of intraoral lesions of histoplasmosis. Here, we discussed the role of the dentist in the diagnosis of these infectious diseases, highlighting the importance of anamnesis and the histopathology/immunohistochemistry exams.

1. Introduction

H. capsulatum infects the human host and grows in yeast form [1–7]. The disease may be self-limiting or asymptomatic in healthy individuals, or still to occur in the disseminated form, including the oral cavity [1–7].

In the mouth, the histoplasmosis manifestations may affect any region but are commonly in the tongue, palate, and oropharyngeal mucosa [7, 8]. Furthermore, the oral lesions present from granulomatous nodules to painful shallow or deep ulcers with symptoms of odynophagia and dysphagia [7].

The single oral manifestation of histoplasmosis in immunosuppressed individuals is rare and the diagnosis is challenging [3, 9]. In addition, at the time of diagnosis of oral histoplasmosis, the health professional should investigate the presence of concomitant diseases, such as malignant neoplasms or other infections as tuberculosis [10].

The occurrence of oral histoplasmosis in patients with pulmonary tuberculosis has been reported in some studies mainly due to immunosuppression and physical weakness caused by bacterial disease [8, 10, 11]. The tuberculosis has been concomitantly diagnosed in approximately 10% of Brazilians with histoplasmosis [12]. Antonello et al. [8] showed that 36% of patients with oral histoplasmosis had concomitant active pulmonary tuberculosis, 18% had malignant neoplasia, 9% had chronic obstructive pulmonary disease, and 9% had no other disease at the time of diagnosis of fungal infection.

Here, we report a case of oral histoplasmosis in a patient with a diagnosis of pulmonary tuberculosis. The role of the dentist in the diagnosis of this infectious disease including the importance of detailed anamnesis and the histopathology/immunohistochemistry exams is discussed.

2. Case Report

A 46-year-old man was attended in the dental clinic complaining of symptomatic oral lesions with two months in duration. The intraoral physical examination revealed diffuse, friable, vegetative areas on the right upper alveolar ridge, hard palate, and left inferior alveolar ridge (Figures 1(a) and 1(b)). His medical history revealed a diagnosis of tuberculosis about a month ago in which the

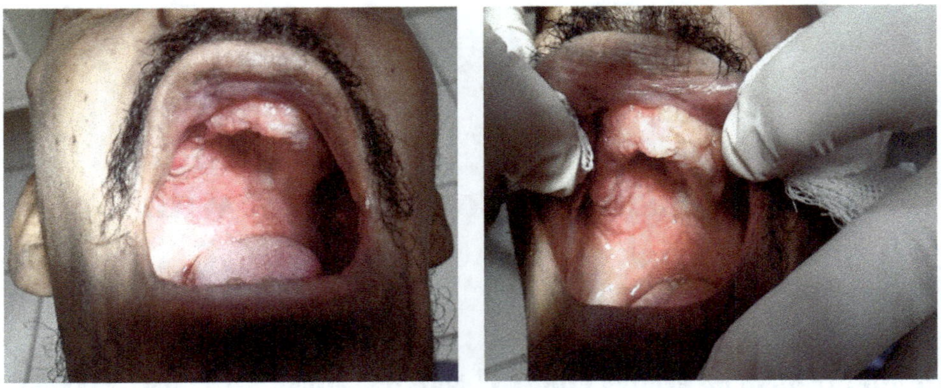

(a) (b)

Figure 1: Clinical aspect of intraoral lesions in the palate and alveolar ridge regions (a, b).

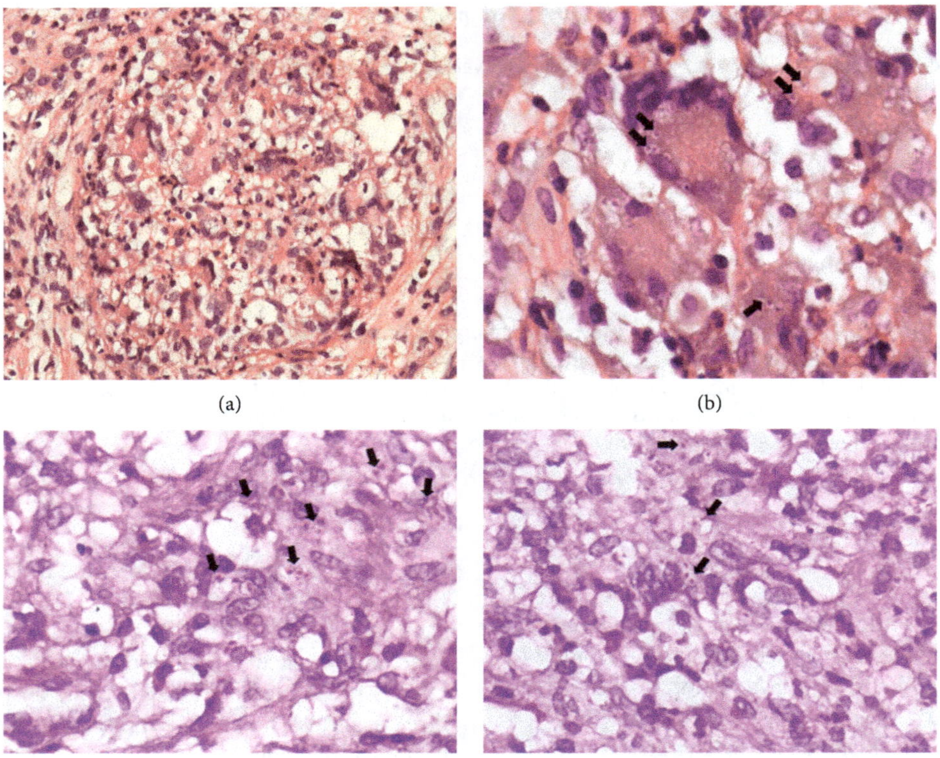

(a) (b) (c) (d)

Figure 2: Connective tissue with intense inflammatory infiltrate with a granulomatous pattern, consisting of giant multinucleated inflammatory cells and vacuolated macrophages, with several fungi suggestive of *H. capsulatum*—(hematoxylin-eosin stain; (a) ×200, (b) ×400). In (c) and (d), the periodic acid-Schiff (PAS) staining showed vacuolated macrophage with positivity for *H. capsulatum* ((c d) ×400). Note the numerous small rosy dots (arrow).

expectorated sputum smears were positive for bacteria and acid-fast bacilli. In addition, at the time of diagnosis of tuberculosis, the patient had a significant weight loss and asthenia. The patient was under antibacterial therapy (oral isoniazid (INH) 225 mg/day, rifampicin (RFP) 450 mg/day, pyrazinamide 1,200 mg/day, and ethambutol (EB) 825 mg/day). Testing for human immunodeficiency virus (HIV) infection was negative. Furthermore, the patient confirmed smoking and chronic alcoholism. He worked as a night flow controller on the side of a highway and lived very close to the countryside. After knowing the patient's medical history, the main hypothesis for oral lesions was tuberculosis.

An incisional biopsy of the right upper alveolar ridge showed connective tissue with intense inflammatory infiltrate with a granulomatous pattern, consisting of giant multinucleated inflammatory cells and vacuolated macrophages, with innumerable fungi suggestive of *H. capsulatum* (Figures 2(a) and 2(b)). Staining slides with periodic acid-Schiff (PAS) (Figures 2(c) and 2(d)) and Grocott-Gomori methenamine silver were positive for the morphological

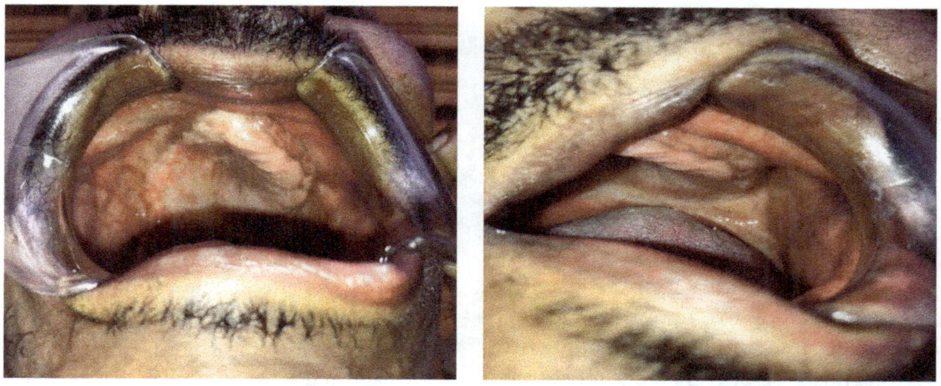

(a) (b)

FIGURE 3: After twelve months, the clinical regression of oral histoplasmosis lesions.

characteristics of *H. capsulatum*. In addition, the immunohistochemical reactivity to Histoplasma using polyclonal antibody was positive; for polyclonal *P. brasiliensis, Leishmania spp.* and Calmette-Guérin bacillus were negative. The diagnosis of oral histoplasmosis was established. We did not search for fungi in other biological samples.

Initially, the drug was maintained for tuberculosis and prescribed fluconazol (400 mg/day) for seven months for treatment of oral histoplasmosis. During the follow-up, when a gradual increase in body weight was noted, fluconazole was substituted for itraconazole 200 mg/day for eight months with the resolution of oral histoplasmosis lesions. The clinical control one year after initiation of itraconazole treatment can be seen in Figures 3(a) and 3(b). One year after the initial treatment of tuberculosis, the patient was cured.

3. Discussion

Tuberculosis remains a public health problem in many countries including Brazil; and with the immunosuppression resulting from the disease, some opportunistic infections may develop, especially in cases associated positive HIV [10, 13]. In the present case reported, a 46-year-old man who presented to her dentist with superficial lesions located in several intraoral sites was in treatment for tuberculosis. The detailed clinical investigation showed that our patient was HIV negative and the oral histoplasmosis diagnosis was established after laboratory exams excluding other infections. The immunosuppression caused by tuberculosis in our patient probably had an important role in the development of intraoral lesions of histoplasmosis.

Sometimes, the diagnosis of intraoral histoplasmosis is challenging because the lesions can be mimicking malignancies, other fungal diseases, or traumatic ulcers, and the biopsy has been a useful resource to establish the final diagnosis [1, 2, 14]. In routine staining (hematoxylin and eosin), PAS and Grocott-Gomori silver methylamine staining can identify fungi within prominent macrophages and giant Langhans-type giant cells. In summary, initially, the histopathology directed our diagnostic hypotheses and, finally, the use of immunohistochemistry was essential to eliminate other oral infectious diseases and establish the final diagnosis. Although we used polyclonal antibodies in our pathological investigation, the analysis made it possible to eliminate the possibility of other infections, including oral tuberculosis and paracoccidioidomycosis. Besides, serology and culture tests may assist in establishing the diagnosis of this fungal disease [1].

Tuberculosis mainly affects the lungs and can present several complications in its clinical course causing weakness, cough, weight loss, shortness of breath, among other signs and symptoms, and the possibility of concomitant infections [1, 10]. As shown in our case, weight loss and asthenia are common clinical signs in patients with concomitant active pulmonary tuberculosis and histoplasmosis [8]. In addition, dysphagia and fever can also be found among these patients [8]. Interestingly, at the time of diagnosis, our patient had several complications but the laboratory tests were negative for HIV. In case a similar to ours, the main suspect has been of oral tuberculosis [2]. All these clinical characteristics and information collected during the anamnesis become the diagnostic process challenging.

Initially, our patient could not be treated with itraconazole. The physician instituted this medicament after effective response to tuberculosis treatment. This decision was also made due to the drug interaction between rifampicin and itraconazole, where itraconazole levels significantly decrease in the presence of the other, so these two drugs should not be administered concomitantly [15, 16]. Additionally, amphotericin B deoxycholate is another medicament that can be used to treat acute and chronic cavitary pulmonary histoplasmosis [17].

H. capsulatum has been considered a fungus endemic in the Mississippi and Ohio River Valleys, also in Central and South America, Asia, and Australia [3, 6, 7, 14]. In all Brazilian regions, this infectious disease has been very common in men between the fourth and fifth decades of life with a high mortality rate; this data may be underestimated due to the lack of mandatory reporting [12]. Moreover, in Brazil, oral lesions of histoplasmosis may lead the dentist to suspect of other infections such as the paracoccidioidomycosis [3, 7].

Although the number of fungal oral lesions diagnosed in Brazilian Referral Centers is relatively low [7, 18], the cases of disseminated histoplasmosis with oral manifestation have increased in recent years, especially in South American men

[1] and consequently has caused concern. Then, the biopsy for histopathology and culture of oral suspected lesions by dentists, particularly in immunosuppressed patients, is mandatory for establishing the diagnosis of this fungal infection.

4. Conclusion

In summary, it is prudent for the dentist to investigate the patient's health status considering the opportunistic oral mucosal infections, especially in immunosuppressed patients. The clinical diagnosis of oral histoplasmosis can be challenging, and a detailed anamnesis associated with complementary laboratory tests are required. Correct therapeutic indication and prolonged follow-up are essential for patient healing to avoid recurrence of this fungal infection.

Acknowledgments

The authors declare that the paper-processing charges were supported by Conselho Nacional de Desenvolvimento Científico e Tecnológico (CNPq; No. 155359/2016-9).

References

[1] T. Pincelli, M. Enzler, M. Davis, A. J. Tande, N. Comfere, and A. Bruce, "Oropharyngeal histoplasmosis: a report of 10 cases," *Clinical and Experimental Dermatololy*, vol. 44, no. 5, pp. e181–e188, 2019.

[2] D. Chatterjee, A. Chatterjee, M. Agarwal et al., "Disseminated histoplasmosis with oral manifestation in an immunocompetent patient," *Case Reports in Dentistry*, vol. 2017, Article ID 1323514, 4 pages, 2017.

[3] I. P. Klein, M. A. Martins, M. D. Martins, and V. C. Carrard, "Diagnosis of HIV infection on the basis of histoplasmosis-related oral ulceration," *Special Care in Dentistry*, vol. 36, no. 2, pp. 99–103, 2016.

[4] M. T. Brazão-Silva, G. W. Mancusi, F. V. Bazzoun, G. Y. Ishisaki, and M. Marcucci, "A gingival manifestation of histoplasmosis leading diagnosis," *Contemporary Clinical Dentistry*, vol. 4, no. 1, pp. 97–101, 2013.

[5] S. Vidyanath, P. Shameena, S. Sudha, and R. G. Nair, "Disseminated histoplasmosis with oral and cutaneous manifestations," *Journal of Oral and Maxillofacial Pathology*, vol. 17, no. 1, pp. 139–142, 2013.

[6] D. Sharma, A. McKendry, S. Nageshwaran, and J. Cartledge, "A case of oral ulceration and disseminated histoplasmosis in HIV infection," *International Journal of STD & AIDS*, vol. 23, no. 7, pp. 522-523, 2012.

[7] O. G. Ferreira, S. V. Cardoso, A. S. Borges, M. S. Ferreira, and A. M. Loyola, "Oral histoplasmosis in Brazil," *Oral Surgery, Oral Medicine, Oral Pathology, Oral Radiology, and Endodontology*, vol. 93, no. 6, pp. 654–659, 2002.

[8] V. S. Antonello, V. F. Zaltron, M. Vial, F. M. Oliveira, and L. C. Severo, "Oropharyngeal histoplasmosis: report of eleven cases and review of the literature," *Revista da Sociedade Brasileira de Medicina Tropical*, vol. 44, no. 1, pp. 26–29, 2011.

[9] G. Fortuna and M. D. Mignogna, "Oral histoplasmosis of a healthy man in a non-endemic area," *Infection*, vol. 39, no. 5, pp. 497-498, 2011.

[10] Z. Cui, M. Lin, S. Nie, and R. Lan, "Risk factors associated with tuberculosis (TB) among people living with HIV/AIDS: a pair-matched case-control study in Guangxi, China," *PLoS One*, vol. 12, no. 3, article e0173976, 2017.

[11] C. Nabet, C. Belzunce, D. Blanchet et al., "*Histoplasma capsulatum* causing sinusitis: a case report in French Guiana and review of the literature," *BMC Infectious Diseases*, vol. 18, no. 1, article 595, pp. 1–7, 2018.

[12] M. A. Almeida, F. Almeida-Silva, A. J. Guimarães, R. Almeida-Paes, and R. M. Zancopé-Oliveira, "The occurrence of histoplasmosis in Brazil: a systematic review," *International Journal of Infectious Diseases*, vol. 86, pp. 147–156, 2019.

[13] A. Kritski, K. B. Andrade, R. M. Galliez et al., "Tuberculosis: renewed challenge in Brazil," *Revista da Sociedade Brasileira de Medicina Tropical*, vol. 51, no. 1, pp. 2–6, 2018.

[14] N. Hendren, C. Yek, J. Mull, and J. B. Cutrell, "Disseminated histoplasmosis presenting as multiple oral ulcers," *BMJ Case Reports*, vol. 2017, 2017.

[15] S. M. Moon, H. Y. Park, B. H. Jeong, K. Jeon, S. Y. Lee, and W. J. Koh, "Effect of rifampin and rifabutin on serum itraconazole levels in patients with chronic pulmonary aspergillosis and coexisting nontuberculous mycobacterial infection," *Antimicrobial Agents and Chemotherapy*, vol. 59, no. 1, pp. 663–665, 2015.

[16] M. Blomley, E. L. Teare, A. de Belder, Y. Thway, and M. Weston, "Itraconazole and anti-tuberculosis drugs," *The Lancet*, vol. 336, no. 8725, article 1255, 1990.

[17] V. K. Mahajan, R. K. Raina, S. Singh et al., "Case report: histoplasmosis in Himachal Pradesh (India): an emerging endemic focus," *The American Journal of Tropical Medicine and Hygiene*, vol. 97, no. 6, pp. 1749–1756, 2017.

[18] A. C. Vasconcelos, C. Aburad, I. F. P. Lima et al., "A scientific survey on 1550 cases of oral lesions diagnosed in a Brazilian referral center," *Anais da Academica Brasileira de Ciências*, vol. 89, no. 3, pp. 1691–1697, 2017.

19

Concentrated Growth Factors as an Ingenious Biomaterial in Regeneration of Bony Defects after Periapical Surgery: A Report of Two Cases

Nivedhitha Malli Sureshbabu[1] **Kathiravan Selvarasu,**[2] **Jayanth Kumar V,**[3] **Mahalakshmi Nandakumar,**[1] **and Deepak Selvam**[1]

[1]*Department of Conservative Dentistry and Endodontics, Saveetha Dental College, Saveetha Institute of Medical and Technical Sciences, Saveetha University, 162, Poonamallee High Road, Chennai, 600077 Tamil Nadu, India*
[2]*Department of Oral and Maxillofacial Surgery, Saveetha Dental College, Saveetha Institute of Medical and Technical Sciences, Saveetha University, 162, Poonamallee High Road, Chennai, 600077 Tamil Nadu, India*
[3]*Department of Oral Medicine and Radiology, Saveetha Dental College, Saveetha Institute of Medical and Technical Sciences, Saveetha University, 162, Poonamallee High Road, Chennai, 600077 Tamil Nadu, India*

Correspondence should be addressed to Nivedhitha Malli Sureshbabu; nivea16@hotmail.com

Academic Editor: Pia L. Jornet

The overall success of a periapical surgery is assessed in terms of regeneration of functional periradicular tissues. The regenerative potential of platelets has been well documented. This article describes the use of concentrated growth factors (CGF), a new family of autologous platelet concentrates, as a sole material for bone regeneration after periapical surgery. 32- and 35-year-old female patients diagnosed with Ellis Class IV, an open apex in 11 with apical periodontitis in 11 and 12 and previously root canal-treated 31 and 41 with a chronic apical abscess, respectively, were managed with endodontic surgery. Subsequent to apicectomy and retrograde filling, the CGF fibrin block and membrane were used before suturing. There was uneventful healing during the immediate post-op and the subsequent follow-up periods. CGF is produced by a differential centrifugation process that results in the formation of a denser fibrin matrix richer in growth factors than those observed in PRF. Reasonable osseous healing was seen as early as 6-month follow-up, thereby recommending the use of CGF as an alternative to bone grafts and membranes in extensive periapical lesions to enhance bone regeneration and to decrease the healing time.

1. Introduction

Periapical surgery is the treatment of choice for teeth with persistent apical periodontitis when the conventional non-surgical method fails to achieve the principal objectives [1]. It has been predicted that the smaller defect heals around one year, whereas for the larger defects, the healing time may be more than two years [2]. However, recently, Lin et al. have demonstrated that the healing of periapical tissues is a "programmed event." More than the size of the lesion, it is the microenvironment consisting of the progenitor/stem cells, extracellular matrix, and bioactive molecules that plays a crucial role in tissue regeneration or scar formation during wound healing [3].

Platelet-rich plasma (PRP) and plasma rich in growth factors (PRGF) classified as the first generation of autologous platelet concentrates (APCs) have demonstrated promising results in the management of extensive periapical lesions, apicomarginal defects, and combined endo-perio lesions and also improved the quality of life of patients undergoing endodontic surgery [4]. However, both have several drawbacks like use of anticoagulant, artificial polymerization, and a time-consuming two-step centrifugation process.

Platelet-rich fibrin (PRF), considered as the second generation platelet concentrate and classified into L-PRF, A-PRF, i-PRF, CGF, PRFM, and Vivostat PRF [5]. A systematic review reported that APCs have a favourable effect on patients' quality of life and are supportive for bone regeneration after endodontic surgery [6].

Concentrated growth factor (CGF) is a newer second generation platelet concentrate that is prepared by centrifuging blood samples at alternating and controlled speeds using a special centrifuge. Differential centrifugation results in the formation of a denser fibrin matrix richer in growth factors than those observed in the PRF and PRP. To our knowledge, this is the first case report for the use of CGF alone in endodontic surgery. For describing the case reports, we have followed the checklist given in CARE guidelines (http://www.care-statement.org/) [7].

2. Case Presentation

2.1. Case Report 1. A 32-year-old female patient was referred to the Department of Conservative Dentistry and Endodontics with chief complaint of discolouration of the upper right front tooth (tooth 11) for the past 6 months. Past dental history revealed a traumatic fall 5 years ago which involved the upper front teeth for which no dental treatment was sought for. Recently, as the discolouration gradually worsened, the patient sought dental treatment to restore esthetics.

Intraoral clinical examination revealed a slightly discoloured 11 and chipping of the incisal edge with no presenting symptoms (Figure 1(a)). Both 11 and 12 responded negatively to the electric pulp tester (Gentle Pulse™ Pulp Vitality Tester, Parkell, USA) and elicited mild tenderness on percussion.

On radiographic examination (VistaScan Mini, UK), extensive periapical radiolucency involving the roots of 11 and 12 and an open apex of 11 was revealed (Figure 1(b)). CBCT for this case (Dentsply Sirona, Orthophos XG 3D) was taken at standardized settings (90 kV, 6 mA, 5 × 5.5 cm, 160 μm, and 14 s) to assess the exact location, size, and extent and proximity of the lesion to anatomical structures.

The preoperative measurements of the lesion as seen in CBCT in different planes can be seen in Figures 1(g), 1(i), 1(k). According to the CBCT-PAI scores, it was graded as a 5D lesion [8]. The score 5 indicates that the diameter of the periapical lesion is greater than 8 mm, and D represents destruction of the periapical cortical bone in the palatal region.

A tentative diagnosis of an Ellis Class IV fracture and open apex in 11 with apical periodontitis in 11 and 12 was made. The differential diagnosis could be a chronic periapical abscess, periapical cyst, and periapical granuloma. The treatment plan was root canal treatment for 11 and 12. The patient was informed about the risks and benefits of the procedure and a written consent was taken.

Under local anaesthesia (2% lignocaine in 1 : 200,000 dilution adrenaline, Neon Laboratories Ltd.) and rubber dam isolation, an access cavity was prepared in 11 and 12 with an Endo access bur (Dentsply Maillefer, Switzerland). The working length was determined with an apex locator (Propex Pixi, Dentsply Maillefer, Switzerland) and confirmed with radiograph. Cleaning and shaping was initiated with 45 K file (Mani, Inc. Japan), and apical preparation was performed till size 80 K file in 11. In 12, apical preparation was done till size 45 K file to full working length, after which step-back preparation was done till 80 K file. Routine root canal-shaping procedure was done along with copious irrigation using 3% sodium hypochlorite (VIP, Vensons, India) and final flush with 0.9% physiologic saline (acuLIFE, India). Calcium hydroxide medicament (RC Cal, Prime Dental Products, India) was placed thrice for a period of 1 week each. As the root canals exhibited persistent discharge of exudates and due to two prognostic factors (size of the lesion which was more than 10 mm and the thinning or destruction of the palatal bone) which were unfavourable for this case [9], periapical surgery was planned following the recommendation given by the Spanish Society of Oral Surgery (point 3: a radiotransparent lesion measuring over 8 to 10 mm in diameter).

The root canals were obturated a day before the surgery using custom-made roll cone technique for 11 and conventional cold lateral compaction technique for 12.

During surgery, after achieving adequate anaesthesia, a crevicular incision was placed from 22 to 14 with a vertical releasing incision on the mesial aspect of 14 to reflect a full thickness mucoperiosteal triangular flap. Cortical softening of the periapical bone was noted from regions 11 to 13. A bony window was created and thorough curettage was done (Figure 1(c)).

Apicoectomy was performed extending 3 mm into the canal space using no.702 tapered fissure burs (SS White burs) in 12. Apicoectomy was not done in 11 because of the presence of an open apex. Root end cavity preparation was done using zirconium nitride ultrasonic retro-tips (Dentsply Maillefer, Switzerland) in 11 and 12. Subsequently, retrograde filling was done with Mineral Trioxide Aggregate (MTA Angelus® Brazil) (Figure 1(d)). Later, the surgical site was prepared for placement of CGF fibrin gel and CGF membrane.

A standard, disposable, two 10 mL nonanticoagulant glass tubes and a matching centrifuge device (MEDIFUGE, Silfradent s.r.l., S. Sofia, Italy) were used. 20 mL of intravenous blood sample from the patient was placed in centrifuge tubes without anticoagulants and accelerated for 30 s, centrifuged at 2700 rpm for 2 min, 2400 rpm for 4 min, 2700 rpm for 4 min, and 3000 rpm for 3 min, and decelerated for 36 s to stop. All of these processes are adjusted automatically by "preprogramming" in the machine.

From the three layers formed, the uppermost platelet-deprived fraction was removed with a sterile syringe. The layer in the form of a fibrin gel containing the CGF was separated from the red blood cell layer. The prepared CGF fibrin gel was placed inside the surgical site and covered with CGF membrane. The layer in the form of a membrane containing the concentrated growth membrane was held with a hemostatic clamp and separated from the RBC layer by using microsurgical scissors. The CGF layer is then placed in a condensing disc and compressed to convert to CGF membrane. (Figures 1(e), 1(f)).

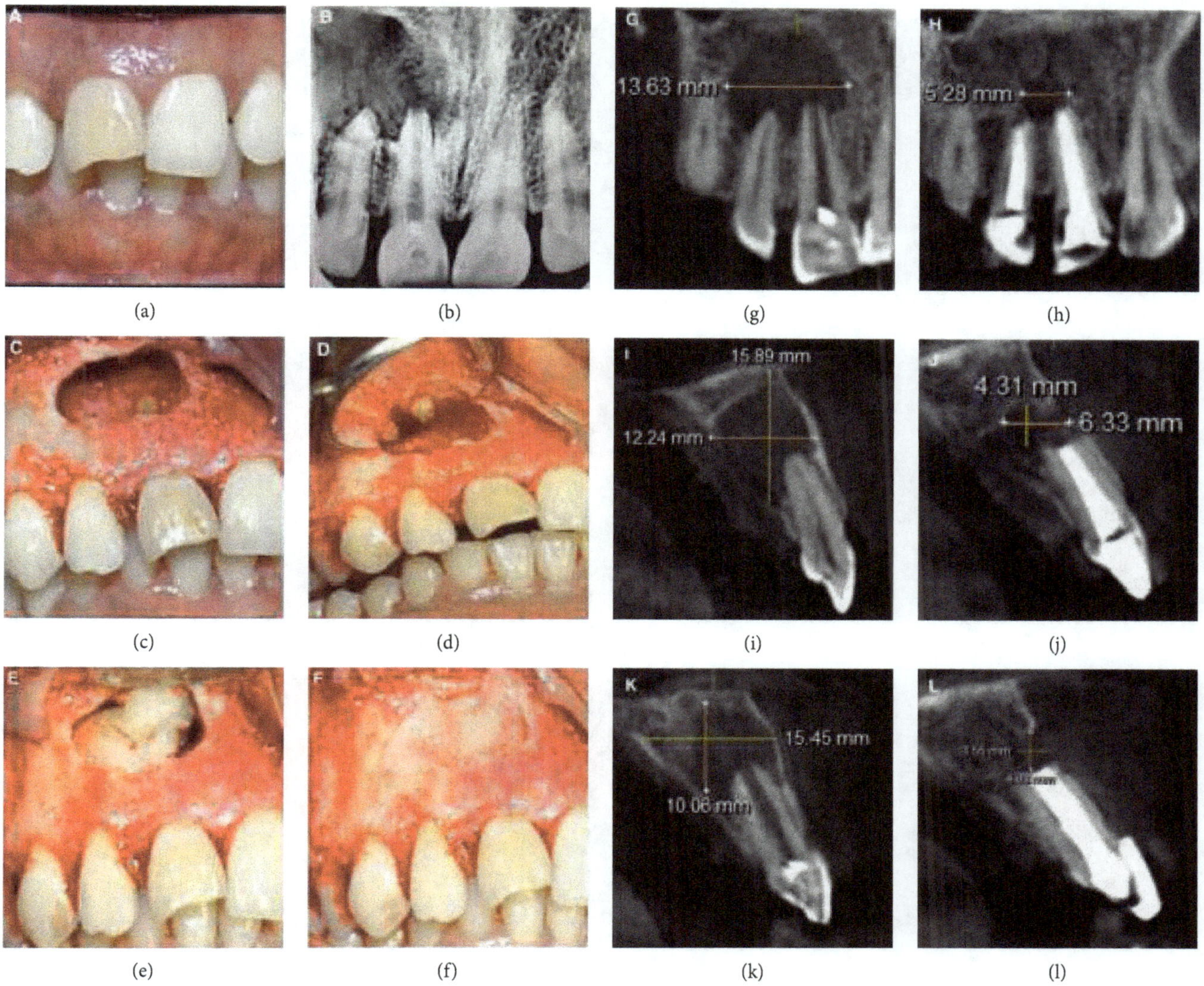

FIGURE 1: Preoperative clinical and surgical procedure and radiographic images: IOPA and CBCT images (Case Report 1). (a) Pre-op clinical photograph showing discoloured 11 with chipping of the incisal edge of the crown. (b) Preoperative IOPA showing the periapical lesion involving the apices of 11 and 12 and extending to the mesial margin of 13. (c) Complete curettage of the lesion and apicectomy done in 12. (d) Retrograde preparation and filling with MTA in 11 and 12. (e) CGF fibrin block placed in the bony cavity. (f) CGF membrane placed to cover the bone defect. (g) Pre-op CBCT image showing the lesion measurement in the coronal slice. (h) Post-op CBCT image showing the lesion measurement in the coronal slice. (i) Pre-op CBCT image showing the lesion measurement in sagittal slice corresponding to 12. (j) Post-op CBCT image showing the lesion measurement in sagittal slice corresponding to 12. (k) Pre-op CBCT image showing the lesion measurement in sagittal slice corresponding to 11. (l) Post-op CBCT image showing the lesion measurement in sagittal slice corresponding to 11.

Subsequent to CGF placement, the flap was closed with 3-0 vicryl sutures (Ethicon Inc. Piscataway, USA). Postoperative instructions were given and systemic antibiotics, analgesics, and supplemental 0.2% chlorhexidine mouthwash were prescribed.

The postoperative CBCT at 1-year follow-up showed satisfactory healing with evident reduction in lesion size as shown in Figures 1(h), 1(j), 1(l), and the patient was asymptomatic at all the recall periods, suggesting a successful treatment outcome. The patient is kept under review, to be followed up after 18 months, 24 months, and 36 months.

2.2. Case Report 2. A 35-year-old female patient reported mild swelling and pus discharge in the lower front region of the mouth for the past 2 months. Past dental history revealed trauma to lower anterior teeth 4 years ago, following which she underwent endodontic treatment. History suggested that there were multiple retreatments in the past for the current chief complaint.

On clinical examination, 31 was discoloured with mild swelling on the labial aspect (Figure 2(a)). Radiographic examination revealed a well-obturated 31 and 41 with large periapical radiolucency (Figure 2(b)). The CBCT-PAI score was 5D (Figures 2(g), 2(i), 2(k)). Based on the above findings, a diagnosis of previously root canal-treated 31 and 41 with a chronic apical abscess was made. History suggested that there were multiple retreatments in the past for the current chief complaint, with presenting complaint of recurring,

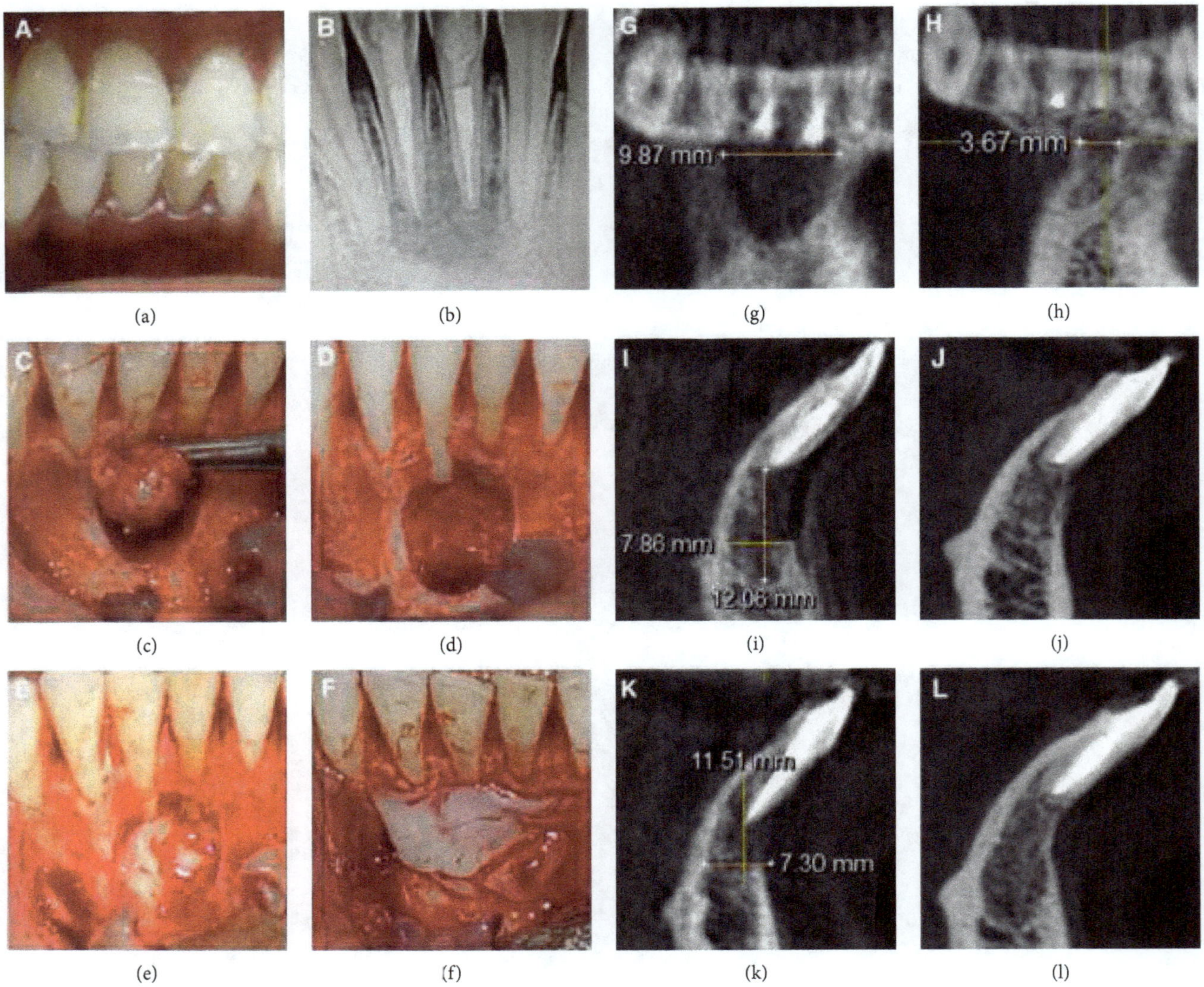

FIGURE 2: Preoperative clinical and surgical procedure and radiographic images: IOPA and CBCT images (Case Report 2). (a) Pre-op clinical photograph shows discoloured 31. (b) Preoperative IOPA showing the periapical lesion involving the apices of 11 and 12 and extending to the mesial margin of 13. (c) Complete curettage of the lesion. (d) Apicectomy done and MTA retrograde filling given in 31 and 41. (e) CGF fibrin-rich block placed in the bony defect. (f) CGF membrane placed before suturing of the flap. (g) Pre-op CBCT image showing the lesion measurement in the coronal slice. (h) Post-op CBCT image showing the lesion measurement in coronal slice. (i) Pre-op CBCT image showing the lesion measurement in sagittal slice corresponding to 41. (j) Post-op CBCT image showing the lesion measurement in sagittal slice corresponding to 41. (k) Pre-op CBCT image showing the lesion measurement in sagittal slice corresponding to 31. (l) Post-op CBCT image showing the lesion measurement in sagittal slice corresponding to 31.

intermittent swelling with pus discharge in the lower front region. And radiographic examination revealed adequate obturation and apical seal, with nonhealing chronic periapical radiolucency. The treatment plan of periapical surgery was decided in accordance with the indications given by the European Society of Endodontology, 2006 (point 3: presence of persisting periapical disease after root canal retreatment).

Under local anaesthesia, the full thickness trapezoidal mucoperiosteal flap was reflected with vertical releasing incisions taken from the mesial aspect of 43 and 33. The surgical site was flushed with sterile saline after thorough curettage of the lesion (Figure 2(c)). Following which, apicectomy and retrograde MTA filling were done (Figure 2(d)). The CGF preparation was similar as described in Case Report 1, and the prepared CGF was placed inside the surgical site and covered with CGF membrane (Figures 2(e), 2(f)). The flap was approximated with interrupted sutures. Follow-up CBCT at 1 year revealed complete healing with complete bone repair, evidently seen in coronal and sagittal views (Figures 2(h), 2(j), 2(l)).

At 1-year follow-up with CBCT, livewire segmentation using OSIRIX Version 9.5 (PIXMEO, Geneva, Switzerland) was done to delineate the lesion from the healthy bone. In case 1, the preoperative and postoperative volume calculations were $0.7862\,cm^3$ and $0.08\,cm^3$, respectively. The lesion size reduction was found to be 89.2%. In case 2, the preoperative and postoperative volume calculations were $0.1358\,cm^3$ and $0.0101\,cm^3$, respectively. The lesion size reduction was found to be 92.5%.

3. Discussion

Our case reports are unique in that CGF was produced using the recommended centrifuge, and it was used as a sole material to understand its exclusive role in repair and regeneration after periapical surgery.

During the preparation of APCs, the quality of the resultant product is greatly influenced by centrifugal characteristics like rotational speed (rpm), time (min), and centrifugation protocols. The centrifugation method for CGF is "preprogrammed" and the resultant CGF is stronger, thicker, and abundant with growth factors. The centrifuge is equipped with self-ventilation that prevents the temperature rise which helps to maintain the viability of enmeshed cells in the fibrin matrix. The dense three-dimensional network of the fibrin ensures slow release of growth factors. Park et al. affirmed that CGF consisted of thicker fibrinogen fibres per area unit and regular fibrinogen structures compared to PRF [10].

The presence of growth factors and leucocytes including also the few CD34+ circulating cells that are concentrated in a small volume is the probable reason for this success, since all the elements have been demonstrated to play an important role in vascular maintenance, angiogenesis, and neovascularization. Park et al. reported that TGF-β1 was released for one week whereas PDGF-BB for 3 weeks and identified that VEGF was one and a half times more in CGF than PRF [10]. However, Qin et al. showed that TGF-β1 had a slow release for 13 days [11]. In a contrasting study, the levels of growth factors released (except bFGF) did not differ significantly among PRP, PRF, and CGF [12].

Growth factors act on target tissues and regulate a variety of cellular events including cell migration, proliferation, and differentiation. Borsani et al. have ascertained that CGF addition enhanced cell proliferation of fibroblasts, endothelial cells, and osteoblasts which are involved in angiogenesis, tissue remodelling and regeneration [13].

There are two case reports in the literature which describe the utilization of CGF in periapical surgery. In the first, CGF was not prepared with the special centrifuge [14]. In the second, CGF was used along with the sticky bone and Mphi laser [15]. Even though both the cases had unfavourable prognostic factors, the follow-up has affirmed the encouraging effect of CGF which has shortened the healing time of extensive periapical lesions to 6 months. This finding corroborates with the outcome of the case reports by Sohn which described two cases of sinus augmentation in which CGF alone was used as a substitute for bone graft and the results established that healing was reduced to half the average healing period without bone graft placement [16]. The benefits of CGF are that it is autologous, can be easily prepared, and cost-effective than bone grafts and membranes in extensive periapical lesions. Taking into account the above benefits, CGF can be earmarked as an ingenious biomaterial for bone regeneration.

4. Conclusion

Considering the encouraging result of these case reports, concentrated growth factors could be recommended as an alternative to bone grafts and membranes in extensive periapical lesions to enhance bone regeneration and to decrease the healing time. However, this case series is an initiative for application of CGF in endodontic surgery. The utilization of CGF in endodontics can be extended to revascularization procedures and endo-perio lesions also. However, the major limitation is that according to the CEBM level of evidence, the case reports have the lowest level of evidence. A well-designed randomized clinical trial is recommended to comprehend the long-term risks and benefits of using CGF in regenerative endodontics.

Acknowledgments

We thank Dr. Sri Prakash for CGF preparation and Dr. Susila for helping during manuscript preparation.

References

[1] Y.-L. Ng, V. Mann, S. Rahbaran, J. Lewsey, and K. Gulabivala, "Outcome of primary root canal treatment: systematic review of the literature–part 1. Effects of study characteristics on probability of success," *International Endodontic Journal*, vol. 40, no. 12, pp. 921–939, 2007.

[2] W. H. Archer, *Oral and Maxillofacial Surgery*, WB Saunders Company, 1975.

[3] L. M. Lin, D. Ricucci, and T. von Arx, "Guided tissue regeneration in endodontic surgery: principle, efficacy, and complications," in *Complications in Endodontic Surgery*, Springer, 2014.

[4] M. Del Fabbro, V. Ceresoli, A. Lolato, and S. Taschieri, "Effect of platelet concentrate on quality of life after periradicular surgery: a randomized clinical study," *Journal of Endodontia*, vol. 38, no. 6, pp. 733–739, 2012.

[5] T. Kawase and T. Tanaka, "An updated proposal for terminology and classification of platelet-rich fibrin," *Regenerative Therapy*, vol. 7, pp. 80-81, 2017.

[6] N. Meschi, A. B. Castro, K. Vandamme, M. Quirynen, and P. Lambrechts, "The impact of autologous platelet concentrates on endodontic healing: a systematic review," *Platelets*, vol. 27, no. 7, pp. 613–633, 2016.

[7] the CARE Group, J. J. Gagnier, G. Kienle et al., "The CARE guidelines: consensus-based clinical case reporting guideline development," *Journal of Medical Case Reports*, vol. 7, no. 1, p. 223, 2013.

[8] C. Estrela, M. R. Bueno, B. C. Azevedo, J. R. Azevedo, and J. D. Pécora, "A new periapical index based on cone beam computed tomography," *Journal of Endodontia*, vol. 34, no. 11, pp. 1325–1331, 2008.

[9] M. Serrano-Giménez, A. Sanchez-Torres, and C. Gay-Escoda, "Prognostic factors on periapical surgery: a systematic review," *Medicina Oral Patología Oral y Cirugia Bucal*, vol. 20, no. 6, pp. e715–e722, 2015.

[10] H. C. Park, S. G. Kim, J. S. Oh et al., "Early bone formation at a femur defect using CGF and PRF grafts in adult dogs: a comparative study," *Implant Dentistry*, vol. 25, no. 3, pp. 387–393, 2016.

[11] J. Qin, L. Wang, L. Zheng et al., "Concentrated growth factor promotes Schwann cell migration partly through the integrin β1-mediated activation of the focal adhesion kinase pathway," *International Journal of Molecular Medicine*, vol. 37, no. 5, pp. 1363–1370, 2016.

[12] L. F. Rodella, G. Favero, R. Boninsegna et al., "Growth factors, CD34 positive cells, and fibrin network analysis in concentrated growth factors fraction," *Microscopy Research and Technique*, vol. 74, no. 8, pp. 772–777, 2011.

[13] E. Borsani, V. Bonazza, B. Buffoli et al., "Biological characterization and in vitro effects of human concentrated growth factor preparation: an innovative approach to tissue regeneration," *Biology and Medicine*, vol. 7, no. 5, p. 726, 2015.

[14] S. Mirković, T. Đurđević-Mirković, and T. Puškar, "Application of concentrated growth factors in reconstruction of bone defects after removal of large jaw cysts: the two cases report," *Vojnosanitetski Pregled*, vol. 72, no. 4, pp. 368–371, 2015.

[15] N. Doan, L. Nguyen-Pham, C. Liang, and Q. T. Duong, "A review on the application of concentrated growth factors and MPhi laser to regenerate oral defects in the oral and maxillofacial region and a two cases report," *International Journal of Oral and Maxillofacial Surgery*, vol. 46, Supplement 1, pp. 203-204, 2017.

[16] D. S. Sohn, *The Use of Concentrated Growth Factors as Alternative to Bone Substitutes for Sinus Augmentation*, Dental Inc., 2009.

20

Intramuscular Myxoma of the Intrinsic Muscles of the Tongue: A Case Report with Literature Review

Naoko Tsunoda,[1] Kei Onodera,[1] Yu Ohashi,[1] Tadashi Kawai,[1] Ikuya Miyamoto,[1] Yasunori Takeda,[2] and Hiroyuki Yamada[1]

[1]*Division of Oral and Maxillofacial Surgery, Department of Oral and Macillofacial Reconstructive Surgery, School of Dentistry, Iwate Medical University, Morioka 020-8505, Japan*
[2]*Division of Clinical Pathology, Department of Oral and Maxillofacial Reconstructive Surgery, School of Dentistry, Iwate Medical University, Morioka 020-8505, Japan*

Correspondence should be addressed to Hiroyuki Yamada; yamadah@iwate-med.ac.jp

Academic Editor: Darko Macan

Myxoma is a benign tumor of mesenchymal origin. It frequently occurs in the muscles of the hip and extremities; however, it rarely occurs in the head and neck region. This report describes the second case of an intramuscular myxoma of the tongue. A 23-year-old woman was referred to our institution for the diagnosis and treatment of a left tongue lesion. T2-weighted magnetic resonance imaging revealed an 8×6-mm mass in the tongue. Based on a clinical diagnosis of a tongue tumor, excisional biopsy was performed under general anesthesia. The histopathological diagnosis was an intramuscular myxoma. The postoperative course was uneventful, and there was no evidence of tumor recurrence 3 years after surgery.

1. Introduction

Myxoma is a benign tumor of mesenchymal origin. It frequently occurs in the muscles of the hip and extremities; however, it rarely occurs in the head and neck region [1]. The symptoms of myxoma include indolent swelling and a slowly growing mass. Myxomas show a female predilection, and most cases are diagnosed between 40 and 70 years of age [1]. No reports have described malignant transformation or metastasis of a myxoma.

In the head and neck region, odontogenic myxomas develop in the maxilla or mandible. They are neoplasms of odontogenic origin and thus differ from soft tissue myxoma, which is classified as a tumor of uncertain differentiation [2]. Because of the rarity of soft tissue myxomas, most clinicians are unfamiliar with their clinic findings.

We herein report the second case of an intramuscular myxoma of the tongue, together with a literature review.

2. Case Presentation

A 23-year-old woman was referred to our institution for the diagnosis and treatment of a left tongue lesion. She had first noticed the lesion approximately 1 month earlier. The patient's medical and family histories were unremarkable. Intraoral examination revealed a 10-mm-diameter elastic soft mass in the left tongue. The overlying mucosa was normal (Figure 1). There was no evidence of cervical lymphadenopathy.

Magnetic resonance imaging (MRI) was performed with a 3.0-Tesla system (MR750; General Electric Company, Boston, MA, USA). On T1-weighted axial images, the mass in the left tongue showed low signal intensity relative to muscle. On T2-weighted images, increased signal intensity was noted within the lesion (Figure 2). The lesion showed a homogeneous appearance. The size of the mass was 8×6 mm. No tumorous lesion was obvious in either the maxilla or mandible.

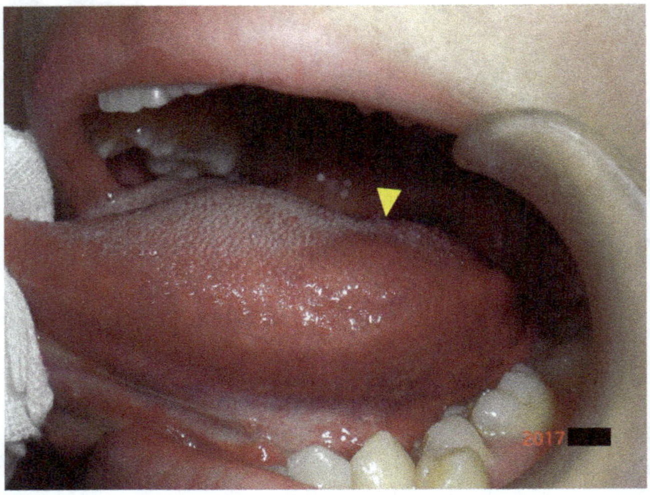

Figure 1: Intraoral photograph showing an elastic soft mass measuring 10 mm in diameter in the left tongue (arrowhead). The overlying mucosa is normal.

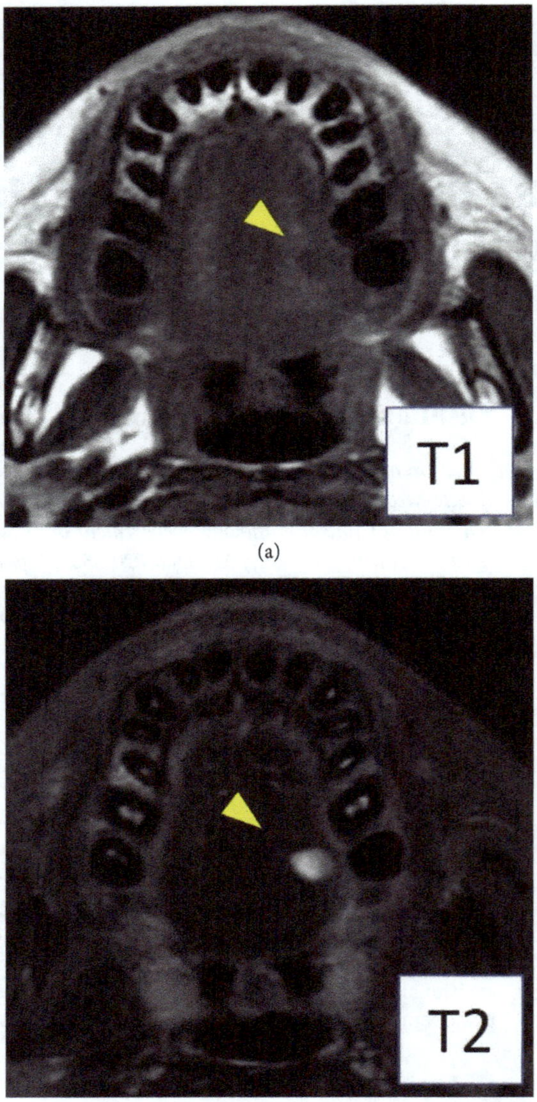

(a)

(b)

Figure 2: Magnetic resonance imaging findings. (a) T1-weighted axial image showing low signal intensity within the lesion (arrowhead). (b) T2-weighted axial image showing increased signal intensity within the lesion (arrowhead).

Based on a clinical diagnosis of a benign tongue tumor, excisional biopsy was performed under general anesthesia. A spindle-shaped incision was made on the lateral surface of the left tongue. The specimen was pulled outward with slight lateral traction and cut using a surgical scalpel. Finally, the whole tumor with surrounding soft tissue was obtained as a surgical specimen (Figure 3). Histopathological examination of the resected tumor revealed that the tumor within the muscle was encapsulated by fibrous connective tissue. Stellate and spindle-shaped cells with no atypia were observed within an abundant myxoid extracellular matrix (Figure 4). No mitotic figures were present. Immunohistochemical analysis revealed that the tumor cells were positive for vimentin (Figure 5) and negative for desmin and cyclin-dependent kinase 4. Thus, the histopathological diagnosis was an intramuscular myxoma.

The postoperative course was uneventful. There was no evidence of tumor recurrence 3 years after surgery.

3. Discussion

Intramuscular myxomas in the head and neck are rare. To the best of our knowledge, 33 cases of intramuscular myxomas in the head and neck, including the present case, have been reported in the literature to date [3–34]. These cases are summarized in Table 1. The patients comprised 14 men and 19 women, and their mean age was 49.0 years (range, 2–86 years). The most frequently involved site was the posterior neck in nine patients, followed by the masseter muscle in four patients. Most cases were sporadic; however, one patient had multiple lesions [10]. The maximum length of the tumor ranged from 0.6 to 15.0 cm, and the tumor in the present case was the second smallest.

Typical MRI findings of intramuscular myxomas are homogeneous low signal intensity in T1-weighted images and high signal intensity in T2-weighted images [35]. Luna et al. [36] reported that 7 of 18 intramuscular myxomas showed an inhomogeneous appearance in T2-weighted images, probably because fibrous internal septa are sometimes seen in intramuscular myxomas. MRI was performed in 12 of 33 intramuscular myxomas in the head and neck region. Nine of these 12 cases showed low to intermediate signal intensity in T1-weighted images and high signal intensity in T2-weighted images [20, 22, 24, 26, 27, 29, 31, 33]. In addition, internal septa were recognized in two large tumors [20, 22]. However, these findings are nonspecific; therefore, no cases were diagnosed as an intramuscular myxoma on MRI.

Preoperative fine needle aspiration cytology was performed in 8 of 33 intramuscular myxomas in the head and neck. Only one case was correctly diagnosed as a myxoma [13]. A diagnosis of myxoma was not reached in the remaining seven cases [12, 15, 18, 20, 23, 26, 34]. Therefore, it is

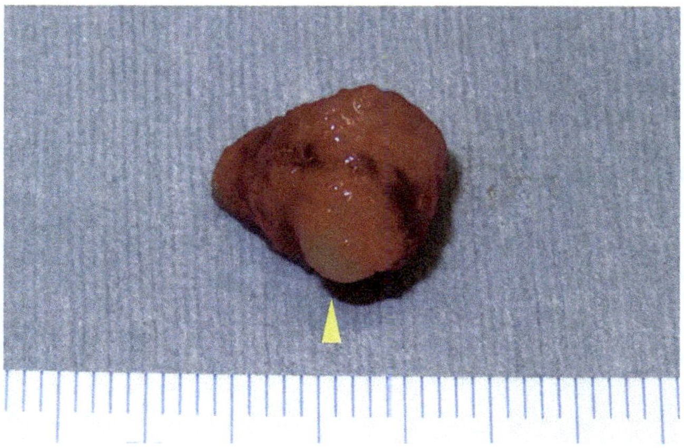

FIGURE 3: Photograph showing the resected tumor (arrowhead) surrounded by the muscle of the tongue.

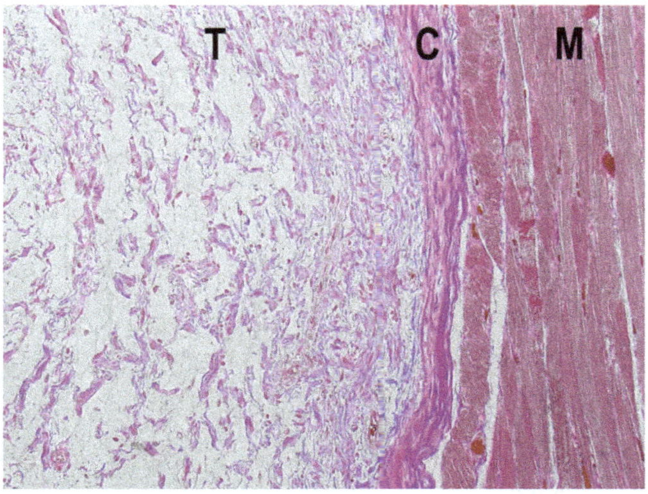

FIGURE 4: Photomicrograph showing stellate and spindle-shaped cells with no atypia in the abundant myxoid extracellular matrix (hematoxylin–eosin stain, ×100). T: tumor, C: fibrous capsule, M: muscle of the tongue.

difficult to achieve the correct diagnosis of myxoma by fine needle aspiration cytology.

The histopathological differential diagnoses of intramuscular myxoma include low-grade myxofibrosarcoma, myxoid liposarcoma, nerve sheath myxoma, and oral focal mucinosis. Low-grade myxofibrosarcoma exhibits infiltrative behavior [2]; however, the tumor in the present case was encapsulated by fibrous connective tissue. Although myxoid liposarcoma contains a prominent myxoid stroma, its characteristic findings of moderate cellularity and lobulated morphology are not seen in intramuscular myxoma [2]. Nerve sheath myxoma is a benign peripheral nerve sheath tumor composed of small epithelioid, ring-like, and spindled Schwann cells [2]. The findings of a multinodular growth pattern and epithelioid Schwann cells arranged in cords can distinguish nerve sheath myxoma from intramuscular myxoma. Oral focal mucinosis is non-neoplastic lesion that likely develops secondary to overproduction of hyaluronic acid by fibroblasts [37]. Fragmented and randomly arranged ropey collagen fibers seen in oral focal mucinosis can help to differentiate it from intramuscular myxoma. In the present case, the encapsulated tumor in the muscle was composed of stellate and spindle-shaped cells with no atypia within an abundant myxoid extracellular matrix. In addition, the tumor cells were negative for desmin and cyclin-dependent kinase 4. These findings were consistent with the diagnosis of intramuscular myxoma.

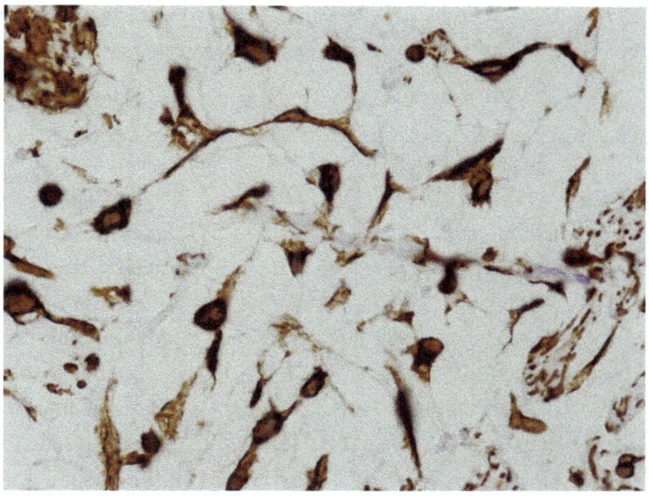

FIGURE 5: Histopathologic photograph showing the results of immunohistochemical analyses for vimentin, which is positive in the tumor cells (vimentin, ×400).

Mazabraud syndrome, which was first reported by the French physician Mazabraud [38] in 1967, is characterized by the combination of multiple intramuscular myxomas and fibrous dysplasia. Care should be taken to avoid overlooking this lesion because Fu et al. [39] reported a sporadic intramuscular myxoma of the masseter muscle with mandibular fibrous dysplasia. In the present case, the MRI findings ruled out fibrous dysplasia in the head and neck; however, other bone sites were not screened because of the absence of clinical symptoms. Therefore, the possibility of Mazabraud syndrome was not completely excluded in the present case.

An intramuscular myxoma in the head and neck region is treated by surgical excision. Recurrence is rare; only two myxomas in the posterior neck [9] and in the lip [14] recurred after surgery. In the case of the posterior neck myxoma [9], the tumor recurred 2 months after the operation because of an inadequate margin of resection as evident by microscopic examination. Reoperation with a wider margin of resection resulted in no evidence of recurrence during 16 years of follow-up. In the other case involving the lip [14], the reason for the recurrence was explained by the absence of a fibrous capsule with tumor infiltration to the surrounding muscle. Reoperation was performed, and no recurrence was reported for 2 years thereafter. Preoperative diagnosis of intramuscular myxoma is difficult, and inadequate resection is associated with recurrence. Because complete resection of intramuscular myxoma is required, some

Table 1: Reported cases of intramuscular Myxoma in the head and neck.

No.	Author, year	Age/ gender	Location	Preoperative examination	Size (cm)	Recurrence (postoperative months)	Follow-up period (months)
1	Enzinger, 1965 [3]	55/F	Sternocleidomastoid muscle	N/A	2.5 × 1.5 × 1.3	Absent	48
2	Rosin, 1973 [4]	44/M	Geniohyoid muscle	N/A	2.0	Absent	18
3	Kindblom et al., 1974 [5]	42/F	Occipitofrontalis muscle	N/A	N/A	Absent	144
4	Canalis et al., 1976 [6]	46/F	Lateral part of neck	N/A	N/A	Absent	24
5	Feldman, 1979 [7]	62/F	Posterior neck	N/A	3.0	Absent	120
6	Bedrosian et al., 1984 [8]	43/F	Masseter muscle	N/A	1.0	Absent	N/A
7	Wood, 1985 [9]	51/M	Posterior neck	N/A	N/A	Present (2)	192
8	Nisijima et al., 1985 [10]	16/F	Digastric muscle	US, CT	1.5, 1.5	Absent	120
9	Hashimoto et al., 1986 [11]	43/F	Massester muscle	N/A	2.0 × 1.0	Absent	55.2
10	Shugar et al., 1987 [12]	68/F	Levator scapulae muscle	CT, FNAC	4.0	Absent	12
11	Mockli et al., 1993 [13]	60/F	Tongue	FNAC	2.0	Absent	N/A
12	Orlandi et al., 1995 [14]	46/M	Orbicularis muscle	X-ray	3.0	Present (5)	24
13	Serrat et al., 1998 [15]	62/M	Temporalis muscle	CT, FNAC	5.0 × 4.0	Absent	9
14	van Roggen et al., 2001 [16]	56/M	Cheek	N/A	3.0	Absent	49
15	Crankson et al., 2002 [17]	5/F	Posterior triangle	US, CT	4.0	Absent	12
16	Robin et al., 2004 [18]	43/F	Temporalis muscle	CT, FNAC	3.5 × 2.6 × 2.0	Absent	18
17	Ozawa et al., 2004 [19]	22/M	Scalene muscle	US, CT	7.0 × 4.0 × 3.0	Absent	48
18	Ishoo, 2007 [20]	2/F	Posterior cervical triangle	CT, MRI, FNAC	5.0 × 4.0	Absent	24
19	Carlson et al., 2009 [21]	15/M	Stapedius muscle	MRI	0.6 × 0.4	N/A	N/A
20	Falavigna et al., 2009 [22]	64/F	Paraspinal muscle	CT, MRI	15.0	Absent	12
21	Papadogeorgakis, 2009 [23]	74/M	Masseter muscle	CT, FNAC	3.0 × 2.0	Absent	26
22	Patsiaoura et al., 2010 [24]	52/M	Mimetic muscle	MRI	2.0 × 1.3	Absent	8
23	Li et al., 2012 [25]	45/F	Posterior neck	US,CT	4.1 × 2.8 × 4.9	Absent	12
24	Kalshi et al., 2013 [26]	70/F	Sternocleidmastoid muscle	CT, MRI, FNAC	2.0 × 1.2 × 1.6	Absent	60
25	Higashida, 2014 [27]	51/M	Temporalis muscle	CT, MRI	6.5 × 4.0 × 3.0	Absent	6
26	Li et al., 2014 [28]	74/M	Hyoglossus muscle	CT	7.9 × 7.9	Absent	36
27	Tataryn et al., 2015 [29]	57/F	Cervical paraspinal musclature	MRI	2.0	Absent	N/A
28	Egami et al., 2015 [30]	76/M	Frontalis muscle	US	2.0	Absent	12
29	Rachidi et al., 2016 [31]	45/M	Levator scapulae and scalane	US, CT, MRI	2.7 × 2.5 × 1.4	Absent	30
30	Custódio et al., 2020 [32]	60/F	Masseter muscle	MRI	N/A	Absent	N/A
31	Nishi et al., 2021 [33]	59/M	Medial pterygoid muscle	MRI	1.75 × 1.36 × 0.71	Absent	6
32	Mijalis et al., 2021 [34]	86/F	Sternocleidmastoid muscle	CT, MRI, FNAC	3.5 × 3.4 × 4.8	Absent	0.25
33	Present case	23/F	Tongue	MRI	0.8 × 0.6	Absent	36

N/A: not applicable, CT: computed tomography, MRI: magnetic resonance imaging, FNAC: fine needle aspiration cytology.

surrounding soft tissue resection is advisable rather than injuring the fibrous capsule of the tumor.

In conclusion, this is the second reported case of an intramuscular myxoma of the tongue [13]. A correct preoperative diagnosis could not be obtained; however, typical findings of an intramuscular myxoma were seen on MRI. The clinical course of such lesions is not fully understood because of their rarity; therefore, long-term clinical follow-up is necessary.

Acknowledgments

We thank Angela Morben, DVM, ELS, from Edanz (https://jp.edanz.com/ac), for editing a draft of this manuscript.

References

[1] M. Miettinen, J. F. Fetsch, C. R. Antonescu, A. L. Folpe, and P. E. Wakely, *Tumors of the Soft Tissues. Nonmalignant Fbro-*

blastic and Myofiblastic Tomors and Tumor-Like Lesions, American Registry of Pathology, Silver Spring, 2015.

[2] WHO Classification of Tumours Editorial Board, *Soft Tissue and Bone Tumours*, World Health Organization, Lyon, 5th ed. edition, 2020.

[3] F. M. Enzinger, "Intramuscular Myxoma; a review and follow-up study of 34 cases," *American Journal of Clinical Pathology*, vol. 43, no. 2, pp. 104–113, 1965.

[4] R. D. Rosin, "Intramuscular myxomas," *British Journal of Surgery*, vol. 60, no. 2, pp. 122–124, 2005.

[5] L. G. Kindblom, B. Stener, and L. Angervall, "Intramuscular myxoma," *Cancer*, vol. 34, no. 5, pp. 1737–1744, 1974.

[6] R. F. Canalis, G. A. Smith, and H. R. Konrad, "Myxomas of the head and neck," *Archives of Otolaryngology*, vol. 102, no. 5, pp. 300–305, 1976.

[7] P. S. Feldman, "A comparative study including ultrastructure of intramuscular myxoma and myxoid liposarcoma," *Cancer*, vol. 43, no. 2, pp. 512–525, 1979.

[8] S. A. Bedrosian, R. L. Goldman, and M. J. Pearl, "Intramuscular myxoma of the masseter," *Journal of Oral and Maxillofacial Surgery*, vol. 42, no. 10, pp. 684–686, 1984.

[9] W. J. Wood Jr., "Intramuscular myxoma: report of two cases and review of the literature," *Arizona Medicine*, vol. 42, no. 7, pp. 417–419, 1985.

[10] W. Nishijima, N. Tokita, I. Watanabe, and S. Takooda, "Intramuscular myxoma of the neck," *Archives of Otorhinolaryngology*, vol. 111, no. 10, pp. 699–701, 1985.

[11] H. Hashimoto, M. Tsuneyoshi, Y. Daimaru, M. Enjoji, and N. Shinohara, "Intramuscular myxoma. A clinicopathologic, immunohistochemical, and electron microscopic study," *Cancer*, vol. 58, no. 3, pp. 740–747, 1986.

[12] J. M. Shugar, P. M. Som, R. J. Meyers, and B. T. Schaeffer, "Intramuscular head and neck myxoma: report of a case and review of the literature," *The Laryngoscope*, vol. 97, no. 1, pp. 105–107, 1987.

[13] G. C. Mockli, B. M. Ljung, and R. L. Goldman, "Fine needle aspiration of intramuscular myxoma of the tongue. A case report," *Acta Cytologica*, vol. 37, no. 2, pp. 226–228, 1993.

[14] A. Orlandi, L. Bianchi, B. Marino, L. G. Spagnoli, and G. Nini, "Intramuscular myxoma of the face: an unusual localization. A clinicopathological study," *Dermatologic Surgery*, vol. 21, no. 3, pp. 251–254, 1995.

[15] A. Serrat, A. Verrier, A. Espeso, and J. Martín, "Intramuscular myxoma of the temporalis muscle," *Journal of Oral and Maxillofacial Surgery*, vol. 56, no. 10, pp. 1206–1208, 1998.

[16] J. F. van Roggen, M. E. McMenamin, and C. D. Fletcher, "Cellular myxoma of soft tissue: a clinicopathological study of 38 cases confirming indolent clinical behaviour," *Histopathology*, vol. 39, no. 3, pp. 287–297, 2001.

[17] S. J. Crankson, M. Al Namshan, K. Al Mane, and H. Bamefleh, "Intramuscular myxoma: a rare neck mass in a child," *Pediatric Radiology*, vol. 32, no. 2, pp. 120–122, 2002.

[18] C. Robin, J. A. Bastidas, and B. Boguslaw, "Case report: myxoma of the temporalis muscle," *Oral Surgery, Oral Medicine, Oral Pathology, Oral Radiology, and Endodontology*, vol. 97, no. 5, pp. 620–624, 2004.

[19] H. Ozawa, M. Fujii, T. Tomita, and K. Ogawa, "Intramuscular myxoma of scalene muscle: a case report," *Auris Nasus Larynx*, vol. 31, no. 3, pp. 319–322, 2004.

[20] E. Ishoo, "Intramuscular myxoma presenting as a rare posterior neck mass in a young child: case report and literature review," *Archives of Otorhinolaryngology-Head & Neck Surgery*, vol. 133, no. 4, pp. 398–401, 2007.

[21] M. L. Carlson, M. J. Shinners, and R. S. Haberman, "Pathology quiz case 2. Intramuscular myxoma of the stapedius muscle," *Archives of Otorhinolaryngology-Head & Neck Surgery*, vol. 135, no. 2, pp. 217, 219–220, 2009.

[22] A. Falavigna, O. Righesso, D. Volquind, and A. R. Teles, "Intramuscular myxoma of the cervical paraspinal muscle," *European Spine Journal*, vol. 18, Suppl 2, pp. 245–249, 2009.

[23] N. Papadogeorgakis, V. Petsinis, N. Nikitakis, L. Goutzanis, and C. Alexandridis, "Intramuscular myxoma of the masseter muscle. A case report," *Oral and Maxillofacial Surgery*, vol. 13, no. 1, pp. 37–40, 2009.

[24] K. Patsiaoura, E. Anagnostou, and N. Benis, "Intramuscular myxoma of the nasal vestibule," *Auris Nasus Larynx*, vol. 37, no. 1, pp. 100–102, 2010.

[25] J. Li, J. Wang, and Z. Shi, "Intramuscular myxoma of trapezius in an adult woman," *The American Surgeon*, vol. 78, no. 3, pp. E135–E136, 2012.

[26] J. S. Kalsi, M. Pring, C. Hughes, and A. Fasanmade, "Presentation of intramuscular myxoma as an unusual neck lump," *Journal of Oral and Maxillofacial Surgery*, vol. 71, no. 5, pp. e210–e214, 2013.

[27] T. Higashida, "Radiological characteristics and management of intramuscular myxoma of the temporal muscle: case report," *Neurologia Medico-Chirurgica*, vol. 54, no. 12, pp. 1022–1025, 2014.

[28] G. Li, W. Jiang, W. Li, and J. Li, "Intramuscular myxoma of the hyoglossus muscle: a case report and literature review," *Oncology Letters*, vol. 7, no. 5, pp. 1679–1682, 2014.

[29] Z. Tataryn, J. Tracy, C. Tsang, J. Wu, C. B. Heilman, and R. O. Wein, "Intramuscular myxoma of the cervical paraspinal musculature: case report and review of the literature," *American Journal of Otolaryngology*, vol. 36, no. 2, pp. 273–276, 2015.

[30] S. Egami, H. Honda, T. Yokoyama, and M. Sugiura, "Intramuscular myxoma on the forehead: an unusual localization with useful sonographic findings," *The Journal of Dermatology*, vol. 42, no. 11, pp. 1111–1112, 2015.

[31] S. Rachidi, A. J. Sood, T. Rumboldt, and T. A. Day, "Intramuscular myxoma of the paraspinal muscles: a case report and systematic review of the literature," *Oncology Letters*, vol. 11, no. 1, pp. 466–470, 2016.

[32] M. Custódio, E. S. Antunes, G. B. M. Alves, and P. H. Braz-Silva, "Unexpected diagnosis of an intramuscular myxoma arising from the masseter muscle," *The British Journal of Oral & Maxillofacial Surgery*, vol. 58, no. 1, pp. 109–111, 2020.

[33] M. Nisi, R. Izzetti, M. Gabriele, and A. Pucci, "Oral intramuscular myxoma: case report and brief review of the literature," *Oral Surgery, Oral Medicine, Oral Pathology, Oral Radiology*, vol. 131, no. 2, pp. e52–ee8, 2021.

[34] E. M. Mijalis, B. Manzi, H. Cuellar, and C. A. O. Nathan, "Intramuscular myxoma of the longus colli mistaken for a cervical rootlet schwannoma," *BMJ Case Reports*, vol. 14, no. 2, 2021.

[35] L. W. Bancroft, M. J. Kransdorf, D. M. Menke, M. I. O'Connor, and W. C. Foster, "Intramuscular myxoma: characteristic MR imaging features," *American Journal of Roentgenology*, vol. 178, no. 5, pp. 1255–1259, 2002.

[36] A. Luna, S. Martinez, and E. Bossen, "Magnetic resonance imaging of intramuscular myxoma with histological compari-

son and a review of the literature," *Skeletal Radiology*, vol. 34, no. 1, pp. 19–28, 2005.

[37] J. L. Silva Cunha, A. A. Leite, A. T. de Castro, L. P. Vervloet, T. M. de Lima Morais, G. de Oliveira Paiva Neto et al., "Oral focal mucinosis: a multi-institutional study and literature review," *Journal of Cutaneous Pathology*, vol. 48, no. 1, pp. 24–33, 2021.

[38] A. Mazabraud, P. Semat, and R. Roze, "Apropos of the association of fibromyxomas of the soft tissues with fibrous dysplasia of the bones," *Presse Médicale*, vol. 75, no. 44, pp. 2223–2228, 1967.

[39] S. Fu, Z. Tian, C. Zhang, and Y. He, "Monosotic fibrous dysplasia and solitary intramuscular myxoma of the head and neck: a unique presentation of Mazabraud's syndrome and a literature review," *Oncology Letters*, vol. 10, no. 5, pp. 3087–3094, 2015.

21

Natural Tooth Pontic using Recent Adhesive Technologies: An Esthetic and Minimally Invasive Prosthetic Solution

Davide Augusti, Gabriele Augusti, Andrei Ionescu, Eugenio Brambilla, and Dino Re

Department of Biomedical, Surgical and Dental Sciences, University of Milan, Italy

Correspondence should be addressed to Gabriele Augusti; g.augusti@libero.it

Academic Editor: Mariano A. Polack

An implant-supported crown represents an established and validated option for single-tooth replacement; however, a restorative solution should be selected according to a wide number of factors including patient's desire, expectations, specific clinical conditions, and financial possibilities. The aim of this case report is to describe a conservative rehabilitation strategy for the replacement of a periodontally compromised mandibular incisor: the extracted natural tooth was used as a pontic bonded to adjacent elements with polyethylene fiber and resin composite. This way, a chairside fabrication of a resin-bonded fiber-reinforced prosthesis is possible, using the patient's own tooth. After showing a satisfactory functional and esthetic result, advantages and pitfalls of this technique along with available data on the literature regarding the natural tooth pontic are addressed. Both patients and clinicians should be aware of minimally invasive, successful solutions for single-tooth replacement; whether indicated or necessary, the natural tooth pontic technique leaves open other treatment options for the future.

1. Introduction

The replacement of a single missing or failing tooth presents one of the greatest challenges in restorative dentistry, especially when the esthetic zone is considered [1]. Nowadays, the main available treatment options to this clinical problem include the use of traditional fixed dental prostheses (FDPs), implant-supported single crowns (SCI), and resin-bonded FDPs (RBFPDs) [2, 3].

Resin-bonded fixed partial dentures (RBFPDs) were first introduced into dentistry in the 1970s [4]: their primary objective was to splint periodontally compromised teeth along with substitution of one or more missing anterior teeth. The application of RBFPDs was extended to posterior areas about ten years later [5]. Compared to implant-supported solutions, RBFPDs are linked to short treatment times and lower postoperative morbidity and costs; surgical procedures are also avoided [6]. With respect to traditional fixed prostheses, RBFPDs can be delivered by minimal or no preparation of natural abutments: this way, an excellent preservation of tooth structure (with reduction of pulpal morbidity) might be achieved [6–8]. The expected survival for indirect (lab-fabricated) RBFPD is relatively high [9]: according to a recent study by Thoma et al., a 91.4% and 82.9% rates were reported after 5 and 10 years of observation, respectively; overcoming complications were mainly related to debonding (15%) and chipping of veneering material (4%). According to a recent systematic review, clinicians should consider using RBFPDs more often because their clinical performance is similar to those of conventional FPDs and implant-supported crowns [10].

Historically, cast RBFPDs were produced exclusively using noble metals like high-gold alloys [5]; nowadays, a wide range of new materials is available: fiber-reinforced composites [11], ceramics with a high content of glass particles (i.e., lithium disilicate, glass-infiltrated zirconia, or alumina) [7, 12], or high-strength ceramics (densely sintered zirconia/alumina polycristal) might be used as frameworks for subsequent veneering or to fabricate monolithic restorations [8, 13].

Fiber-reinforced resin composites (FRC) have been widely adopted in dentistry [14], as direct materials to fabricate periodontal, posttraumatic, or orthodontic splints to stabilize teeth, and for indirect restorative purposes as well. FRC materials consist of glass, carbon, or polyethylene fibers contained within a resin matrix; the type of fiber, its architecture (i.e., spatial arrangement), and the quality of the fiber/matrix coupling determine the mechanical properties of the material [14, 15]. Laboratory studies have shown that FRC materials exhibit a flexural strength that is greater than unreinforced flow or traditional composite materials [15, 16]. By using FRCs, both FDP and RBFDP frameworks can be realized in a minimal invasive fashion, utilizing combinations of various kinds of adhering and retentive elements (like surface bonding wings on anterior areas of the mouth) [11]. A direct, intraoral fabrication of an anterior resin-bonded FRC prosthesis is possible using prefabricated pontics, a denture tooth, or an extracted natural tooth [17].

The immediate bonding of a natural tooth to adjacent elements presents a low-cost alternative for direct tooth replacement [6, 17–19]; this technique enables the original tooth anatomy to be replaced, providing excellent function and esthetics (size, shape, and color) at the same time. Use of patient's own tooth as pontic represents a conservative restorative solution with no laboratory procedures involved; it is well-suited for patients who ask for an immediate replacement of a hopeless tooth in the esthetic zone [20, 21] and are not candidates for implant therapy. The use of a natural tooth as pontic (NTP) provides promising results by means of a combined application of fiber-reinforced materials and adhesive technologies.

The aim of this study is to describe a conservative rehabilitation strategy for the replacement of a periodontally compromised mandibular incisor: the extracted natural tooth was used as pontic, precisely repositioned with a customized index, and finally bonded to adjacent elements with polyethylene ribbon and resin composite. After case illustration, an analysis of available data in the literature related to NTP and associated outcomes will be addressed.

2. Case Presentation

2.1. Patient Presentation and Chief Complaint. A male, 55-year-old Caucasian patient presented at our private practice seeking treatment for increased tooth mobility at the lower right central incisor (tooth number 4.1). The medical history revealed a longstanding, drug-controlled type II diabetes mellitus and single-episode acute pancreatitis. The patient was a nonsmoker and had received some previous treatments in our office in the past; however, he demonstrated poor adherence to follow-up visits and maintenance care. Two panoramic radiographs (Figures 1(a) and 1(b)) were available to evaluate intraoral changes developed during a timespan of approximately ten years (2008-2017). An overall periodontal breakdown was noted with horizontal bone loss, especially at upper and lower anterior areas; upper first premolars and second molars had been extracted, and traditional fixed dental prostheses had been used to replace elements 1.4 and 2.4. In the lower arch, angular bony defects were present at mesial surfaces of teeth 4.7, 4.3, and 3.7/occlusion/overjet/overbite.

Clinically, tooth 4.1 exhibited a deep probing pocket depth (PPD > 10 mm) on both mesial and distal sides, in association with class 2 mobility according to Miller's index (i.e., the tooth is held between the metallic handles of two instruments and moved in the buccolingual or buccopalatal direction; the moved distance is visually estimated by the person carrying out the examination: a score of 2 means a detectable horizontal mobility superior to 1 mm) [22]. Gingival margin inflammation and recession (2 mm) and loss of interdental papilla between lower incisors and supragingival calculus were noted (Figures 2(a) and 2(b)). A periapical radiograph revealed more than 80% of bone support loss and subgingival calculus along the root surface (Figure 3). A poor periodontal prognosis was assigned to the tooth.

2.2. Treatment Plan. During consultation, clinical problems related to the tooth and side effects associated to extraction without replacement were explained to the patient; his main desire was to preserve function and receiving at the same time a cost-effective treatment. In addition, the immediate prosthetic replacement at the stage of surgery was not a priority for the patient: an agreement for a delayed approach was reached (see next). Due to systemic and dental local conditions, a surgical plan based on implant-supported prosthesis (either immediate or delayed) was discarded; adjacent teeth were not affordable abutments for a traditional, fixed, definitive dental bridge.

Despite a poor periodontal prognosis, the color, shape, and position of the lower central incisor were considered acceptable (i.e., good esthetic integration with adjacent teeth). According to the above considerations, a chairside fiber-reinforced composite bridge using the patient's own natural tooth as pontic was the selected therapeutic approach; informed consent was obtained.

2.3. Silicone Index and Tooth Extraction. A preliminary prophylaxis for supra- and subgingival calculus debridement was scheduled: a single session, full-mouth disinfection with mechanical scaling and root planing was carried out one week before extraction. The spatial relationship of the hopeless tooth with adjacent incisors was recorded: a silicone-based, medium-consistency bite registration material (Glassbite® Clear, 80shore; Detax, Ettlingen, Germany) was directly applied on the lower anterior teeth (from canine to canine) and allowed to set (Figure 4(a)). A transparent rigid matrix was finally obtained for accurate repositioning of the lower central incisor after extraction (Figure 4(b)). Customized resin splints have been also suggested for the same purpose [18, 23].

Under local anesthesia, the lower central incisor was atraumatically extracted with forceps; the alveolar socket was carefully debrided/degranulated (with the aid of hand excavators) and finally rinsed with saline solution. 4-0 silk

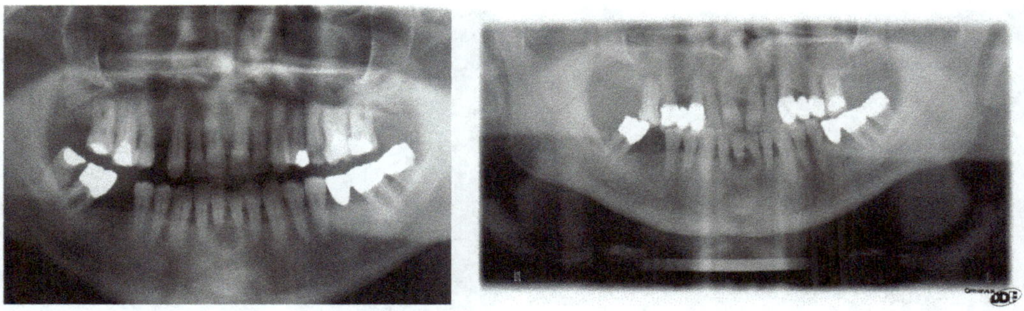

(a) (b)

FIGURE 1: Panoramic radiographs of the patient exposed at year 2008 (a) and 2017 (b): loss of teeth and periodontal breakdown are visible.

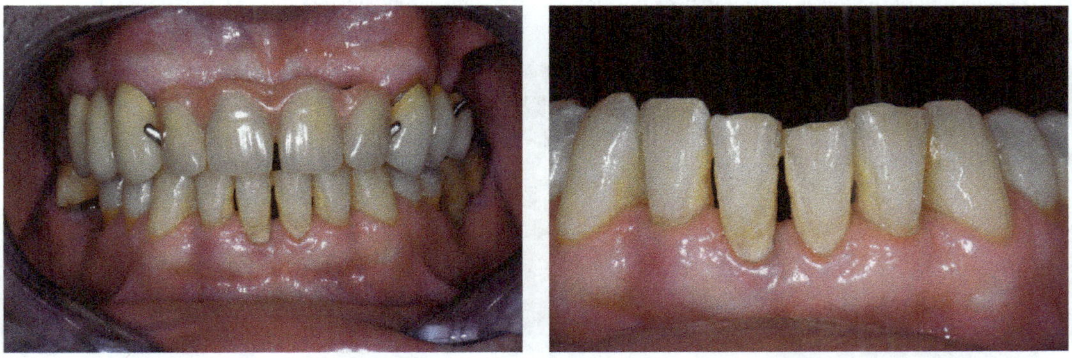

(a) (b)

FIGURE 2: Clinical presentation of the patient at initial examination: (a) full-mouth and (b) frontal lower incisors views.

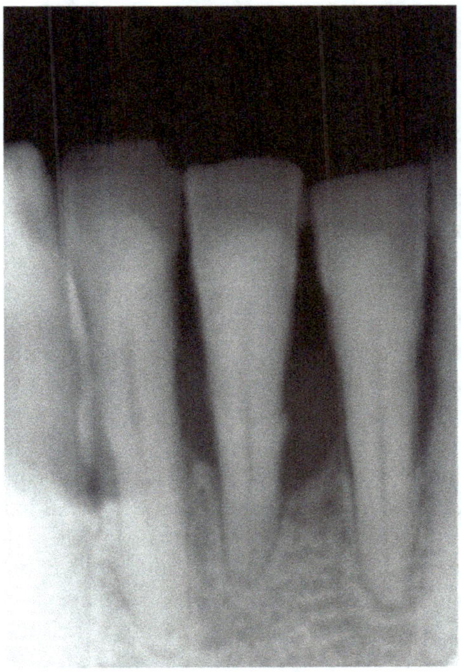

FIGURE 3: A poor periodontal prognosis was assigned to the lower central incisor, showing more than 80% of bone support loss.

crossed sutures were used for gingival and clot stabilization; a postextraction radiograph was exposed (Figures 5(a) and 5(b)). After surgery, initial soft tissue closure and remodeling were deemed necessary for two main reasons: (1) an unpredictable socket healing due to systemic conditions of the patient, suboptimal hygiene control, and periodontal disease affecting the tooth [24]and (2) to provide a more accurate trimming of the extracted crown-root complex following the initial apical repositioning of soft tissues. In the meantime, proper treatment and storage of the extracted tooth was carried out.

2.4. Treatment of the Extracted Tooth and Storage. A traditional endodontic access cavity was prepared; coronal pulp tissue was mechanically removed and chemically dissolved from the chamber to avoid later discoloration through decomposing of organic remnants. The root canal was instrumented using stainless steel manual K-files (up to ISO size #25), along with 5.25% NaOCL and EDTA irrigations. To prevent dehydration, the tooth was kept in saline solution until any further manipulation.

2.5. Try-In. Seven weeks after the extraction procedure, an uneventful healing of soft tissues was confirmed (Figure 6). The root of the extracted tooth was shortened (Figure 7(a)); resection was carried out to produce slight compression and transient ischemia (within three minutes) to the surrounding gingiva (Figures 7(b) and 7(c)). The root canal was irrigated and dried with standardized paper points; a universal adhesive (Scotchbond™ Universal Adhesive, 3M ESPE) was applied with a microbrush along the root canal/pulp chamber walls and photoactivated. Flowable resin composite

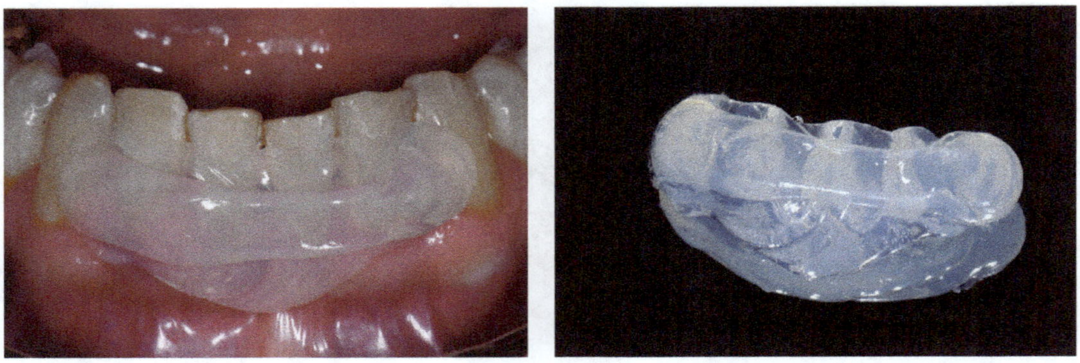

(a) (b)

FIGURE 4: (a) Recording of the lower central incisor position using a transparent silicone index; (b) extraoral view of the matrix.

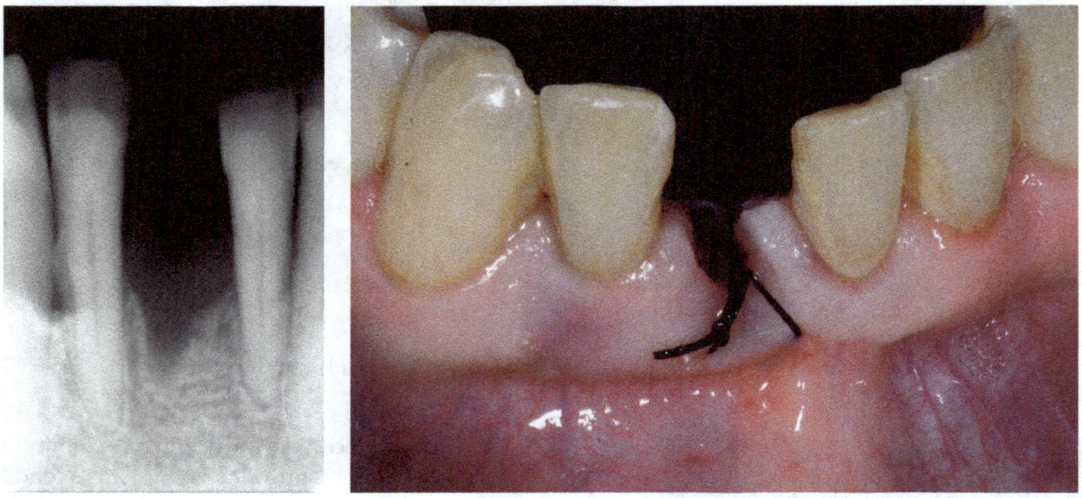

(a) (b)

FIGURE 5: (a) The hopeless tooth was extracted; (b) a cross-suture was useful for clot stabilization.

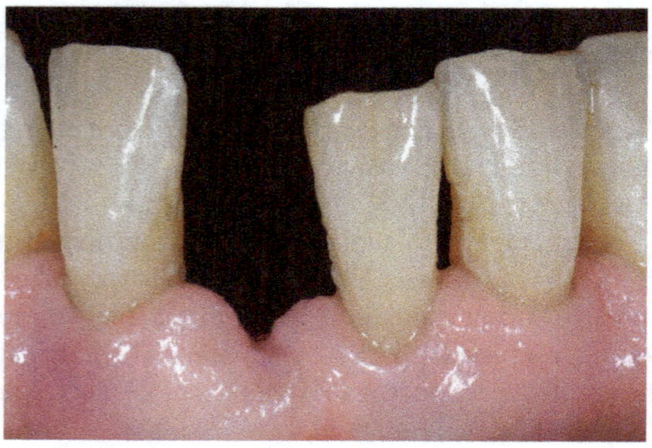

FIGURE 6: Soft tissue healing seven weeks after tooth extraction.

(Clearfil™ Majesty ES Flow, Kuraray Noritake Dental Inc.) was used for sealing of both the access cavity and the root-end preparation; complete light-curing polymerization of 20 s per surface was performed (light unit Bluephase C8, Ivoclar Vivadent). The sealed root-end was shaped to obtain an ovate pontic configuration: the surface was finished to have a smooth and convex contour; final polishing was carried out using pumice paste (coarse/fine grit, Kerr). Steps for the preparation of the extracted tooth are illustrated in Figure 8.

2.6. Splinting of the Natural Tooth Pontic. Proper seating and proximal contacts of the natural tooth pontic were checked, along with the correct shade and texture integration before rubber dam application. The length of the polyethylene fiber (Ribbond™ Ultra, 2 mm width; Ribbond Inc., Seattle, WA, US) required for splinting was measured (with the aid of the previously fabricated silicone index) and cut: all four lower incisors were included. A relative coronal insertion of the fiber was selected to ensure adequate interdental cleaning (with interproximal brushes) of periodontally compromised teeth. Following rubber dam isolation, a superficial groove was prepared on the lingual surfaces of the incisors (coronal third) to inlay the splint (Ribbond™ Ultra thickness: 0.12 mm); a corresponding slot preparation was carried out on the natural tooth pontic at the same level of adjacent teeth. The lingual and proximal surfaces were conditioned with 35% phosphoric acid, rinsed, and dried thoroughly; a single-bottle, multipurpose, light-curing universal adhesive resin ((Scotchbond™ Universal Adhesive, 3M ESPE) was applied to etched preparations according to manufacturer

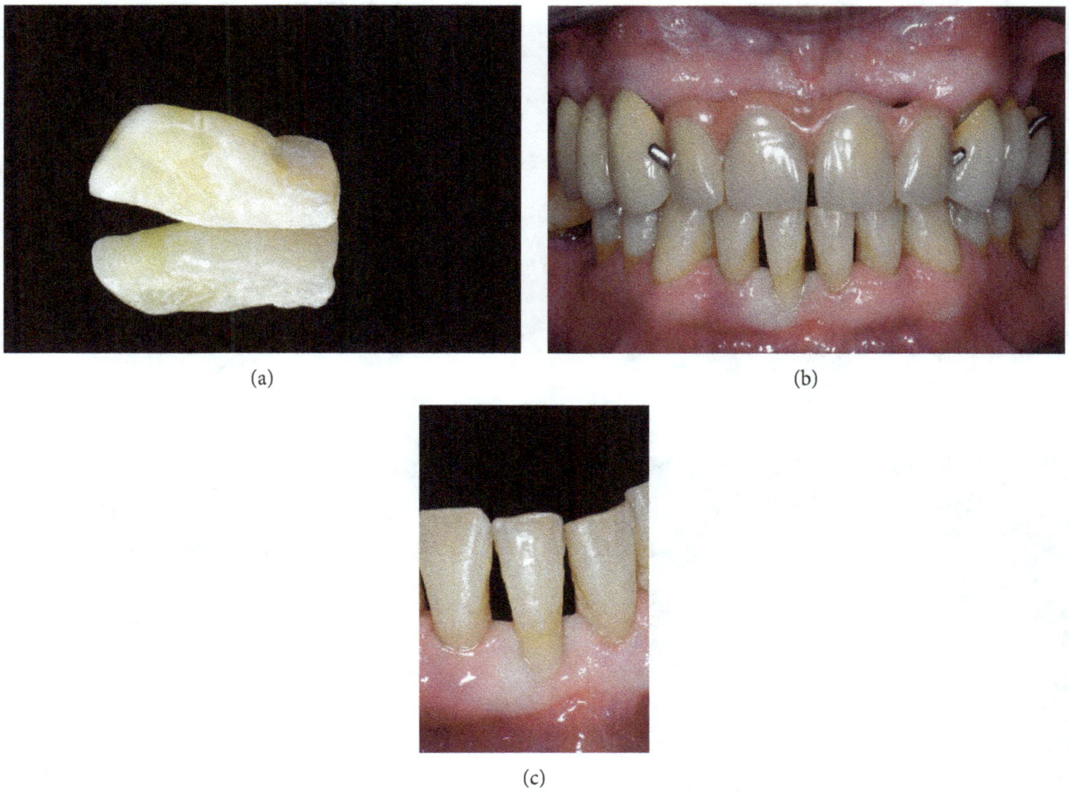

FIGURE 7: (a) Partial resection of the root portion; clinical try-in of the extracted and trimmed tooth revealed slight compression of gingival tissues (b, c).

instructions and light cured for 40 seconds. A thin layer of flowable composite resin (Clearfil™ Majesty ES Flow, Kuraray Noritake Dental Inc.) was applied to the grooves and proximal surfaces of adjacent teeth. Just before placement, the fiber was impregnated with the adhesive bonding agent; then, it was precisely adapted to the preparations with hand instrument—in order to obtain an excellent fit into the slots—and light cured from multiple directions (20 s per surface). The polyethylene fiber is adapted easily to dental contours and can be manipulated during the bonding process; a passive application prevented unintentional orthodontic movement of involved teeth. During flow and fiber placement, the pontic was maintained in a correct spatial relationship with adjacent teeth using the silicone index. A direct composite resin was finally placed and photopolymerized to completely cover the fiber and restore the lingual anatomy of the incisors (Figure 9). All margins were carefully refined and polished using silicon carbide brushes (Jiffy Brushes, Ultradent), until smooth lingual surfaces were obtained. The completed restoration is shown at rubber dam removal (Figures 10(a) and 10(b)); centric and excursive occlusion was verified with articulating papers; premature contacts were eliminated. A final radiograph of the bonded natural tooth pontic was exposed (Figure 11); oral hygiene instructions were given to the patient for proper interdental and under-the-pontic cleanings.

2.7. Follow-Up. The patient was recalled six months later; no fractures of the splint or pontic failure (partial or full debonding) were recorded during this period. A satisfactory esthetic integration with adjacent lower incisors is shown (Figure 12).

3. Discussion

When facing a lost mandibular anterior tooth, alveolar defects of the edentulous area, and/or periodontal disease of adjacent teeth might be present, making implant-supported or traditional FPD restorations more difficult. Our case report demonstrated the chairside fabrication of an FRC-prosthesis, using a natural tooth as pontic, that solution represents a minimally invasive approach for tooth replacement. In addition, the glass fiber composite splint was simultaneously used for stabilization of adjacent teeth with reduced periodontal support [25]. According to current indications [26, 27], splinting of periodontally compromised mobile incisors is an option in case of advanced horizontal bone loss, to improve the patient's comfort (including speaking, biting, and chewing) and to provide better control of occlusion. Statistically significant changes of bone level at splinted teeth over a 10-year period were not observed when active and regular maintenance therapies were undertaken [27]; this way, splinting (that in our case was associated with tooth replacement) can be considered an adjunctive measure to maintain periodontally compromised mobile anterior mandibular teeth in patients attending regular supportive care [27].

Li et al. evaluated indirect (lab fabricated) glass fiber-reinforced RBFPD as periodontal splints to replace lost anterior teeth: a survival rate of 89% at the fourth year was found;

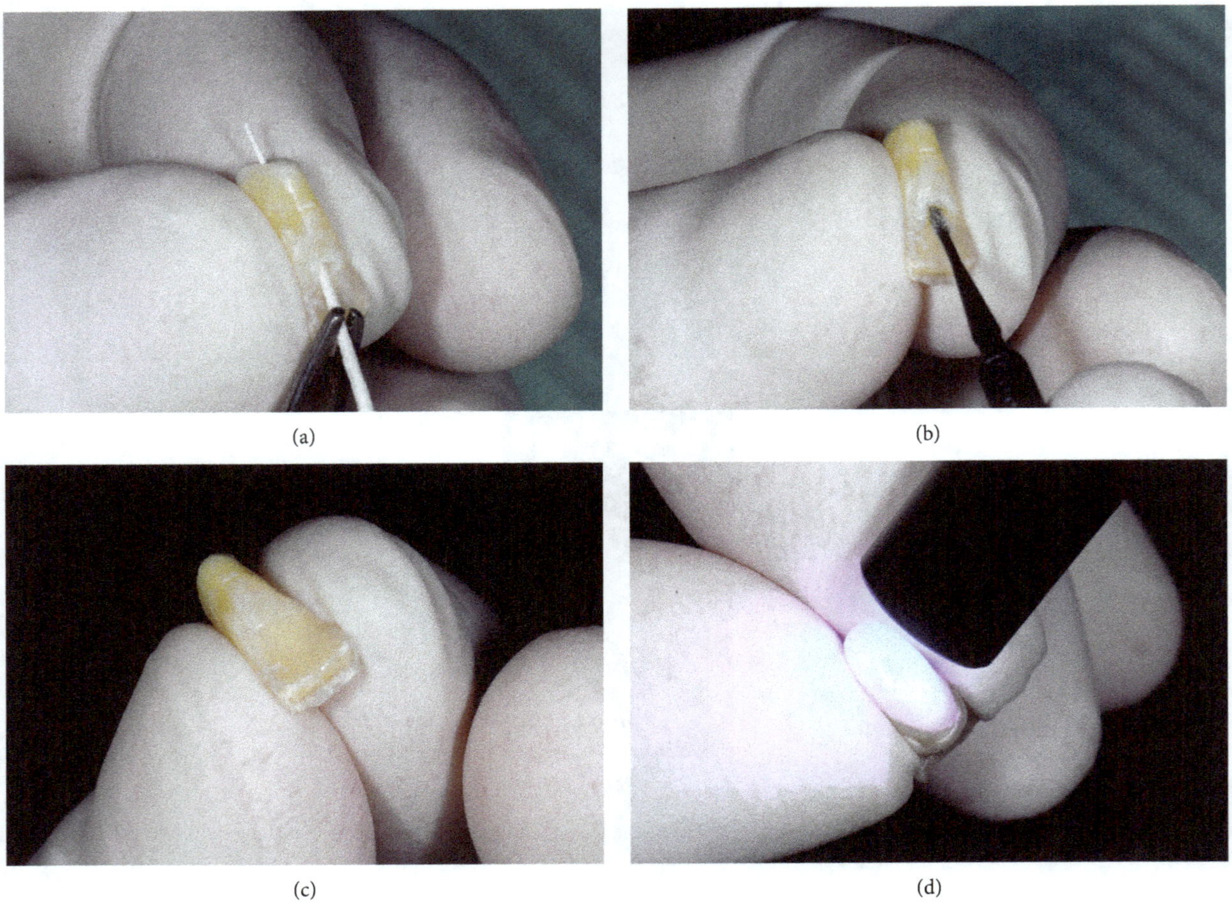

Figure 8: (a) After preliminary etching and rinsing, the tooth canal and pulp chamber were carefully dried with paper points. (b) A single-component, light-curing universal adhesive was applied using a narrow microbrush. (c) Flowable resin composite was used for sealing of both the access cavity and the root-end preparation. (d) Light-curing activation at the pontic surface.

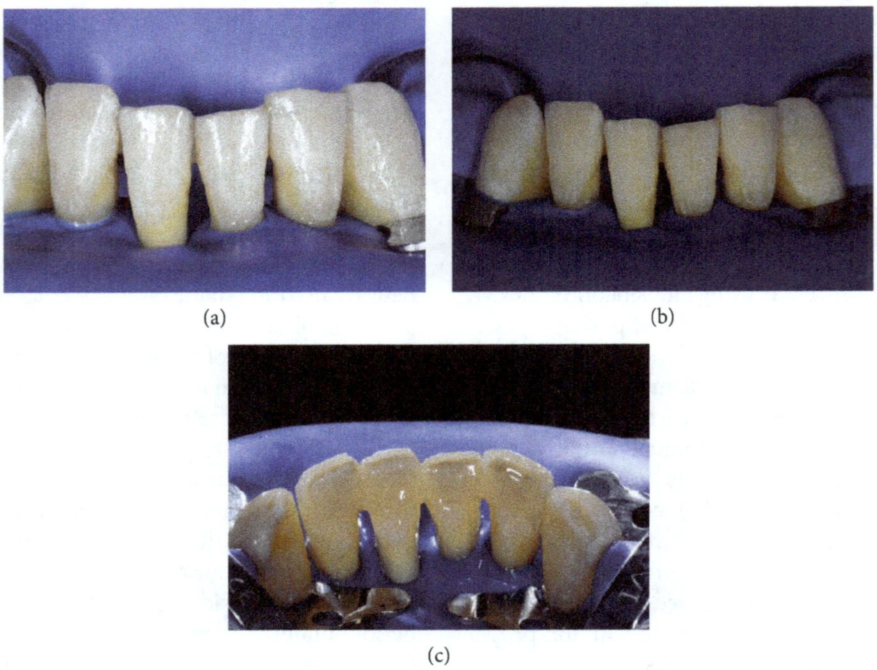

Figure 9: (a) Vestibular view of completed restoration under rubber dam isolation using (a) standardized flash-ring illumination and (b) cross-polarized exposures. (c) Lingual view showing resin composite fully covering the polyethylene fiber.

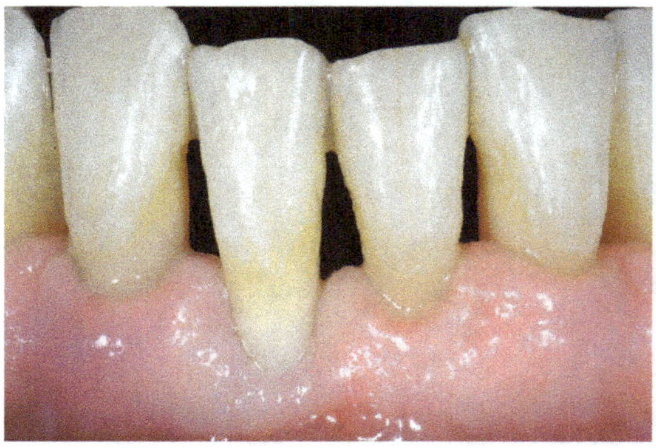

(a)

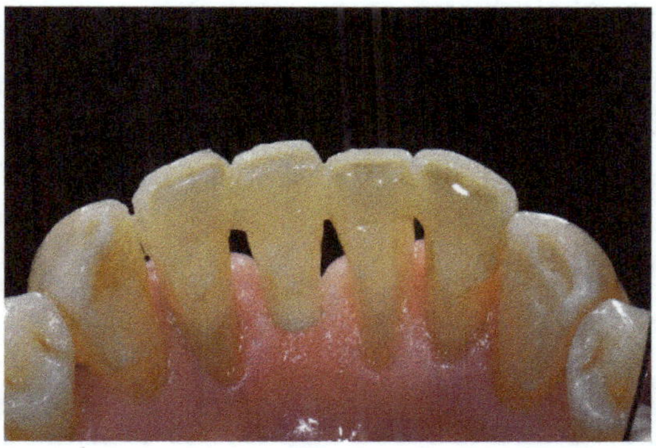

(b)

FIGURE 10: Intraoral (a) vestibular and (b) lingual views of the restoration immediately after rubber dam removal.

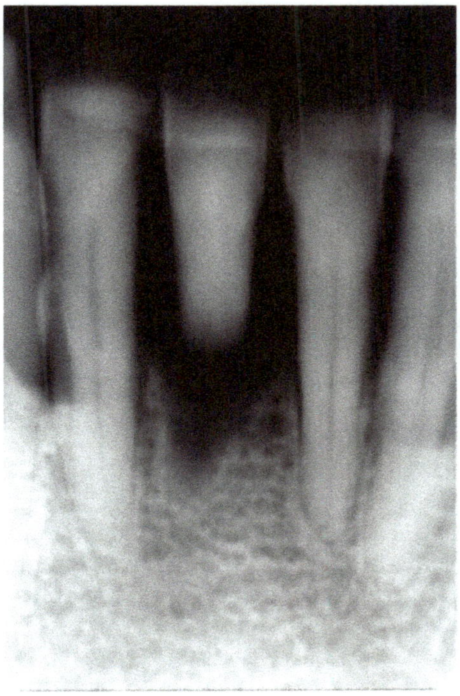

FIGURE 11: Periapical radiograph showing the natural tooth pontic bonded to adjacent elements; the radiopaque fiber extending to all lower incisors can be appreciated.

the bleeding index scores and probing depths (mm) of adjacent teeth significantly improved from 1 year after the restoration to the end of the observation period [25]. A chairside direct prosthesis fabricated using the patient's own natural tooth might offer an economical advantage when looking at clinical/laboratory costs and number of appointments: in contrast to the development of classic RBFPDs, like those described by Li et al. [25], traditional impressions and working models are avoided, and time for indirect fabrication is saved.

Few data is available for the long-term survival/success of natural tooth pontic prosthesis. The mean follow-up period of published case reports on that topic is 1 year [19, 20]; however, other authors demonstrated excellent functional and esthetic results for longer time intervals, at two- [18] and six-year [17] follow-ups, for example. Quirynen et al. carried out a long-term evaluation of composite-bonded natural teeth as replacement of lower incisors with terminal periodontitis [28]: they found a survival rate of 80% after 5 years of function: the abutment teeth also showed stable probing depths and a negligible loss in attachment (0.1 mm/year). Among other factors, the improved condition of abutment teeth might also be explained by a supragingival placement of prosthetic or composite margins (with traditional RBFPD or natural tooth pontic prosthesis, respectively); in fact, both oral hygiene procedures and long-term maintenance of the restoration are facilitated. According to Sconnenschein et al., the probing depth of splinted mandibular teeth decreased from 3.39 mm to 2.12 mm and remained stable over the 3-year observation period, with the application of a strict supportive periodontal therapy; no splinted tooth was lost within the first 3 years after splinting [27].

A single-retainer, cantilever design has been suggested for traditional and all-ceramic anterior RBFPDs [8]; in fact, a recent systematic review has highlighted a significant lower survival rate for two-retainer (inlay or surface-only) restorations [9]. Single-retainer RBFPDs might reduce the risk of fracture of the adhesive cement (debonding), induced by unsynchronized movement of the abutment teeth in different directions under functional load [9, 29]. Despite a cantilevered, resin-bonded bridge with a natural tooth pontic might be planned, an optimal periodontal condition of the abutment tooth is recommended [29]; for this reason, a cantilever design was not selected for our patient. Further contraindications for RBFPDs, regardless an artificial or natural pontic, are represented by limited interocclusal space (deep bite), low overjet, parafunctional habits, and short clinical crowns [29]: recurrent debonding or fractures may occur with that unfavourable conditions.

The natural tooth pontic might be seated in a number of ways: flow or restorative composite without any additional reinforcement [18], metal wires, or fiber materials combined with resin composite. A splint made of stainless steel wire (round, twisted, or multistranded) and composite represents an alternative fixation method of the extracted tooth to adjacent elements and also for periodontal stabilization [30, 31]. Splints consisting of metal wire and composite resin have an interface with different elastic moduli and may be more susceptible to fatigue failure initiation [32]. According to

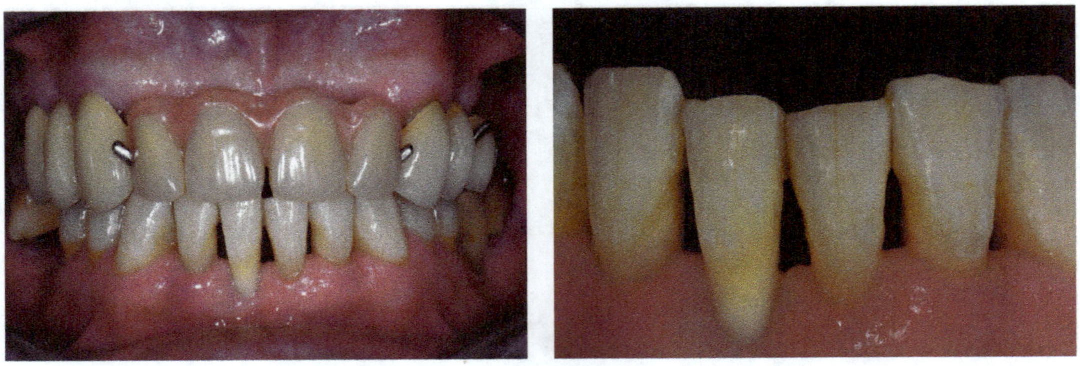

(a) (b)

Figure 12: Postoperative functional and esthetic result at 6 months of follow-up: (a) full-mouth and (b) cross-polarized views of the completed restoration.

Foek et al., specimens of the braided stainless steel wire group frequently failed at the composite-wire interface; on the other hand, the debonding forces were statistically similar to the nonmetal retainers [33]. Ribbond® retainers presented adhesive failure and material breakage in 50% and 40% of the specimens, respectively [33]. Resin adhesion to polyethylene FRCs might be less favorable because of the difficulty in plasma coating, silanization, and impregnation of the polyethylene fibers; such combinations of failure types may not cause direct enamel damage but will necessitate removal of the attached retainers and renewal of the bonding procedure [33]. Insights regarding the biomechanical behavior of teeth splinted using different materials have been also reported: according to Soares et al., periodontal splints with composite and adhesive systems were more effective than a rigid fixation method (stainless steel wire) in reducing the mandibular bone strain levels during occlusal function [32]. According to Sfondrini et al., the maximum load resistance of full-bonded fiber-reinforced composite splint is higher than a fixation obtained using metal wires combined with traditional composite [34]: despite an optimal splinting material has not been identified yet, to improve the mechanical strength of our direct prosthesis, a ribbon-based splint was chosen. Inlay-like retentions, slots, or groove preparation of abutment teeth is possible. Despite a slot-type preparation (or its size) of abutment teeth might have limited influence on the strength of the bonded bridge [35], that specific design was selected for two main reasons: (1) coverage of the fiber with an increased amount of composite, to avoid long-term exposure of fiber itself, and (2) patient's comfort, in order to minimize the thickness of incisors' surfaces at the lingual side.

Known limitations of resin-bonded prosthesis (including a natural pontic, as in our case) are related to fractures of the framework/splint, exposures of the fiber, and partial/full debonding of the attached tooth; long-term wear, discoloration, microleakage, or secondary caries at the tooth-restorative interface are also possible. Despite common adhesive techniques can be used for intraoral repairings or reluting, these complications imply additional interventions (repairings or substitution), costs, and sometimes unscheduled appointments at the office. According to Graetz et al., 75.3% of splinted teeth in periodontitis patients required repair (from zero up to three repairs/splint/year), highlighting potential frequent interventions in the long term [31]. Next studies should be focused on long-term evaluations of natural tooth pontic prosthesis; the soft and hard tissues behavior or modifications under the pontic site should be further clarified. Current ridge preservation techniques using biomaterials, membranes, or a partial extraction approach could be enhanced by the immediate insertion of a natural or artificial tooth pontic [36]: new insights are necessary when a combination of these procedures is adopted.

Despite the limitations of our study, an excellent functional, esthetic, mid-term result has been achieved adopting a minimally invasive restorative solution for single-tooth replacement; whether indicated or necessary, the natural tooth pontic technique leaves open other treatment options for the future.

References

[1] S. Elangovan and G. Avila-Ortiz, "Case selection is critical for successful outcomes following immediate implant placement in the esthetic zone," *Journal of Evidence Based Dental Practice*, vol. 17, no. 2, pp. 135–138, 2017.

[2] D. Augusti, G. Augusti, and D. Re, "Prosthetic restoration in the single-tooth gap: patient preferences and analysis of the WTP index," *Clinical Oral Implants Research*, vol. 25, no. 11, pp. 1257–1264, 2014.

[3] R. Kuijs, A. van Dalen, J. Roeters, and D. Wismeijer, "The resin-bonded fixed partial denture as the first treatment consideration to replace a missing tooth," *The International Journal of Prosthodontics*, vol. 29, no. 4, pp. 337–339, 2016.

[4] A. L. Rochette, "Attachment of a splint to enamel of lower anterior teeth," *The Journal of Prosthetic Dentistry*, vol. 30, 4, Part 1, pp. 418–423, 1973.

[5] V. P. Thompson and G. J. Livaditis, "Etched casting acid etch composite bonded posterior bridges," *Pediatric Dentistry*, vol. 4, no. 1, pp. 38–43, 1982.

[6] W. F. Vasques, F. V. Martins, J. C. Magalhaes, and E. M. Fonseca, "A low cost minimally invasive adhesive alternative for maxillary central incisor replacement," *Journal of Esthetic and Restorative Dentistry*, vol. 30, no. 6, pp. 469–473, 2018.

[7] C. A. Barwacz, M. Hernandez, and R. H. Husemann, "Minimally invasive preparation and design of a cantilevered, all-ceramic, resin-bonded, fixed partial denture in the esthetic zone: a case report and descriptive review," *Journal of Esthetic and Restorative Dentistry*, vol. 26, no. 5, pp. 314–323, 2014.

[8] M. Kern, "Single-retainer resin-bonded fixed dental prostheses as an alternative to orthodontic space closure (and to single-tooth implants)," *Quintessence International*, vol. 49, no. 10, pp. 789–798, 2018.

[9] D. S. Thoma, I. Sailer, A. Ioannidis, M. Zwahlen, N. Makarov, and B. E. Pjetursson, "A systematic review of the survival and complication rates of resin-bonded fixed dental prostheses after a mean observation period of at least 5 years," *Clinical Oral Implants Research*, vol. 28, no. 11, pp. 1421–1432, 2017.

[10] I. A. Alraheam, C. N. Ngoc, C. A. Wiesen, and T. E. Donovan, "Five-year success rate of resin-bonded fixed partial dentures: a systematic review," *Journal of Esthetic and Restorative Dentistry*, vol. 31, no. 1, pp. 40–50, 2019.

[11] K. E. Ahmed, K. Y. Li, and C. A. Murray, "Longevity of fiber-reinforced composite fixed partial dentures (FRC FPD)—Systematic review," *Journal of Dentistry*, vol. 61, pp. 1–11, 2017.

[12] M. Kern, "Fifteen-year survival of anterior all-ceramic cantilever resin-bonded fixed dental prostheses," *Journal of Dentistry*, vol. 56, pp. 133–135, 2017.

[13] D. Augusti, G. Augusti, A. Borgonovo, M. Amato, and D. Re, "Inlay-retained fixed dental prosthesis: a clinical option using monolithic zirconia," *Case Reports in Dentistry*, vol. 2014, Article ID 629786, 7 pages, 2014.

[14] A. Scribante, P. K. Vallittu, M. Ozcan, L. V. J. Lassila, P. Gandini, and M. F. Sfondrini, "Travel beyond clinical uses of fiber reinforced composites (FRCs) in dentistry: a review of past employments, present applications, and future perspectives," *BioMed Research International*, vol. 2018, Article ID 1498901, 8 pages, 2018.

[15] Y. Maruo, G. Nishigawa, M. Irie, K. Yoshihara, and S. Minagi, "Flexural properties of polyethylene, glass and carbon fiber-reinforced resin composites for prosthetic frameworks," *Acta Odontologica Scandinavica*, vol. 73, no. 8, pp. 581–587, 2015.

[16] J. Juloski, M. Beloica, C. Goracci et al., "Shear bond strength to enamel and flexural strength of different fiber-reinforced composites," *The Journal of Adhesive Dentistry*, vol. 15, no. 2, pp. 123–130, 2013.

[17] H. Kermanshah and F. Motevasselian, "Immediate tooth replacement using fiber-reinforced composite and natural tooth pontic," *Operative Dentistry*, vol. 35, no. 2, pp. 238–245, 2010.

[18] B. Dimaczek and M. Kern, "Long-term provisional rehabilitation of function and esthetics using an extracted tooth with the immediate bonding technique," *Quintessence International*, vol. 39, no. 4, pp. 283–288, 2008.

[19] J. H. Jang, S. H. Lee, J. Paek, and S. Y. Kim, "Splinted porcelain laminate veneers with a natural tooth pontic: a provisional approach for conservative and esthetic treatment of a challenging case," *Operative Dentistry*, vol. 40, no. 6, pp. E257–E265, 2015.

[20] K. P. Kumar, S. K. Nujella, S. S. Gopal, and K. K. Roy, "Immediate esthetic rehabilitation of periodontally compromised anterior tooth using natural tooth as pontic," *Case Reports in Dentistry*, vol. 2016, Article ID 8130352, 4 pages, 2016.

[21] R. Raj, K. Mehrotra, I. Narayan, T. M. Gowda, and D. S. Mehta, "Natural tooth pontic: an instant esthetic option for periodontally compromised teeth—a case series," *Case Reports in Dentistry*, vol. 2016, Article ID 8502927, 6 pages, 2016.

[22] C. P. Wu, Y. K. Tu, S. L. Lu, J. H. Chang, and H. K. Lu, "Quantitative analysis of miller mobility index for the diagnosis of moderate to severe periodontitis - a cross-sectional study," *Journal of Dental Sciences*, vol. 13, no. 1, pp. 43–47, 2018.

[23] M. Stimmelmayr, M. Stangl, J. Kremzow-Stangl et al., "Precise placement of single-retainer resin-bonded fixed dental prostheses with an innovative splint design," *Journal of Prosthodontics*, vol. 26, no. 5, pp. 359–363, 2017.

[24] J. H. Kim, K. T. Koo, J. Capetillo et al., "Periodontal and endodontic pathology delays extraction socket healing in a canine model," *Journal of Periodontal & Implant Science*, vol. 47, no. 3, pp. 143–153, 2017.

[25] J. Li, T. Jiang, P. Lv, X. Fang, Z. Xiao, and L. Jia, "Four-year clinical evaluation of GFRC-RBFPDs as periodontal splints to replace lost anterior teeth," *The International Journal of Prosthodontics*, vol. 29, no. 5, pp. 522–527, 2016.

[26] R. Kathariya, A. Devanoorkar, R. Golani, N. Shetty, V. Vallakatla, and M. Y. Bhat, "To splint or not to splint: the current status of periodontal splinting," *Journal of the International Academy of Periodontology*, vol. 18, no. 2, pp. 45–56, 2016.

[27] S. K. Sonnenschein, C. Betzler, M. A. Rutters, J. Krisam, D. Saure, and T. S. Kim, "Long-term stability of splinted anterior mandibular teeth during supportive periodontal therapy," *Acta Odontologica Scandinavica*, vol. 75, no. 7, pp. 475–482, 2017.

[28] M. Quirynen, C. Mongardini, P. Lambrechts et al., "A long-term evaluation of composite-bonded natural/resin teeth as replacement of lower incisors with terminal periodontitis," *Journal of Periodontology*, vol. 70, no. 2, pp. 205–212, 1999.

[29] M. Kern, "Clinical long-term survival of two-retainer and single-retainer all-ceramic resin-bonded fixed partial dentures," *Quintessence International*, vol. 36, no. 2, pp. 141–147, 2005.

[30] L. C. Sekhar, V. P. Koganti, B. R. Shankar, and A. Gopinath, "A comparative study of temporary splints: bonded polyethylene fiber reinforcement ribbon and stainless steel wire + composite resin splint in the treatment of chronic periodontitis," *The Journal of Contemporary Dental Practice*, vol. 12, no. 5, pp. 343–349, 2011.

[31] C. Graetz, F. Ostermann, S. Woeste, S. Salzer, C. E. Dorfer, and F. Schwendicke, "Long-term survival and maintenance efforts of splinted teeth in periodontitis patients," *Journal of Dentistry*, vol. 80, pp. 49–54, 2019.

[32] P. B. Soares, A. J. Fernandes Neto, D. Magalhaes, A. Versluis, and C. J. Soares, "Effect of bone loss simulation and periodontal splinting on bone strain: periodontal splints and bone strain," *Archives of Oral Biology*, vol. 56, no. 11, pp. 1373–1381, 2011.

[33] D. L. Foek, E. Yetkiner, and M. Ozcan, "Fatigue resistance, debonding force, and failure type of fiber-reinforced composite, polyethylene ribbon-reinforced, and braided stainless steel wire lingual retainers in vitro," *The Korean Journal of Orthodontics*, vol. 43, no. 4, pp. 186–192, 2013.

[34] M. F. Sfondrini, P. Gandini, P. Tessera, P. K. Vallittu, L. Lassila, and A. Scribante, "Bending Properties of Fiber-Reinforced Composites Retainers Bonded with Spot- Composite Coverage," *BioMed Research International*, vol. 2017, Article ID 8469090, 6 pages, 2017.

[35] G. Aktas, E. G. Basara, E. Sahin, S. Uctasli, P. K. Vallittu, and L. V. Lassila, "Effects of different cavity designs on fracture load of fiber-reinforced adhesive fixed dental prostheses in the anterior region," *The Journal of Adhesive Dentistry*, vol. 15, no. 2, pp. 131–135, 2013.

[36] M. Bakshi, D. Tarnow, and N. Bittner, "Changes in ridge dimension with pontics immediately placed at extraction sites: a pilot study," *The International Journal of Periodontics & Restorative Dentistry*, vol. 38, no. 4, pp. 541–547, 2018.

22

A Rare Case of Single-Rooted Mandibular Second Molar with Single Canal

Abdulmohsen Alfadley[1,2] **Ahmad Alquraishi,**[3] **Yaser Almazrou,**[4] **and Fahd Aljarbou**[5]

[1]*Department of Restorative and Prosthetic Dental Sciences, College of Dentistry, King Saud bin Abdulaziz University for Health Sciences, Riyadh, Saudi Arabia*
[2]*King Abdullah International Medical Research Center, Ministry of National Guard Health Affairs, Riyadh, Saudi Arabia*
[3]*Internship Unit, College of Dentistry, King Saud bin Abdulaziz University for Health Sciences, Ministry of National Guard Health Affairs, Riyadh, Saudi Arabia*
[4]*Presidency of State Security, Department of Medical Services, Riyadh, Saudi Arabia*
[5]*Department of Restorative Dental Sciences, Division of Endodontics, College of Dentistry, King Saud University, Riyadh, Saudi Arabia*

Correspondence should be addressed to Abdulmohsen Alfadley; fadleya@ksau-hs.edu.sa

Academic Editor: Gavriel Chaushu

The root canal anatomy of mandibular second molar teeth is known to be highly variable. Whilst the most frequently seen configuration is two mesial canals and one distal canal, other variations such as four canals, two canals, and C-shaped canal system do also exist. This case report describes the diagnosis and management of unusual root canal configuration of a mandibular second molar, with one canal in a single conical root, using the contemporary advancements in endodontics. Following clinical and radiographic examinations of the case, a diagnosis of symptomatic irreversible pulpitis with symptomatic apical periodontitis of tooth #47 was established, and root canal treatment followed by composite buildup and crown were planned. Clinicians should be aware of the different anatomic variants each tooth may exhibit. Furthermore, clinicians need to possess the proper knowledge and skills that allow them to utilize the diagnostic and therapeutic tools available at their disposal in order to optimize the quality of care provided to their patients.

1. Introduction

The principal objective of endodontic treatment is to prevent and, when needed, to treat endodontic disease, apical periodontitis [1]. In order to accomplish this objective, high-quality chemomechanical cleaning and shaping of the intricate root canal system are required in order to eradicate intracanal microorganisms [2, 3]. This task requires elaborate knowledge of pulp space anatomy, including expected and less usual canal morphology. Variations such as additional canals, bi/trifurcations, lateral and furcal canals, apical deltas, and canal ramifications are frequently encountered during root canal treatment, and their incidence and clinical significance have been reported before [4, 5]. Due to the complex and highly variable pulp space anatomy, it is not uncommon to overlook part of this anatomy during the debridement phase [6] resulting in the emergence or persistence of endodontic disease [7].

The root canal morphology of mandibular second molars has been elegantly evaluated in landmark studies by Vertucci and Weine et al. using clearing and radiographic techniques, respectively [8, 9]. Similar to the mandibular first molar, this tooth most commonly has two roots; mesial and distal, with two mesial canals (mesiobuccal and mesiolingual) and one distal canal [8–10]. Nevertheless, other configurations have been reported in mandibular second molar teeth such as four canals, two canals, C-shaped canal, taurodontism, and one canal in a single root [8–12]. Previously published articles agree on the rare occurrence of one canal in a single-rooted (Vertucci Type I) mandibular second molars. For instance,

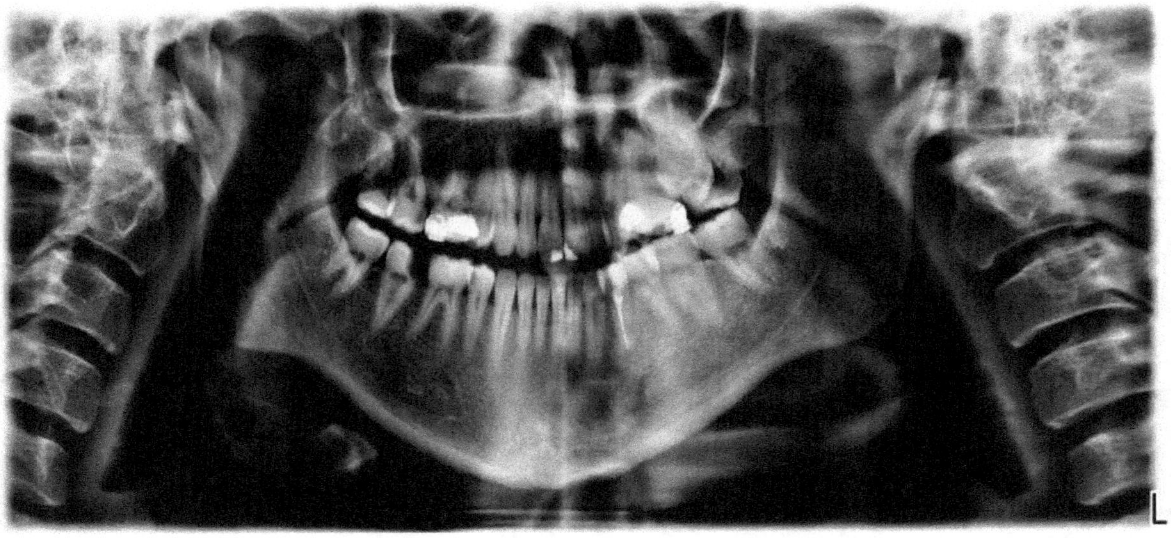

Figure 1: Panoramic radiograph of presenting patient confirms the lack of symmetry between single-rooted tooth #47 and contralateral tooth #37 which presents with two distinct roots.

Weine et al. reported that only 1.3% of mandibular second molars had a single canal configuration all the way from an orifice to an apex [9]. In line with that, Demirbuga et al. used advanced imaging technique and found the prevalence of such anatomic variant to be close to 2% [13]. Such high variability in the root canal anatomy of this tooth emphasizes the importance of properly integrating theoretical knowledge of dental morphology with the information obtained from pretreatment radiographs. Furthermore, additional exploration of internal anatomy should be made during treatment in order to avoid the possibility of untreated canal system. Several of the recent advances in endodontics have contributed to safe, predictable, and efficient root canal treatment. Such developments include digital radiography, cone beam computed tomography (CBCT), microcomputed tomography (micro-CT), dental operating microscope (DOM), thermomechanically treated nickel-titanium files, and improved obturation devices [14–17]. The aim of this case report was to describe the diagnosis and management of rare root canal configuration of a mandibular second molar, showing one canal in a single conical root, using the contemporary advancements in endodontics.

2. Case Report

A 25-year-old Saudi Arabian man presented to the dental clinic with a chief complaint of "severe pain to cold water" in the lower right side of the jaw. The history revealed that pain started about three weeks ago and has increased in intensity over the past five days with occasional spontaneous symptoms. The patient had several dental treatments done in the past such as periodontal scaling, restorations, root canal treatment, and extractions, without any complications. The patient denied having any relevant medical condition such as chronic illness, use of medication, allergy, or previous hospitalization.

Upon extraoral examination, no significant findings were noted. Intraoral examination showed tooth #47 with deep occluso-mesial caries. On application of the cold test to the tooth, the patient responded with severe prolonged pain compared to adjacent teeth. Tooth #47 was tender to percussion but responded normally to palpation and bite tests. Periodontal probing generally ranged from 2 to 3 mm, without any increase in tooth mobility. The health of the surrounding mucogingival tissues was within normal limits. Radiographic assessment commenced by systematic evaluation of the already available panoramic radiograph (Figure 1). The obtained preoperative periapical radiographs (Figures 2(a) and 2(b)) demonstrated the presence of one large canal along with one conical root and slight widening of the periodontal ligament space around the apex of tooth #47. A diagnosis of symptomatic irreversible pulpitis with symptomatic apical periodontitis of tooth #47 was established, and root canal treatment followed by composite buildup and crown were planned. Prior to treatment, CBCT (Planmeca Promax, Planmeca, Finland) was obtained in order to enable three-dimensional assessment of pulp space morphology. Further evaluation of sagittal, coronal, and axial slices confirmed the presence of one large round-oval canal extending from the orifice level to the root apex without any evidence of additional canals (Figures 2(a)–2(g)).

Local anesthesia was administered through inferior alveolar nerve block using one carpule (1.8 ml) of 2% lidocaine with 1 : 100,000 of epinephrine (Lidocaine HCl, Huons Co., Seoul, Korea). Another carpule was added for buccal and lingual infiltrations. Following rubber dam isolation, caries excavation and access cavity preparation were accomplished using size 6 long shank round bur in a high-speed handpiece. Then, pulp extirpation was performed using barbed broach. The dental operating microscope (OPMI Pico, Carl Zeiss Surgical, Oberkochen, Germany) showed the presence of a large round canal orifice located in the center of the pulp chamber floor (Figure 3(a)). Following irrigation with 5.25% NaOCl, shaping of the coronal two-thirds of the canal was performed using ProTaper Gold rotary files (Dentsply Maillefer) in the following sequence: SX, S1, and S2. Working

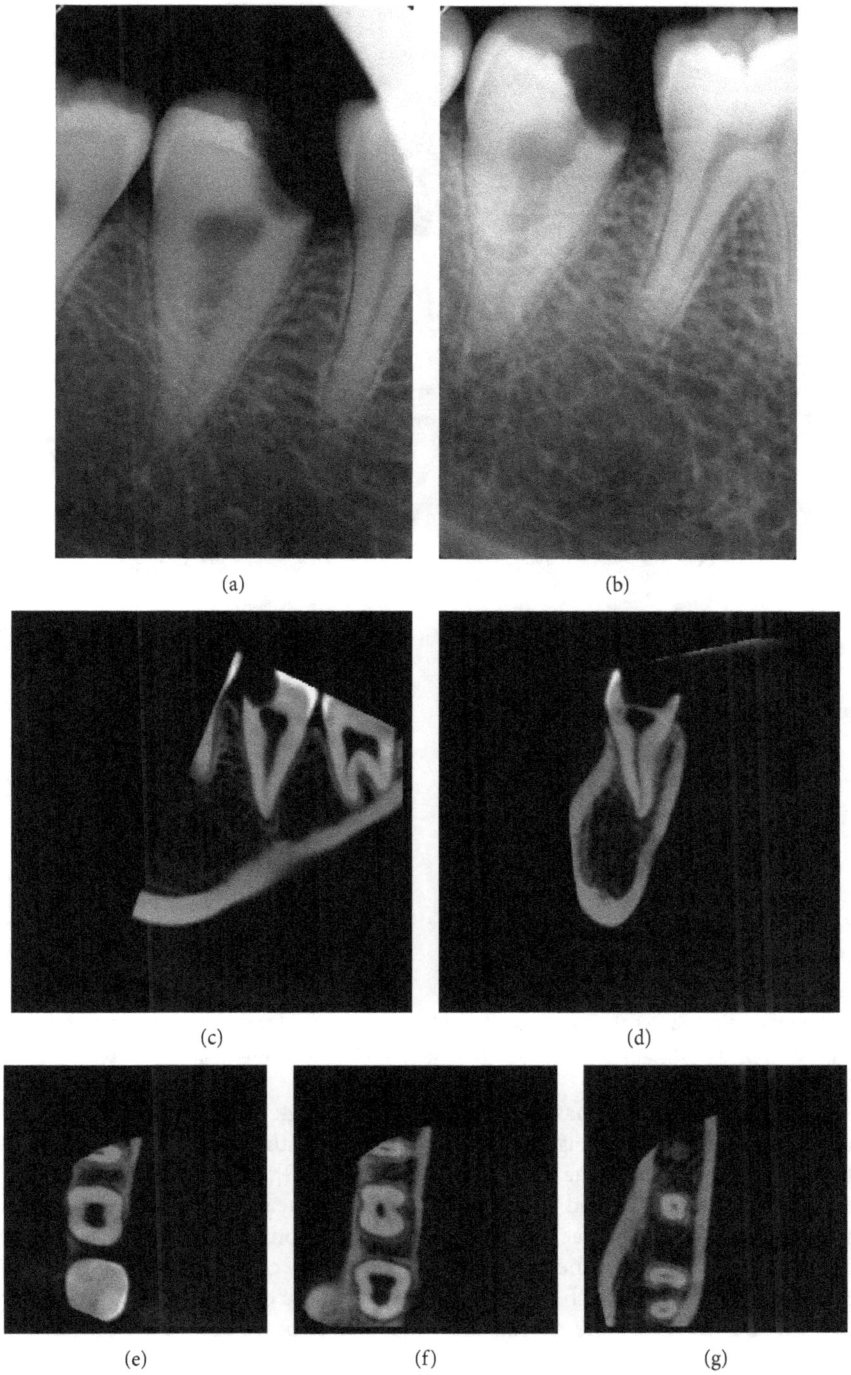

Figure 2: Preoperative radiographic assessment. (a) Straight-on and (b) angulated initial radiographs showing tooth #47 with deep occluso-mesial caries along with large pulp space situated within a single conical root. (c, d) Sagittal and coronal CBCT slices suggest the presence of one root canal configuration. (e–g) Further evaluation of the axial cuts in the coronal, middle, and apical thirds confirms the presence of Vertucci Type I canal system.

length (WL) was determined using a size 20 K file attached to an electronic apex locator and then confirmed using a digital radiograph (Figure 3(b)). After that, size 10 and 15 K files were precurved and placed against the canal walls to further explore the internal anatomy. Root canal shaping was then completed using hybrid instrumentation technique. Canal shaping to WL was first accomplished using S1 and S2 instruments. After that, apical enlargement was performed using Vortex Blue rotary files (Dentsply Tulsa Dental Specialties, Tulsa, OK) in the following sequence: 25/0.06, 30/0.06, 35/0.06, and 40/0.06. During the shaping procedure, EDTA gel (Glyde File Prep; Dentsply Maillefer, Ballaigues, Switzerland) was utilized as lubricant, and 5.25% NaOCl solution was used to irrigate the canal. Recapitulation and verification of canal patency were frequently performed during the procedure. Final irrigation was performed using 17% EDTA (Meta Biomed Co. Ltd., Mandaluyong, Korea), after which the canal was dried using sterile absorbent paper

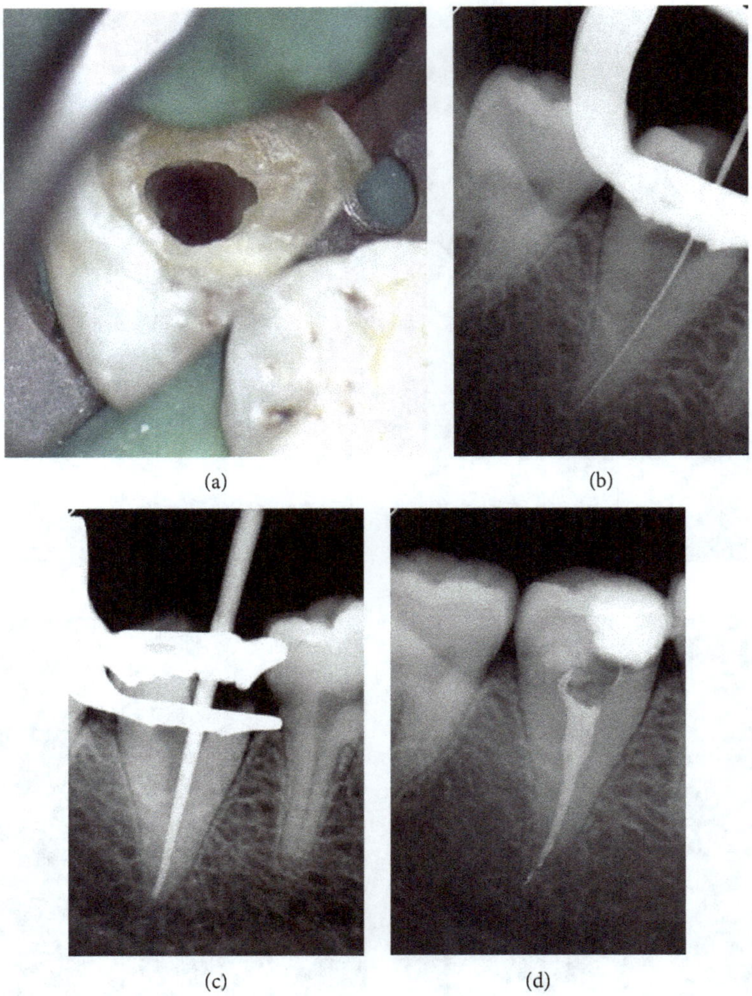

Figure 3: (a) Accessed cavity preparation shows the presence of one large root canal located in the center of the pulp chamber. (b) Working length determination radiograph. (c) Master gutta-percha cone radiograph. (d) Final radiograph showing dense obturation with sealer puffs.

points. The snug fit of a size 40, taper 0.06 master gutta-percha cone was evaluated radiographically (Figure 3(c)). The canal was then obturated with gutta-percha cone and AH26 sealer (Dentsply Maillefer) using a hybrid technique combing cold lateral and warm vertical compaction techniques (Figure 3(d)). The pulp chamber was then cleaned using alcohol-moistened cotton pellet, after which the access cavity was temporized with Cavit. After one week, the patient reported complete resolution of the symptoms. The tooth was restored using post-retained composite buildup and then referred for the fabrication of a full coverage restoration. The patient gave his informed consent for the publication of this case.

3. Discussion

This case report describes the endodontic management of a mandibular second molar tooth with a single root canal aided by the contemporary advancements in the field. Assessment of preoperative periapical radiographs demonstrated the presence of one root with a large canal space suggesting the likelihood of C-shaped canal configuration. In fact, when only one root is present, the root canal system may contain only a single large canal or two root canals that may or may not join within the canal system or a C-shaped canal configuration [18]. However, systematic evaluation of CBCT slices revealed the presence of one large round canal. This observation was confirmed upon access cavity preparation as careful inspection of the pulpal floor with the dental operating microscope demonstrated the presence of one round orifice.

Cone beam computed tomography (CBCT) is a reliable and noninvasive approach that is often used in the diagnosis and treatment plan of endodontic cases. The American Association of Endodontists and American Academy of Oral and Maxillofacial Radiology published a joint position statement related to the use of CBCT [19]. The need for CBCT should be considered if the evaluation of differently angled periapical radiographs fails to provide conclusive information or if additional information in the buccolingual dimension is required. In cases deemed appropriate for the acquisition of CBCT scan, a narrow field of view which is associated with reduced radiation dose and higher spatial resolution is recommended [19]. The statement states that CBCT should only be used as an adjunctive tool in certain situations such as assessment of teeth with complex or unusual root canal anatomy, identification of calcified canals, evaluation of the outcome of endodontic treatment, and planning of surgical retreatment. Other indications for CBCT acquisition include the diagnosis and management of dentoalveolar trauma, resorptive defects, and dental implants [14, 19, 20].

Previous studies on the root canal anatomy of mandibular second molars confirm the rarity of our reported case. For instance, such observation was not documented in previous studies among American [8], Turkish [21], Thai [22], Malaysian [23], and even Saudi Arabian populations [24]. Furthermore, Weine et al., Demirbuga et al., and Gulabivala et al. reported a low prevalence rate of 1.3%, 2.1%, and 2.2% among American, Turkish, and Burmese populations, respectively [9, 13, 25]. Rahimi et al. evaluated root canal configuration of mandibular second molars among Iranian subpopulations using a clearing technique. In their study, only 6 out of the 139 teeth (4.3%) demonstrated the presence of the Vertucci Type I configuration discussed in this case report [26]. Interestingly, Fava et al. published a case report documenting the presence of one root and one root canal in all maxillary and mandibular second molar teeth of the same patient [11]. The information obtained from the different studies on root canal anatomy of teeth has important clinical implications. Whilst some of the endodontic procedural errors are encountered during the search for missing or additional root canals, such mistakes can be minimized if the clinician has an awareness of the expected location and dimensions of the pulp chamber as well as an understanding of the usual and less frequent root canal configurations. Although additional canals are more common, the clinician should also be aware that in certain situations; there is a probability of fewer root canals than the normally presumed pulp space morphology. This shall minimize the risk caused by injudicious removal of tooth structure and its subsequent effect on the mechanical properties of the tooth.

Recently, several studies have investigated the root canal anatomy of mandibular second molar teeth using CBCT. For instance, Pan et al. examined the root canal morphology in a Malaysian subpopulation and reported that the most common configuration seen in two-rooted mandibular second molars was one distinct distal canal (96.9%) and two separate mesial canals (78.1%) [23]. Furthermore, Mashyakhy and Gambarini evaluated root canal morphology differences between genders in a Saudi Arabian population. In agreement with previously cited studies, the most common configuration seen in mandibular second molars was three root canals in a two-rooted tooth whilst the prevalence of C-shaped canal configuration was found to be 8% of examined teeth. In addition, no significant differences were detected between both genders in terms of number of roots, number of canals, Vertucci types in mesial/distal roots, and prevalence of C-shaped canal configuration [24].

Sabala et al. reported that the rarer the aberration, the more likely that it was bilateral [27]. Moreover, Mashyakhy et al. assessed the bilateral symmetry of roots and root canal systems of mandibular first molars in Saudi Arabian population using CBCT. Their symmetrical analysis revealed 100% symmetry in the number of roots and 56% in the number of root canals between the right and left teeth in the same person [28]. Hence, clinicians should suspect the presence of a similar anatomic configuration on the contralateral tooth when examining the preoperative radiograph of a particular case. In our case, however, careful inspection of a magnified panoramic radiograph has clearly shown the presence of a two-rooted mandibular second molar on the contralateral side.

4. Conclusion

This case report presented the endodontic management of unusual root canal configuration of a mandibular second molar, a single root canal from an orifice to an apex, aided by the contemporary digital advancements in endodontics. This report highlighted the importance of textbook knowledge, radiographic examination, and careful intraoperative exploration as the main cornerstones in investigating pulp space anatomy. Clinicians need to employ the diagnostic and therapeutic tools available at their disposal in order to optimize the quality of care provided to their patients. Furthermore, clinicians should be aware of the various root canal configurations of each tooth, as it may impact subsequent treatment procedures as well as the long-term outcome of the case.

References

[1] D. Ørstavik and T. R. Pitt Ford, "Apical periodontitis. Microbial infection and host responses," in *Essential endodontology: prevention and treatment of apical periodontitis*, D. Ørstavik and T. R. Pitt Ford, Eds., Blackwell Science, Oxford, 1998.

[2] D. Ørstavik, "Time-course and risk analyses of the development and healing of chronic apical periodontitis in man," *International Endodontic Journal*, vol. 29, no. 3, pp. 150–155, 1996.

[3] S. Friedman, "Considerations and concepts of case selection in the management of post-treatment endodontic disease (treatment failure)," *Endod Topics*, vol. 1, no. 1, pp. 54–78, 2002.

[4] I. Jung, M. Seo, A. Fouad et al., "Apical Anatomy in Mesial and Mesiobuccal Roots of Permanent First Molars," *Journal of Endodontia*, vol. 31, no. 5, pp. 364–368, 2005.

[5] B. Marroquin, M. Elsayed, and B. Willershausenzonnchen, "Morphology of the Physiological Foramen: I. Maxillary and Mandibular Molars," *Journal of Endodontics*, vol. 30, no. 5, pp. 321–328, 2004.

[6] M. Song, H. C. Kim, W. Lee, and E. Kim, "Analysis of the cause of failure in nonsurgical endodontic treatment by microscopic inspection during endodontic microsurgery," *Journal of Endodontia*, vol. 37, no. 11, pp. 1516–1519, 2011.

[7] G. Cantatore, E. Berutti, and A. Castellucci, "Missed anatomy: frequency and clinical impact," *Endodontic Topics*, vol. 15, no. 1, pp. 3–31, 2006.

[8] F. J. Vertucci, "Root canal anatomy of the human permanent teeth," *Oral Surgery, Oral Medicine, Oral Pathology, Oral Radiology, and Endodontics*, vol. 58, no. 5, pp. 589–599, 1984.

[9] F. S. Weine, R. A. Pasiewicz, and R. T. Rice, "Canal configuration of the mandibular second molar using a clinically oriented in vitro method," *Journal of Endodontia*, vol. 14, no. 5, pp. 207–213, 1988.

[10] S. Sert and G. Bayirli, "Evaluation of the root canal configurations of the mandibular and maxillary permanent teeth by

gender in the Turkish population," *Journal of Endodontia*, vol. 30, no. 6, pp. 391–398, 2004.

[11] L. R. G. Fava, I. Weinfeld, F. P. Fabri, and C. R. Pais, "Four second molars with single roots and single canals in the same patient," *International Endodontic Journal*, vol. 33, no. 2, pp. 138–142, 2000.

[12] G. Felsypremila, T. S. Vinothkumar, and D. Kandaswamy, "Anatomic symmetry of root and root canal morphology of posterior teeth in Indian subpopulation using cone beam computed tomography: a retrospective study," *Eur J Dent*, vol. 9, no. 4, pp. 500–507, 2015.

[13] S. Demirbuga, A. E. Sekerci, A. N. Dinçer, M. Cayabatmaz, and Y. O. Zorba, "Use of cone-beam computed tomography to evaluate root and canal morphology of mandibular first and second molars in Turkish individuals," *Medicina Oral, Patología Oral y Cirugía Bucal*, vol. 18, no. 4, pp. e737–e744, 2013.

[14] F. Valenti-Obino, D. Di Nardo, L. Quero et al., "Symmetry of root and root canal morphology of mandibular incisors: a cone-beam computed tomography study <i>in vivo</i>," *Journal of Clinical and Experimental Dentistry*, vol. 11, no. 6, pp. e527–e533, 2019.

[15] K. Alfouzan, A. Alfadley, L. Alkadi, A. Alhezam, and A. Jamleh, "Detecting the second mesiobuccal canal in maxillary molars in a Saudi Arabian population: a Micro-CT study," *Scanning*, vol. 2019, 6 pages, 2019.

[16] G. Gambarini, M. Seracchiani, L. Piasecki et al., "Measurement of torque generated during intracanal instrumentation in vivo," *International Endodontic Journal*, vol. 52, no. 5, pp. 737–745, 2018.

[17] A. Jamleh, A. Alghaihab, A. Alfadley, H. Alfawaz, A. Alqedairi, and K. Alfouzan, "Cyclic fatigue and torsional failure of EdgeTaper platinum endodontic files at simulated body temperature," *Journal of Endodontia*, vol. 45, no. 5, pp. 611–614, 2019.

[18] A. Roy, N. Velmurugan, and N. Suresh, "Mandibular second molar with a single root and a single canal: case series," *Journal of Clinical and Diagnostic Research*, vol. 7, no. 11, pp. 2637-2638, 2013.

[19] American Association of Endodontics and American Academy of Oral and Maxillofacial Radiology, "AAE and AAOMR Joint Position Statement: Use of Cone Beam Computed Tomography in Endodontics 2015 Update," *Journal of Endodontics*, vol. 41, no. 9, pp. 1393–1396, 2015.

[20] G. Gambarini, L. Piasecki, G. Miccoli, G. Gaimari, D. D. Nardo, and L. Testarelli, "Cone-beam computed tomography in the assessment of periapical lesions in endodontically treated teeth," *European Journal of Dentistry*, vol. 12, no. 1, pp. 136–143, 2019.

[21] M. K. Caliskan, Y. Pehlivan, F. Sepetcioglu, M. Turkun, and S. S. Tuncer, "Root canal morphology of human permanent teeth in a Turkish population," *Journal of Endodontia*, vol. 21, no. 4, pp. 200–204, 1995.

[22] K. Gulabivala, A. Opasanon, Y. L. Ng, and A. Alavi, "Root and canal morphology of Thai mandibular molars," *International Endodontic Journal*, vol. 35, no. 1, pp. 56–62, 2002.

[23] J. Y. Y. Pan, A. Parolia, S. R. Chuah, S. Bhatia, S. Mutalik, and A. Pau, "Root canal morphology of permanent teeth in a Malaysian subpopulation using cone-beam computed tomography," *BMC Oral Health*, vol. 19, no. 1, p. 14, 2019.

[24] M. Mashyakhy and G. Gambarini, "Root and root canal morphology differences between genders: a comprehensive in-vivo CBCT study in a Saudi population," *Acta Stomatologica Croatica*, vol. 53, no. 3, pp. 231–246.

[25] K. Gulabivala, T. H. Aung, A. Alavi, and Y. L. Ng, "Root and canal morphology of Burmese mandibular molars," *International Endodontic Journal*, vol. 34, no. 5, pp. 359–370, 2001.

[26] S. Rahimi, S. Shahi, M. Lotfi, V. Zand, M. Abdolrahimi, and R. Es'haghi, "Root canal configuration and the prevalence of C-shaped canals in mandibular second molars in an Iranian population," *Journal of Oral Science*, vol. 50, no. 1, pp. 9–13, 2008.

[27] C. L. Sabala, F. W. Benenati, and B. R. Neas, "Bilateral root or root canal aberrations in a dental school patient population," *Journal of Endodontics*, vol. 20, no. 1, pp. 38–42, 1994.

[28] M. Mashyakhy, H. R. Chourasia, E. Halboub, A. A. Almashraqi, Y. Khubrani, and G. Gambarini, "Anatomical variations and bilateral symmetry of roots and root canal system of mandibular first permanent molars in Saudi Arabian population utilizing cone- beam computed tomography," *The Saudi Dental Journal*, vol. 31, no. 4, pp. 481–486, 2019.

23

Application of Platelet-Rich Fibrin as Regeneration Assistant in Immediate Autotransplantation of Third Molar with Unformed Roots: Case Report and Review of Literature

Hamzah Alkofahi,[1] Alaa Maghaireh,[2] Mamoon Fnaish,[2] Mohammad Jarrah,[1] and Mohammad Bataineh[3]

[1]*Department of Oral and Maxillofacial Surgery, Jordanian Royal Medical Services, Irbid, Jordan*
[2]*Department of Periodontics, Jordanian Royal Medical Services, Irbid, Jordan*
[3]*Department of Endodontics, Jordanian Royal Medical Services, Irbid, Jordan*

Correspondence should be addressed to Hamzah Alkofahi; hamzah_kofahi@yahoo.com

Academic Editor: Giuseppe Alessandro Scardina

Background. Autogenous Tooth Transplantation (ATT) is the surgical movement of a maturely or immaturely formed tooth from its original site to another extraction site or a surgically prepared socket in the same individual. The most important factor in the healing process after autotransplantation is the presence of intact and viable periodontal ligament cells, which have the ability to differentiate into osteoblasts and able to induce bone production. ATT can successfully replace removable dentures as a restoration option in a growing patient, while implants can be placed only after skeletal maturity is attained. *Case Presentation.* In this case, we presented an immediate ATT of the third molar with unformed roots to the extraction socket of the first molar with evidence of continued root formation after 2 years of follow-up. *Conclusion.* Platelet-Rich Fibrin (PRF) can induce sustainable and accelerated healing, and it can also induce the regeneration process of the periodontal tissues and pulpal formation. This process plays a key role in future root development and success rate.

1. Background

Autogenous Tooth Transplantation (ATT) is the surgical movement of a maturely or immaturely formed tooth from its original site to another extraction site or a surgically prepared socket in the same individual [1–3]. Vidman et al. in 1915 was the first to report autotransplantation [4]. Since then, the procedure has gained popularity in premolars and canines. Slagsvold and Bjercke in 1974 reported the results of the autotransplantation of 34 premolars with incompletely formed roots done in the period between 1959 and 1970 with a mean follow-up duration of 6 years. He showed a 100% survival rate with the maintained ability of the transplanted teeth to complete root development [5].

The biology of successful autotransplantation depends on the ability of root periodontal (PDL) cells to differentiate and induce dentine and cementum formation. PDL cells have the ability to differentiate into osteoblasts and are able to induce bone formation. Andreasen et al. showed that the presence of intact and viable periodontal ligament cells is considered to be the most important factor to have a successful healing process after autotransplantation [6]. PDL healing has a better prognosis in the case of incomplete roots transplanted in fresh extraction sockets than in the case of surgically formed sockets [7–9].

Many reports have emphasized that the optimum time to achieve a successful ATT is when the tooth root has reached two-thirds to three-quarters of its expected length. However, other factors play an important role including (1) performing atraumatic extraction to preserve Hertwig's root sheath and insure future root growth [10], (2) decreasing the duration of the teeth out of socket before implantation [11], (3) having the apical foramen dimensions > 1 mm to increase the probability of postoperative revascularization [12], and (4) maintaining a good alveolar bone support at the time of ATT [13].

ATT can be a permanent aesthetic restoration for patients who are not suitable for dental implants or fixed prosthesis. It has the advantage of low cost and the ability to move the teeth orthodontically in the future, if needed. Moreover, patients who undergo ATT maintain normal chewing and arch integrity [14], pulpal viability, and preserve periodontal ligament health, maintain normal proprioception reflexes, and stimulate eruption in growing patients [15]. ATT has the ability to preserve bone level and induce alveolar bone formation, which is important to keep the dental implant viable after the patient completes growth, even in the case of failure [7, 13, 16].

There are other types of autotransplantation including intra-alveolar transplantation, i.e., when the position of the tooth is changed within the original socket, e.g., surgical uprighting and intentional replantation, and when the tooth is replanted in the original socket after intentional extraction for treatment of endodontic lesions [17]. ATT is classified based on the time of procedure after the extraction of the recipient tooth, i.e., immediate or delayed transplantation after an initial phase of healing [18].

ATT is indicated to replace missing congenital teeth. In most of these cases, the source of the donor tooth is the crowding in the opposing arch [16]. ATT of lower premolars transplanted in the upper maxillary incisor sockets after traumatic tooth loss were also reported successfully [19]. ATT can be used for the reconstruction of marginal mandibular resection assisted with orthodontic treatment. Osterne et al. reported a successful case of the reconstruction of a mandibular alveolar bone defect in the region of the lower left canine and premolars post ameloblastoma resection with autotransplantation of the immature third molars followed by orthodontic treatment [11].

There is a high incidence of first molar loss in the pubertal patient because of caries and periodontal problems [7, 14, 20]. In these cases, ATT can successfully replace removable dentures, while implants can be placed only after skeletal maturity is attained [21].

In this case report, we present an immediate ATT of the third molar with unformed roots in the extraction socket of a first molar. We used Platelet-Rich Fibrin (PRF) to accelerate the healing and regeneration process of the periodontal tissues and pulpal formation. This process plays key role in future root development and success rate.

1.1. Case Report. A 16-year-old female patient presented in the Oral and Maxillofacial Surgery Clinic at the Royal Medical Services of Jordan-Prince Rashid Hospital. The patient was referred from the Conservative Clinic at the same institution complaining from pain and tenderness on percussion at the area of tooth number 19. The patient's medical records showed no medical history. Dental examination has showed that the patient has extensive class II caries into subgingival level in tooth number 19 with necrotic pulp. Panoramic radiograph showed a periapical condensing osteitis with deep class II caries of tooth number 19 as shown in Figure 1. After

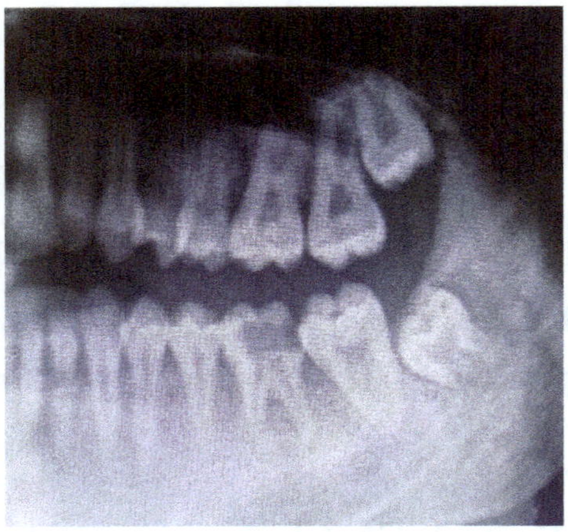

Figure 1: Recipient tooth number 19 with deep caries and donor tooth number 16 with unformed roots.

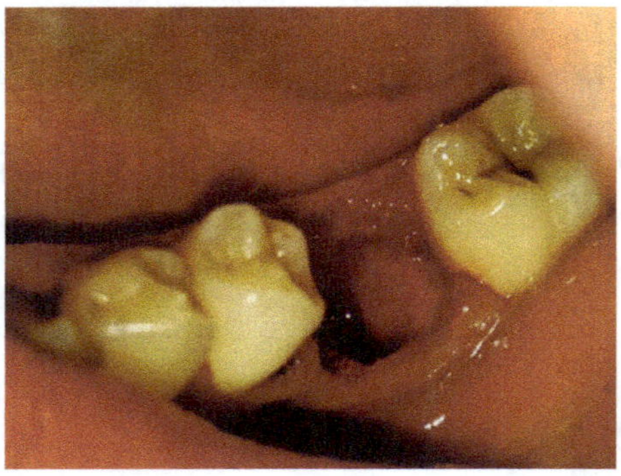

Figure 2: Recipient tooth number 19 with deep caries and donor tooth number 16 with unformed roots.

consulting with the endodontist, several treatment options were presented including root canal treatment with crown lengthening, extraction followed by ATT, or extraction followed by future implant or fixed prosthesis. The patient and her parent were interested in ATT, after considering the low cost in comparison to the implant option. Hence, the decision was made to extract tooth number 19, followed by ATT and application of PRF at time of transplant.

1.2. Treatment. A consent form authorizing the procedure and explaining treatment risks and complications was signed by the patient's parent. On the day of ATT and one hour before the extraction, PRF was prepared according to Choukroun's protocol. Ten cc of venous blood was withdrawn, and blood was centrifuged at 3000 rpm for 10 minutes. The sealed tube was stored at 4°C and ready to use.

1.3. Extraction of Tooth Number 19. The patient underwent local anesthesia of the left inferior alveolar, lingual, and buccal nerves with 2 ampules of 1.8 mm of 2% articaine with 1 : 100,000 epinephrine. Once a profound anesthesia was confirmed, atraumatic extraction of tooth number 19 was done by straight elevator with minimal luxation. Extraction socket walls and apexes were cleaned from any granulation tissue by curettage of the socket and copious irrigation with 0.9% saline (Figure 2).

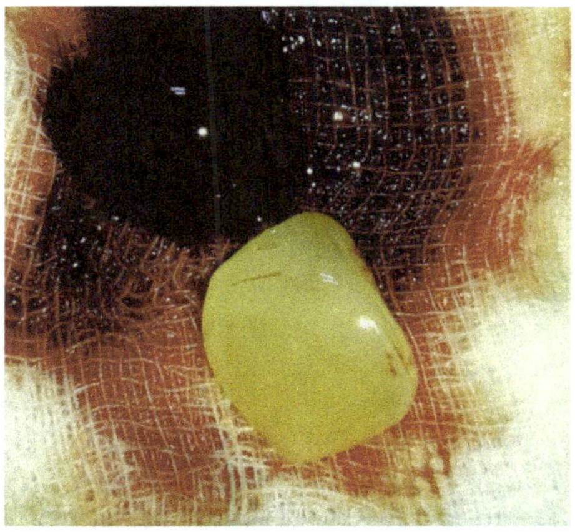

(a)

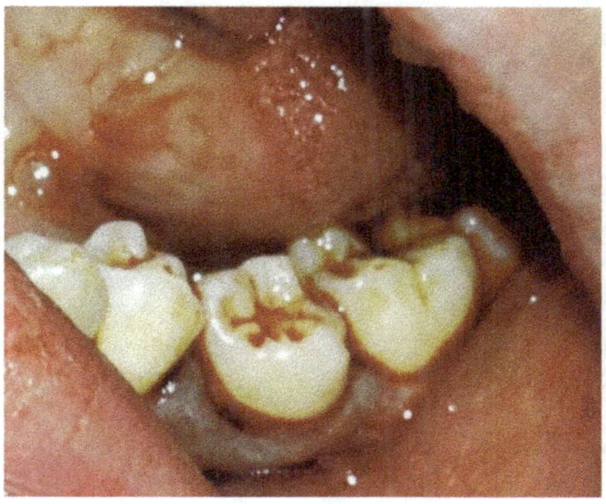

(b)

Figure 3: (a) PRF ready for application. (b) Donor third molar at place ready for splinting.

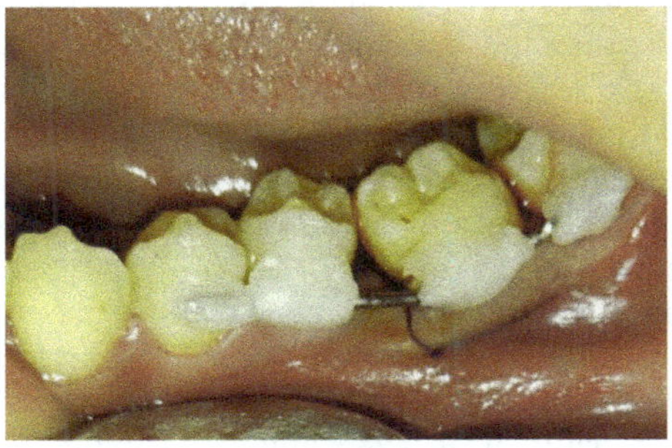

Figure 4: Rigid splinting of third molar.

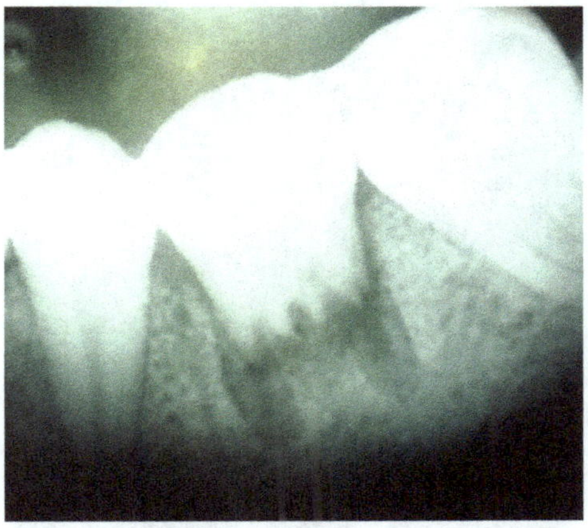

Figure 5: Immediate postoperative radiograph showing third molar fitting well in tooth number 19 socket.

1.4. Extraction of Tooth Number 16. The decision to choose tooth number 16 as donator tooth was done following a radiographic assessment of root development and crown width mesiodistally of all third molars compared to the crown width of tooth number 19. The patient underwent local anesthesia of tooth number 16 through local infiltration of the posterior superior alveolar nerve and the greater palatine nerve with 2 ampules of 2% articaine with 1 : 100,000 epinephrine.

After confirming profound anesthesia, tooth number 16 was exposed using a small mucoperiosteal flap with mesial releasing incision distal to tooth number 15 with minimal bone removal. Tooth number 16 was moved with caution to the attached follicle and was stored in 0.9% saline. Copious irrigation of the transplant socket with 0.9% saline and smooth bony edges were confirmed before closure of the flap with interrupted 4/0 vicryl sutures.

1.5. ATT of Third Molar in Tooth Number 19 Socket. At the transplanted socket, PRF was separated from red corpuscles and placed in the socket. The donator third molar was positioned on the recipient site and adjusted to 1 mm infraocclusion position by trimming interradicular bone, then returning back to saline. The implanted tooth was secured with 0.7 mm wire and composite resin from tooth number 18 to number 20 (Figures 3 and 4).

Immediate postoperative periapical radiograph was taken to ensure the accurate position of the transplanted tooth in the recipient site as shown in Figure 5. In addition to postextraction instructions, the patient was instructed to rinse with 0.12% chlorhexidine gluconate mouthwash two times/day and was prescribed acetaminophen 500 mg tablets three times/day for 3 days, then PRN.

1.6. Postoperative Follow-Up. During the follow-up visit on day 7 postoperatively, the healing of the donor site and the implanted tooth were examined and no issues were reported. Subsequent follow-up was done on a weekly basis. During the 4-week follow-up visit, the splint was changed from nonrigid to flexible orthodontic wire. Subsequent follow-up visits were done at 3, 6, and 12 months.

One year later, the implanted tooth showed continuous root formation as shown in Figure 6, with normal periodontium, tooth mobility, and vital pulp testing. The patient was satisfied and did not report any complaint. On the 2-year follow-up visit, periapical radiograph showed continuous root development reaching >1 root/crown ratio with open apex (Figure 7), and no signs of root resorption confirming the previous findings (Figure 8).

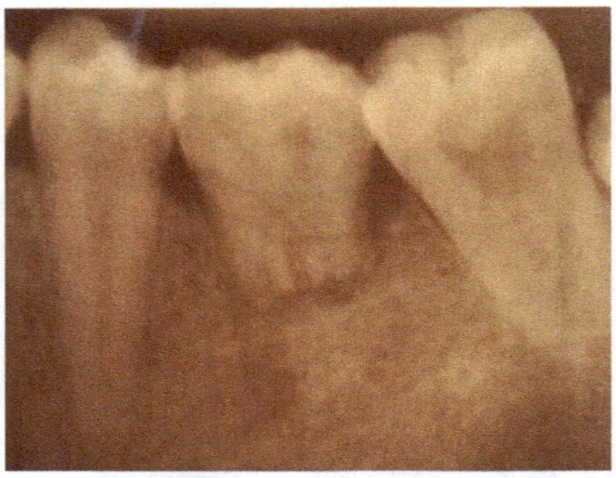

Figure 6: Periapical radiograph showing root formation 1 year after ATT.

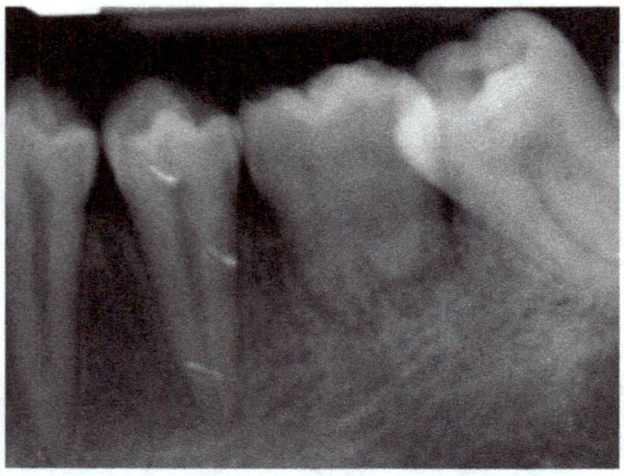

Figure 7: 2-year periapical radiograph showing increased root length and open apex.

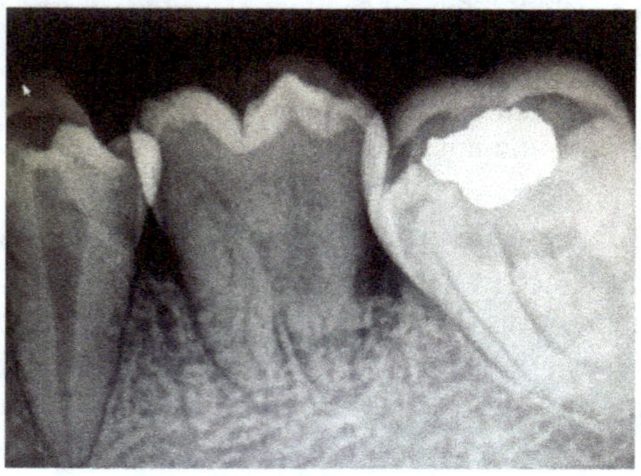

Figure 8: 3-year periapical follow-up radiograph.

2. Discussion

Tooth loss during puberty age especially the first molar is not uncommon. In such cases, limited treatment options are available, such as ATT and implants. Implants are not indicated because they lack the ability to grow and may result in unsightly infraocclusion if placed during growth spurt. Such growth issues warrant the consideration of refined treatment choices with growth-friendly treatment modalities in growing children and/or adolescents.

ATT is considered as a reliable treatment option with proven success. However, for reporting the long-term evaluation of results, the researchers use the survival rate for describing the percentage of transplanted teeth still present at the time of examination [13]. On other hand, successful ATT should fulfil specific criteria including viable tooth with stable occlusion, no pathological mobility or pocket probing depths, and without evidence of ankylosis, root resorption, or infection [22, 23].

Schwartz et al. in 1985 [24] reported the survival rate of 210 autotransplanted teeth and found a 76.2% survival rate following 5 years postoperatively, while the 10-year survival rates dropped to 59.6%. A more recent study by Andreasen et al. [12], evaluating the long-term survival rate and pulpal healing of 370 autotransplanted premolars, with complete and incomplete root formation, has showed that survival rates of the completed root teeth is 98% and 95% for the uncompleted root teeth after an observation period ranging from 1 to 13 years. Andreasen et al. noticed that pulpal healing was highly related to the stage of root development at the time of transplantation. Teeth transplanted with incomplete and complete root formation showed 96% and 15% pulp healing, respectively.

Other studies showed that the ATT success rate may vary between mature and immature teeth. Kugelberg et al. [25] reported a 96% success rate for 23 immature teeth and 82% for 22 mature teeth following 4 years of follow-up. In 2010, Yan et al. [26] and Mensink and Van Merkesteyn [27] reported a 100% success rate of open apex teeth following more than 4 years.

The most recent systemic review and meta-analysis by Rohof et al. [28] in 2018 showed that ATT is a reliable treatment option with survival and success rates of autotransplantation of immature teeth >95% and with complications rates <5% in terms of ankylosis (2.0%), root resorption (2.9%), and pulp necrosis (3.3%).

Meta-analyses, evaluating outcomes of autotransplanted teeth with complete root formation, showed 2% annual failure rate, 2.1% root resorption rate, and 1.2% ankyloses rate with 1- and 5-year survival rates of 98% and 90.5%, respectively [28, 29].

Although ATT of mature and immature teeth is associated with a high success rate, endodontic treatment is usually necessary in mature teeth within 4 weeks to prevent development of pulp-associated lesion. On the other hand, ATT of immature teeth showed the ability of continuous pulp healing and reinnervation. Andreason et al. found that pulpal healing was the usual finding in teeth with immature root formation. He found necrotic pulp that necessitated endodontic treatment in all autotransplanted teeth with completely formed roots. However, according to Denys et al., the teeth with a root length less than half is associated with increased risk for arrested root development rather than more mature ones. His recommendation is that two-thirds to three-quarters of the expected root length is needed to optimize outcomes [30].

PRF was introduced by Choukroun et al. in 2001 as the second generation of platelet concentrates, composed of autologous leukocyte-platelet-rich fibrin matrix and containing various mitogenic factors such as platelet-derived growth factor, vascular endothelial growth factor, and transforming growth factor released by an α granule [31]. According to Choukroun, PRF is prepared simply by centrifuging a patient's own blood at 3000 rpm for 10 minutes without the need for thrombin or anticoagulant additives [31]. After centrifuging, PRF collected as the middle layer containing growth factors [32]. PRF stimulates angiogenesis through migration, division, and phenotypic change of endothelial cells. It also promotes cell mitosis and induces osteogenesis without inflammatory reactions. These effects act in a slow sustained process for at least one week [33] and up to 4 weeks [34, 35]. Dohan Ehrenfest et al. showed that PRF can induce a strong and continuous differentiation and stimulation of osteoblasts for 14 days with fibroblasts [36].

Moreover, PRF has shown successful results when used as a sole agent in periodontal regeneration like clinical attachment loss and intrabony defects [37, 38]. PRF has also shown to be effective in regenerative endodontics. Wang et al. evaluated the effect of PRF in the regenerative therapy of immature permanent canines [39]. PRF was able to increase the thickness of dental-associated mineral tissue. After 12 months follow-up, Bakhtiar et al. reported radiographic evidence of further root development and apical closure in 4 immature teeth with necrotic pulps [40].

Root formation and development are induced by Hertwig's epithelial root sheath (HERS), which is a bilayered epithelium that functions as a stimulator of mesenchymal cell differentiation into odontoblasts and cementoblasts [41]. Within the scope of PRF effects in dental regeneration, the possible mechanism for root development after transplanting third molars with less than a quarter root formed could be explained by the fact that PRF contains a dense fibrin network and a concentration of many growth factors like platelet-derived growth factor and vascular endothelial growth factor in sustainable way. The most important factor is transforming growth factor $\beta 1$ (TGF$\beta 1$), which is also secreted by HERS that induces positively the differentiation of dental papilla cells into odontoblasts ensuring a suitable environment for PDL cells to proliferate and the synthesis of an extracellular matrix [42].

Application of PRF in ATT has been reported successfully in 2 case reports followed for 6 months. Robindro Singh et al. has used PRF in the ATT of an impacted central incisor in a prepared socket as the second stage after the excision of odontoma. He applied the PRF membrane around the tooth at the time of ATT. His 6-month follow-up showed successful results with signs of root developments [42]. Devi et al. reported the immediate ATT of an immature third molar in the socket of an adjacent tooth. Radiographic and clinical examinations have shown successful results [3]. In addition to normal mobility and pocketing examination, two years of radiographic evaluation showed continued root development, as shown in the 3-year follow-up periapical radiograph after transplantation with other favorable clinical measurements.

3. Conclusion

From the presented case, we conclude that the benefits of including PRF in autotransplantation of teeth with immature roots, even when less than a quarter of the roots have formed, acts positively during the immediate and late regeneration process. PRF can eliminate the risk of arrested root formation and the need for pulpal treatment and can decrease the risk of complications.

References

[1] R. A. Mendes and G. Rocha, "Mandibular third molar autotransplantation—literature review with clinical cases," *Journal of the Canadian Dental Association*, vol. 70, no. 11, pp. 761–766, 2004.

[2] C. M. Clokie, D. M. Yau, and L. Chano, "Autogenous tooth transplantation: an alternative to dental implant placement?," *Journal of the Canadian Dental Association*, vol. 67, no. 2, pp. 92–96, 2001.

[3] T. P. Devi, W. T. Singh, N. Sanjeeta, and N. R. Singh, "Immediate autotransplantation of immature third molar with regeneration of recipient site using autologous platelet-rich fibrin," *Journal of Medical Society*, vol. 28, no. 3, pp. 196–199, 2014.

[4] M. Tsukiboshi, "Autogenous tooth transplantation: a reevaluation," *International Journal of Periodontics & Restorative Dentistry*, vol. 13, no. 2, pp. 120–149, 1993.

[5] O. Slagsvold and B. Bjercke, "Autotransplantation of premolars with partly formed roots: a radiographic study of root growth," *American Journal of Orthodontics*, vol. 66, no. 4, pp. 355–366, 1974.

[6] J. O. Andreasen, "Periodontal healing after replantation and autotransplantation of incisors in monkeys," *International Journal of Oral Surgery*, vol. 10, no. 1, pp. 54–61, 1981.

[7] F. Ustad, F. M. Ali, Z. Kota, A. Mustafa, and M. I. Khan, "Autotransplantation of teeth: a review," *American Journal of Medical and Dental Sciences*, vol. 1, no. 1, pp. 25–30, 2013.

[8] T. Nimčenko, G. Omerca, V. Varinauskas, E. Bramanti, F. Signorino, and M. Cicciù, "Tooth auto-transplantation as an alternative treatment option: a literature review," *Dental Research Journal*, vol. 10, no. 1, pp. 1–6, 2013.

[9] T. Shimada, "Effect of periodontal ligament curetted in alveolar socket for autotransplantation of tooth in adult monkeys," *Journal of Japanese Society of Oral Implantology*, vol. 11, pp. 492–500, 1998.

[10] J. O. Andreasen, L. Kristerson, and F. M. Andreasen, "Damage to the Hertwig's epithelial root sheath: effect upon growth after autotransplantation of teeth in monkeys," *Endodontics & Dental Traumatology*, vol. 4, no. 4, pp. 145–151, 1988.

[11] R. L. Osterne, J. J. Moreira Neto, A. D. de Araújo Lima, and R. L. Nogueira, "Autotransplantation of immature third molars and orthodontic treatment after en bloc resection of conventional ameloblastoma," *Journal of Oral and Maxillofacial Surgery*, vol. 73, no. 9, pp. 1686–1694, 2015.

[12] J. O. Andreasen, H. U. Paulsen, Z. Yu, T. Bayer, and O. Schwartz, "A long-term study of 370 autotransplanted premolars. Part II. Tooth survival and pulp healing subsequent to transplantation," *European Journal of Orthodontics*, vol. 12, no. 1, pp. 14–24, 1990.

[13] C. Atala-Acevedo, J. Abarca, M. J. Martínez-Zapata, J. Díaz, S. Olate, and C. Zaror, "Success rate of autotransplantation of teeth with an open apex: systematic review and meta-analysis," *Journal of Oral and Maxillofacial Surgery*, vol. 75, no. 1, pp. 35–50, 2017.

[14] M. Zakershahrak, A. Moshari, M. Vatanpour, Z. Khalilak, and A. Jalali Ara, "Autogenous transplantation for replacing a hopeless tooth," *Iranian Endodontic Journal*, vol. 12, no. 1, pp. 124–127, 2017 Winter.

[15] J. H. Park, K. Tai, and D. Hayashi, "Tooth autotransplantation as a treatment option: a review," *The Journal of Clinical Pediatric Dentistry*, vol. 35, no. 2, pp. 129–135, 2010 Winter.

[16] D. Cross, A. El-Angbawi, P. McLaughlin et al., "Developments in autotransplantation of teeth," *The Surgeon*, vol. 11, no. 1, pp. 49–55, 2013.

[17] M. Tsukiboshi, "Autotransplantation of teeth: requirements for predictable success," *Dental Traumatology*, vol. 18, no. 4, pp. 157–180, 2002.

[18] M. Marques-Ferreira, M. F. Rabaça-Botelho, L. Carvalho, B. Oliveiros, and E. V. Palmeirão-Carrilho, "Autogenous tooth transplantation: evaluation of pulp tissue regeneration," *Medicina Oral, Patología Oral y Cirugía Bucal*, vol. 16, no. 7, pp. e984–e989, 2011.

[19] B. U. Zachrisson, "Planning esthetic treatment after avulsion of maxillary incisors," *Journal of the American Dental Association (1939)*, vol. 139, no. 11, pp. 1484–1490, 2008.

[20] J. Gonzalez-Ocasio and M. Stevens, "Autotransplantation of third molars with platelet-rich plasma for immediate replacement of extracted non-restorable teeth: a case series," *Journal of Oral and Maxillofacial Surgery*, vol. 75, no. 9, pp. 1833.e1–1833.e6, 2017.

[21] R. P. Carmichael and G. K. B. Sàndor, "Dental Implants, Growth of the Jaws, and Determination of Skeletal Maturity," *Atlas of the Oral and Maxillofacial Surgery Clinics*, vol. 16, no. 1, pp. 1–9, 2008.

[22] O. Bauss, W. Engelke, C. Fenske, R. Schilke, and R. Schwestka-Polly, "Autotransplantation of immature third molars into edentulous and atrophied jaw sections," *International Journal of Oral and Maxillofacial Surgery*, vol. 33, no. 6, pp. 558–563, 2004.

[23] P. P. Reich, "Autogenous transplantation of maxillary and mandibular molars," *Journal of Oral and Maxillofacial Surgery*, vol. 66, no. 11, pp. 2314–2317, 2008.

[24] O. Schwartz, P. Bergmann, and B. Klausen, "Autotransplantation of human teeth: A life-table analysis of prognostic factors," *International Journal of Oral Surgery*, vol. 14, no. 3, pp. 245–258, 1985.

[25] R. Kugelberg, U. Tegsjo, and O. Malmgren, "Autotransplantation of 45 teeth to the upper incisor region in adolescents," *Swedish Dental Journal*, vol. 18, no. 5, pp. 165–172, 1994.

[26] Q. Yan, B. Li, and X. Long, "Immediate autotransplantation of mandibular third molar in China," *Oral Surgery, Oral Medicine, Oral Pathology, Oral Radiology, and Endodontics*, vol. 110, no. 4, pp. 436–440, 2010.

[27] G. Mensink and R. Van Merkesteyn, "Autotransplantation of premolars," *British Dental Journal*, vol. 208, no. 3, pp. 109–111, 2010.

[28] E. C. M. Rohof, W. Kerdijk, J. Jansma, C. Livas, and Y. Ren, "Autotransplantation of teeth with incomplete root formation: a systematic review and meta-analysis," *Clinical Oral Investigations*, vol. 22, no. 4, pp. 1613–1624, 2018.

[29] W. C. Chung, Y. K. Tu, Y. H. Lin, and H. K. Lu, "Outcomes of autotransplanted teeth with complete root formation: a systematic review and meta-analysis," *Journal of Clinical Periodontology*, vol. 41, no. 4, pp. 412–423, 2014.

[30] D. Denys, M. Shahbazian, R. Jacobs et al., "Importance of root development in autotransplantations: a retrospective study of 137 teeth with a follow-up period varying from 1 week to 14 years," *European Journal of Orthodontics*, vol. 35, no. 5, pp. 680–688, 2013.

[31] D. M. Dohan, J. Choukroun, A. Diss et al., "Platelet-rich fibrin (PRF): a second-generation platelet concentrate. Part I: technological concepts and evolution," *Oral Surgery, Oral Medicine, Oral Pathology, Oral Radiology, and Endodontics*, vol. 101, no. 3, pp. e37–e44, 2006.

[32] N. K. Kiran, K. S. Mukunda, and T. N. Tilak Raj, "Platelet concentrates: a promising innovation in dentistry," *Journal of Dental Sciences and Research*, vol. 2, no. 1, pp. 50–61, 2011.

[33] Z. Mazor, R. A. Horowitz, M. Del Corso, H. S. Prasad, M. D. Rohrer, and D. M. Dohan Ehrenfest, "Sinus floor augmentation with simultaneous implant placement using Choukroun's platelet-rich fibrin as the sole grafting material: a radiologic and histologic study at 6 months," *Journal of Periodontology*, vol. 80, no. 12, pp. 2056–2064, 2009.

[34] A. Mengji, Subashani, M. Shastri, and R. Anjum, "The clinical application of platelet-rich fibrin (PRF) and allograft in treatment of bony defect—a case report," *IOSR Journal of Dental and Medical Sciences*, vol. 14, no. 12, 2015.

[35] C. H. Tsai, S. Y. Shen, J. H. Zhao, and Y. C. Chang, "Platelet-rich fibrin modulates cell proliferation of human periodontally related cells in vitro," *Journal of Dental Sciences*, vol. 4, no. 3, pp. 130–135, 2009.

[36] D. M. Dohan Ehrenfest, A. Diss, G. Odin, P. Doglioli, M. P. Hippolyte, and J. B. Charrier, "In vitro effects of Choukroun's PRF (platelet-rich fibrin) on human gingival fibroblasts, dermal prekeratinocytes, preadipocytes, and maxillofacial osteoblasts in primary cultures," *Oral Surgery, Oral Medicine, Oral Pathology, Oral Radiology, and Endodontics*, vol. 108, no. 3, pp. 341–352, 2009.

[37] M. Arunachalam, S. J. Pulikkotil, and N. Sonia, "Platelet rich fibrin in periodontal regeneration," *The Open Dentistry Journal*, vol. 10, pp. 174–181, 2016.

[38] A. B. Castro, N. Meschi, A. Temmerman et al., "Regenerative potential of leucocyte- and platelet-rich fibrin. Part A: intrabony defects, furcation defects and periodontal plastic surgery. A systematic review and meta-analysis," *Journal of Clinical Periodontology*, vol. 44, no. 1, pp. 67–82, 2017.

[39] Q. L. Wang, P. P. Yang, L. H. Ge, and H. Liu, "Preliminary evaluation of platelet rich fibrin-mediated tissue repair in immature canine pulpless teeth," *The Chinese Journal of Dental Research*, vol. 19, no. 1, pp. 49–54, 2016.

[40] H. Bakhtiar, S. Esmaeili, S. Fakhr Tabatabayi, M. R. Ellini, M. H. Nekoofar, and P. M. H. Dummer, "Second-generation platelet concentrate (platelet-rich fibrin) as a scaffold in regenerative endodontics: a case series," *Journal of Endodontia*, vol. 43, no. 3, pp. 401–408, 2017.

[41] X. Huang and Y. Chai, "Molecular regulatory mechanism of tooth root development," *International Journal of Oral Science*, vol. 4, no. 4, pp. 177–181, 2012.

[42] W. Robindro Singh, K. Aheibam, and A. Nameirakpam, "Post-odontoma autotransplantation of an impacted tooth: a case report," *Journal of Oral Biology and Craniofacial Research*, vol. 5, no. 2, pp. 120–123, 2015 May-Aug.

24

Management of Discolored Failure Root Canal-Treated Upper Lateral Incisor

Nik Abdul Ghani Nik Rozainah,[1] **Azih Nurul Farah,**[1] **and Mohmed Isaqali Karobari**[2]

[1]*Conservative Department, School of Dental Sciences, Health Campus, Universiti Sains Malaysia, 16150 Kubang Kerian, Kelantan, Malaysia*
[2]*Conservative Unit, School of Dental Sciences, Health Campus, Universiti Sains Malaysia, 16150 Kubang Kerian, Kelantan, Malaysia*

Correspondence should be addressed to Nik Abdul Ghani Nik Rozainah; rozainah@usm.my

Academic Editor: Mine Dündar

Root canal treatment failure can be determined based on a patient's complaint and on the basis of clinical examination and radiographic findings. Most of the signs and symptoms for the failure are pain and discomfort, swelling and sinus formation at the surrounding soft tissue, and discoloration of the subjected tooth. Factors such as mechanical perforation during the procedures, overfilled or underfilled root canal, and missed or unfilled canals are the main factors for the failure outcome. This case report presents a discolored and infected upper lateral incisor which was previously root canal treated. The tooth was successfully managed under nonsurgical and surgical retreatment followed by an internal bleaching and full porcelain veneer. Apical tissue healing and acceptable tooth appearance was observed during a 12-month review.

1. Introduction

The successful outcome of root canal treatment is highly dependent on the elimination of persistent infection and reinfection of the root canal space. Failure can be determined on the patient's complaint, during basic clinical examination, and from radiographic findings. It is more related with the lack of knowledge on the part of the operator and lack of referral for the complex anatomy cases and severe root curvature to be treated by a specialist [1]. Many studies have shown that the failures were related to the presence of extraradicular biofilms, root fracture, mechanical perforations, residual necrotic pulp tissue, broken instruments, periodontal disease, root canal overfilling, root canal underfilling, missed canals or unfilled canals, and insufficient coronal restoration after completion of root canal treatment [2–4]. This clinical report presents a young man who had experienced a root canal treatment failure of his upper left lateral incisor. The tooth had been poorly treated, where the extruded root canal filling had caused a continuous and persistent periapical lesion. At the same time, poorly obturated material had contributed to the tooth discoloration. Root canal retreatment was successfully constructed for the tooth followed by internal bleaching and E-max full porcelain veneer. The successful outcome was observed after a year, where there was evidence of periapical healing and a satisfactory appearance of the tooth.

2. Case Presentation

A 26-year-old man was referred to the Conservative Clinic for the management of the discoloration of a previous root canal treatment for tooth 22. The patient claimed to have had a history of trauma during his teenage years, and the tooth had multiple episodes of pain and swelling. The lesion healed after the completion of root canal treatment which was almost 5 years back. However, for the last few months, the tooth started to cause discomfort with a slight pain during biting or chewing. He also noticed that it became darker and blackish in color. The patient otherwise was cleared from any medical illness, and his health condition was fit and healthy. During an intraoral examination, tooth 22 showed dark discoloration and was tender to palpation and percussion. A 1 mm × 1 mm soft tissue swelling was located at the

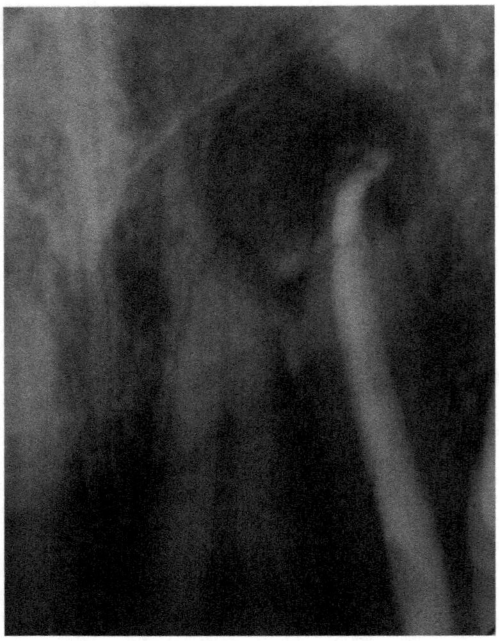

Figure 1: Periapical radiograph showing that tooth 22 had a well-condensed root canal filling, where the gutta percha was overextended with a periapical lesion at the area.

palatal site of the tooth. Thermal test and electronic pulp test indicated a positive response of the adjacent teeth 21 and 23. Periapical radiograph showed that tooth 22 had a well-condensed root canal filling; however, the gutta percha was overextended and there was periapical lesion at the area (Figure 1). Cone Beam Computed Tomography (CBCT) revealed that the size of the lesion was approximately 2 mm × 2 mm (Figure 2). The provisional diagnosis was a failure root canal-treated tooth with chronic apical periodontitis and discolored tooth. After discussion and explanation, the patient agreed for nonsurgical retreatment to remove the infection and extruded gutta percha, thus eliminating and healing the apical periodontitis before undergoing an internal bleaching. The patient was also aware of the possibility of periapical surgery as a complementary approach to resolve the pathology if the conventional retreatment failed to succeed.

2.1. Nonsurgical Root Canal Retreatment. During retreatment, a Dental Operating Microscope (Zeiss OPMI ® pico, Germany) was used to enhance illumination and magnification to reach the apical root and assess the extruded gutta percha. The gutta percha was removed with the use of a chloroform solvent (Sultan Healthcare Inc., USA). Apical gutta percha was hooked and removed with the Hedstrom file #40 and #45 (DiaDent, South Korea) (Figure 3). The canal was rinsed with sodium hypochlorite 2.5% (HUSM Pharmacy, Malaysia) and a new corrected working length was confirmed. No canal preparation was done since it was already shown to have an acceptable diameter and was tapered; furthermore, the apical end showed some root resorption and loss of apical stopper. Nonsetting calcium hydroxide paste (Pulpdent, USA) intracanal medicament was placed into the canal, and the coronal seal was achieved by Fuji IX Glass Ionomer Cement (GC International, Japan). The patient came for a review after 4 weeks; the palatal swelling was completely healed, and he also denied any pain. However, radiographically, the size of the apical lesion remained the same. We discussed with the patient regarding periapical surgery to resolve the pathology and for histopathology biopsy. Verbal and written consent was obtained from the patient. Obturation was performed with F3 ProTaper Gutta Percha (Dentsply Maillefer, USA) as a filling material together with AH plus sealer (Dentsply Maillefer, USA). The root canal was filled up to the new working length 2 mm short from the open apex. The cavity access was sealed with the composite resin Zmack microhybrid (Zhermack SpA, Italy) for a permanent coronal seal.

2.2. Periapical Surgery. During periapical surgery, the operating site was anesthetized with 2% lignocaine containing 1 : 100,000 adrenaline. The Luebke-Oschenbein flap was designed, and once the flap was raised, there was a buccal bone resorption which presented as a small hole measuring 1 mm × 1 mm. Once the lesion was excised, the exposed root tip with an open apex was filled with Mineral Trioxide Aggregate (ProRoot® MTA, Dentsply Sirona, Canada). Freeze-dried cancellous Osteo-Lamb bone graft (USM Tissue Bank, Malaysia) was placed at the bony defect to encourage the growth of key surrounding tissue (Figure 4). Flap closure was carried out with 3-0 VICRYL suture (Ethicon, USA). Oral intake of ibuprofen 600 mg was prescribed when necessary. Histopathological examination revealed fragments of densely collagenous tissue with mature fibroblasts, patchy chronic inflammatory cells, scanty vascular channels, and nerve bundles. A focal area shows a loosely edematous background with admixed hemorrhage, numerous capillaries, and intense inflammatory cells comprising lymphoplasma cells, macrophages, and neutrophils (Figure 5). No epithelial cell lining was observed. The definitive diagnosis was periapical granuloma.

2.3. Nonvital Bleaching. During 6 months of review, the healing was successful and the patient denied any complaint (Figure 6). The tooth was prepared for an internal bleaching under rubber dam isolation. During the procedure, 2 mm gutta percha was cut in the apical direction beyond the cemento-enamel junction. The area was then washed with normal saline, rinsed, and dried. A thin layer of 1 mm Glass Ionomer Fuji II (GC International, Japan) was placed to cover the gutta percha prior to the application of 35% hydrogen peroxide agent (Ultradent Opalescence™ Endo, USA). The bleaching agent was expressed into the open pulp chamber. The cavity was temporarily filled using GC Fuji IX glass ionomer cement (GC International, Japan). The procedure was repeated for every three continuous follow-up visits in three weeks' time until desired results were obtained. Composite resin Zmack microhybrid (Zhermack SpA, Italy) was used as a final and permanent filling.

The patient came back after 2 weeks for an indirect full veneer preparation. Minimal enamel reduction was constructed and an impression taken with light and heavy body

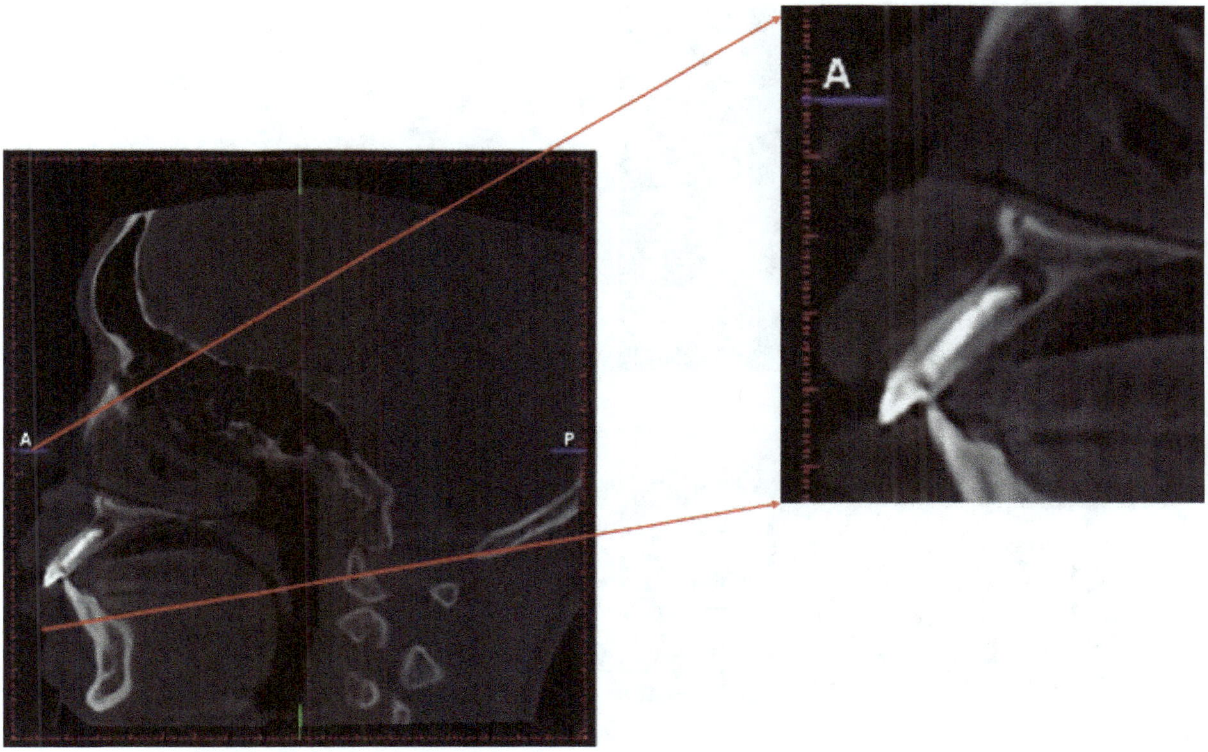

FIGURE 2: Cone Beam Computed Tomography (CBCT) of tooth 22 with a periapical lesion.

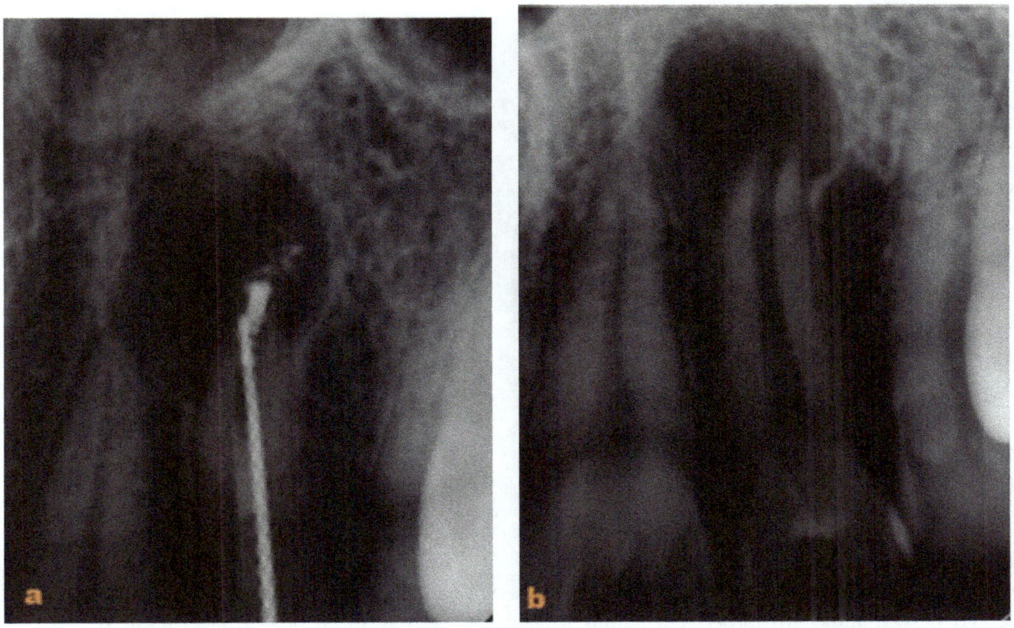

(a) (b)

FIGURE 3: Periapical radiograph of tooth 22 after GP removal with a Hedstrom file.

hydrophilic vinyl polysiloxane material (Examix™ NDS, Japan). Laboratory construction for IPS E-max ceramic (Ivoclar Vivadent, Liechtenstein) was completed after 3 days and the patient was called for full veneer issue. The tooth was adequately isolated by the placement of a rubber dam, and RelyX™ Unicem self-adhesive universal resin cement (3M ESPE, Germany) was used for the cementation. One-year follow-up showed an almost complete healing of the lesion, and acceptable tooth color appearance (Figure 7).

3. Discussion

In the present clinical cases, the quality of the coronal seal and root canal filling was not achieved to a satisfactory

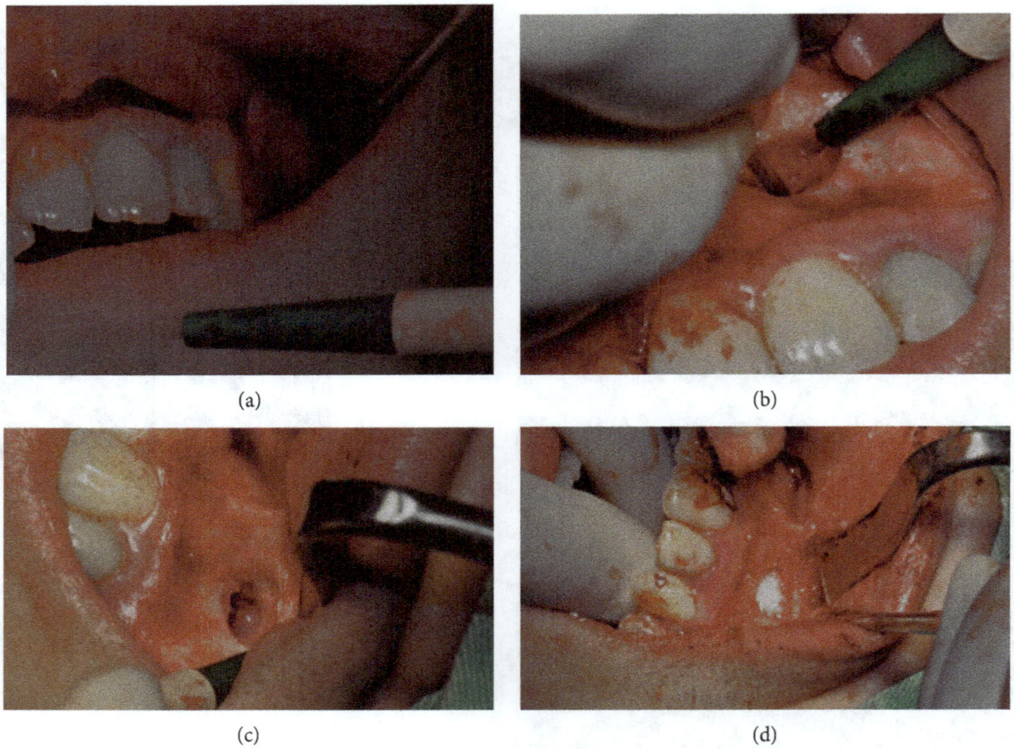

FIGURE 4: Periapical surgery procedure of tooth 22: (a) flap preparation, (b) enucleation of lesion, (c) bone preparation for graft, and (d) bone graft placement.

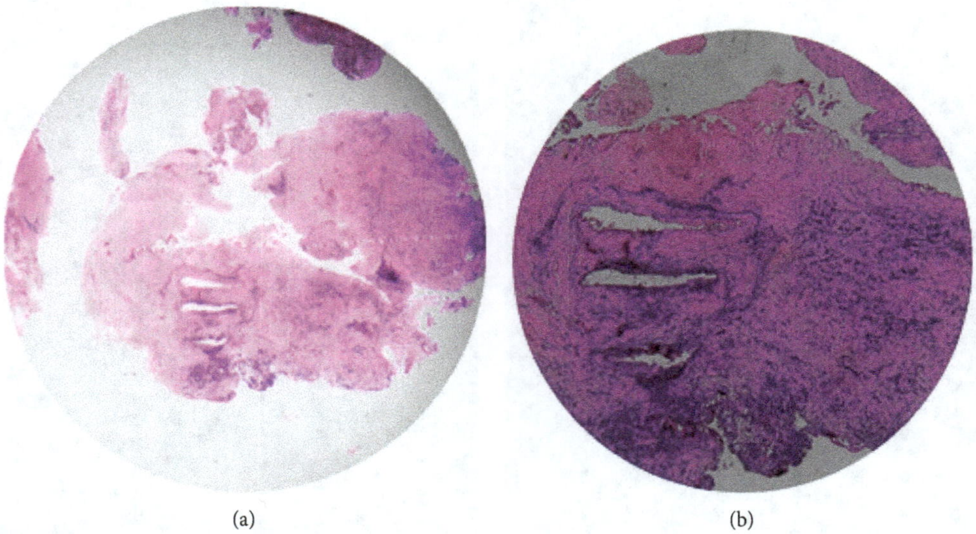

FIGURE 5: Histopathological finding of lesion: (a) collagenous tissue with mature fibroblasts, patchy chronic inflammatory cells, scanty vascular channels, and nerve bundle; (b) loosely edematous background with admixed hemorrhage, numerous capillaries, and intense inflammatory cells comprising lymphoplasma cells, macrophages, and neutrophils.

standard. The extruded gutta percha and the presence of bacterial colonies in the periapical area could be major contribution factors to the inflammatory periapical lesion. Even though the gutta percha for the root canal filling proved to be least toxic and compatible with connective tissue, the studies also revealed that it might cause an early short-term inflammatory tissue reaction [5, 6]. Nonsurgical root canal retreatment is always the first line approach to deal with a failure root canal-treated tooth. In the present clinical cases, nonsurgical retreatment was performed to clean and disinfect the defective canal and to retract the overfilling gutta percha beyond the apical end of the root. Since the patient had suffered for a very long time from the inflammatory lesion and there was still no sign of healing after foreign body removal, we decided to proceed with periapical surgery. The surgery itself is always the last resort, with the main objective

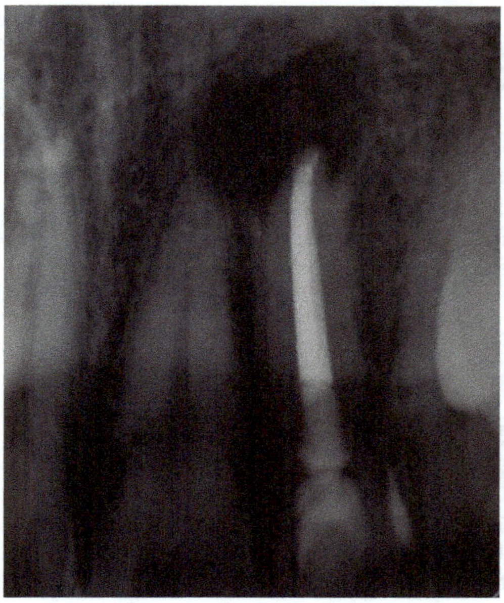

FIGURE 6: Posttreatment radiograph after 6 months.

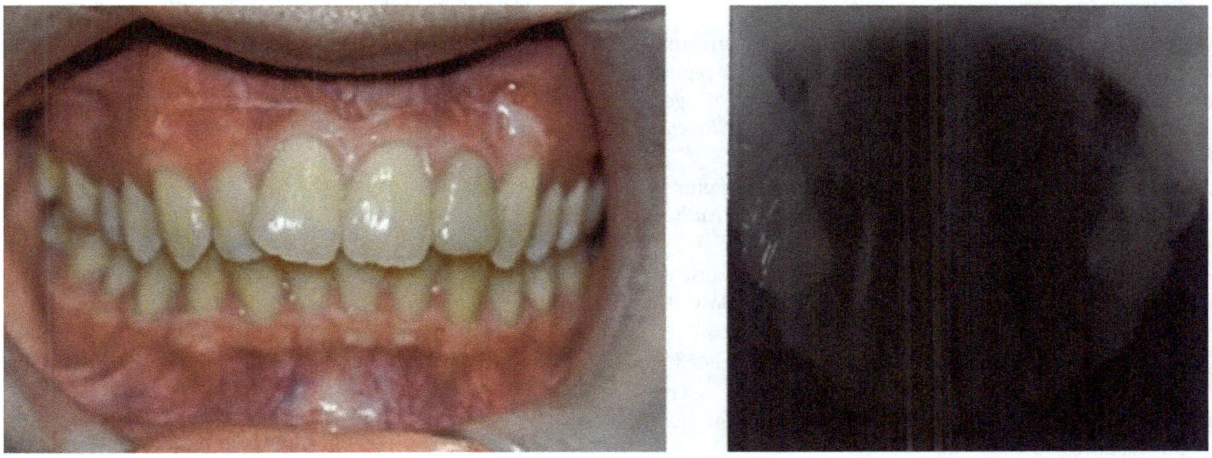

FIGURE 7: One year follow-up in radiograph with patient's tooth color appearance.

of removing the disease of periapical tissues. It is also aimed at sealing the apical root canal system with biocompatible materials in order to facilitate the regeneration of hard and soft tissues, including the formation of new attachment cells [7]. Furthermore, all the endodontic surgery should be undertaken in order for a histopathology assessment to confirm the diagnosis [8]. In the present clinical cases, histopathological biopsy had revealed that the lesion contained condensed fibrous connective tissue which was infiltrated by some hemorrhage and moderate chronic inflammatory cells comprising polymorphonuclear neutrophils, lymphoplasma cells, and macrophages with no epithelium lining detected. Therefore, the diagnosis was confirmed as periapical granuloma. Studies showed that the periapical granuloma contains high inflammatory cell and mediators such as Cyclooxygenase-2 (COX-2) and Tumor Necrosis Factor Alpha (TNF-α). Cytokines Interleukin-33 (IL-33) which belongs to the Interleukin-1 (IL-1) family and its receptor-related ST2 were also present and involved in periapical inflammation [9, 10]. A study revealed that the secretion of TNF-α by macrophages and of COX-2 by several cells was higher in periapical granuloma indicating a greater inflammatory response in these lesions [9]. Furthermore, another study showed increased numbers of IL-33- and ST2-positive fibroblasts in periapical lesions when compared to healthy periapical tissues suggesting that IL-33/ST2 signaling may be involved in periapical inflammation and tissue fibrosis [10]. The formation of new bone had been observed as early as 12 weeks after periapical surgical repair and placement of substitute bone [11]. The use of hydroxyapatite (HA) to fill the osseous defect has been proven to produce a very successful result. HA granules act as a scaffold for blood vessels and migration of osteoblast from surrounding healthy bone, thus promoting differentiation of mesenchymal cells into cartilages and bone. HA will be slowly resorbed and later will be replaced by new bone formation [12, 13]. In our case, freeze-dried cancellous Osteo-Lamb bone graft was used as it was well accepted by the patient and never contradicted with his faith and beliefs. Because of the small anatomical and minimal sound tooth structure, we decided to proceed with a less invasive tooth preparation for the discolored tooth appearance. Nonvital internal bleaching was first constructed for the tooth to achieve acceptable color appearance before proceeding with the indirect full veneer restoration. E-max veneers were chosen since they are made up of porcelain which is highly resistant to stain and only minimal enamel reduction is needed to fit a 0.3 mm thickness of the material [14, 15].

4. Conclusion

A multidisciplinary approach is necessary for a tooth with a previous failure root canal treatment, where consideration for the patient's concern is always prioritized. This case presented with a successful outcome of nonsurgical and surgical root canal retreatment followed by internal bleaching and finally with indirect ceramic veneer restoration.

References

[1] A. Iqbal, "The factors responsible for endodontic treatment failure in the permanent dentitions of the patients reported to the College of Dentistry, the University of Aljouf, Kingdom of Saudi Arabia," *Journal of Clincal and Diagnostic Research*, vol. 10, no. 5, pp. 146–148, 2016.

[2] I. Akbar, "Radiographic study of the problems and failures of endodontic treatment," *International Journal of Health Sciences*, vol. 9, no. 2, pp. 111–118, 2015.

[3] M. Yamaguchi, Y. Noiri, Y. Itoh et al., "Factors that cause endodontic failures in general practices in Japan," *BMC Oral Health*, vol. 18, no. 1, pp. 70–75, 2018.

[4] K. Olcay, H. Ataoglu, and S. Belli, "Evaluation of related factors in the failure of endodontically treated teeth: a cross-sectional study," *Journal of Endodontics*, vol. 44, no. 1, pp. 38–45, 2018.

[5] E. Rosen, T. Goldberger, S. Taschieri, M. del Fabbro, S. Corbella, and I. Tsesis, "The prognosis of altered sensation after extrusion of root canal filling materials: a systematic review of the literature," *Journal of Endodontics*, vol. 42, no. 6, pp. 873–879, 2016.

[6] J. L. Nino-Barrera, L. F. Gamboa-Martinez, H. Laserna-Zuluaga et al., "Factors associated to apical overfilling after a thermoplastic obturation technique—Calamus® or Gutta-core®: a randomized clinical experiment," *Acta Odontológica Latinoamericana*, vol. 31, no. 1, pp. 45–52, 2018.

[7] T. von Arx and M. AlSaeed, "The use of regenerative techniques in apical surgery: a literature review," *The Saudi Dental Journal*, vol. 23, no. 3, pp. 113–127, 2011.

[8] P. A. Rosenberg, J. Frisbie, J. Lee et al., "Evaluation of Pathologists (Histopathology) and Radiologists (Cone Beam Computed Tomography) Differentiating Radicular Cysts from Granulomas," *Journal of Endodontics*, vol. 36, no. 3, pp. 423–428, 2010.

[9] P. R. Álvares, J. A. A. de Arruda, L. V. O. Silva et al., "Immunohistochemical analysis of cyclooxygenase-2 and tumor necrosis factor alpha in periapical lesions," *Journal of Endodontics*, vol. 44, no. 12, pp. 1783–1787, 2018.

[10] M. Velickovic, N. Pejnovic, R. Petrovic et al., "Expression of interleukin-33 and its receptor ST2 in periapical granulomas and radicular cysts," *Journal of Oral Pathology Oral Medicine*, vol. 45, no. 1, pp. 70–76, 2016.

[11] S. Mishra, R. K. Singh, S. Mohammad, R. Pradhan, and U. S. Pal, "A comparative evaluation of decalcified freeze-dried bone allograft, hydroxyapatite and their combination in osseous defects of the jaws," *Journal of Maxillofacial and Oral Surgery*, vol. 9, no. 3, pp. 236–240, 2010.

[12] P. S. Eggli, W. Müller, and R. K. Schenk, "Porous hydroxyapatite and tricalcium phosphate cylinders with two different pore size ranges implanted in the cancellous bone of rabbits. A comparative histomorphometric and histologic study of bony ingrowth and implant substitution," *Clinical Orthopaedics and Related Research*, vol. 232, pp. 127–138, 1998.

[13] J. C. Le Huec, T. Schaeverbeke, D. Clement, J. Faber, and A. Le Rebeller, "Influence of porosity on the mechanical resistance of hydroxyapatite ceramics under compressive stress," *Biomaterials*, vol. 16, no. 2, pp. 113–118, 1995.

[14] L. A. Linhares, L. F. Pottmaier, and G. C. Lopes, "Fracture resistance of veneers in premolars," *European Journal of Dentistry*, vol. 12, no. 2, pp. 191–198, 2018.

[15] A. Tsouknidas, E. Karaoglani, N. Michailidis, D. Kugiumtzis, A. Pissiotis, and K. Michalakis, "Influence of preparation depth and design on stress distribution in maxillary central incisors restored with ceramic veneers: A 3D finite element analysis," *Journal of Prosthodontics*, vol. 29, no. 2, pp. 151–160, 2020.

25

Parathyroidectomy Resolves Tooth Discoloration: A New Presenting Sign of Hyperparathyroidism?

Estella Musacchio,[1] Andrea Piotto,[2] Pierluigi Binotto,[3] Antonio Toniato,[4] and Leonardo Sartori[1]

[1]*Department of Medicine DIMED-Clinica Medica 1-University of Padova, Via Giustiniani 2, 35128 Padova, Italy*
[2]*Department of Surgical, Oncological, and Gastroenterological Sciences-Clinica Chirurgica 3-University of Padova, Via Giustiniani 2, 35128 Padova, Italy*
[3]*Private Dental Practice, Via M. Polo 10, 35123 Padova, Italy*
[4]*Endocrine Surgery Unit, Istituto Oncologico Veneto IOV-IRCCS, Via Gattamelata 64, 35128 Padova, Italy*

Correspondence should be addressed to Estella Musacchio; estella.musacchio@unipd.it

Academic Editor: Hüsamettin Oktay

Introduction. We report the resolution of tooth discoloration following parathyroidectomy in an otherwise asymptomatic woman with primary hyperparathyroidism-associated hypercalcemia. *Case Report.* A 59-year-old Caucasian woman, diagnosed with primary hyperparathyroidism in 2011, nonsmoker with excellent overall oral health. She complained of tooth discoloration starting in 2013. Pigmentation was particularly evident in the necks of the lower central and lateral incisors (Vita Classical score C2). No bleaching was undertaken. Parathyroidectomy was performed five years after primary hyperparathyroidism diagnosis. Six months later, a reduction in pigmentation was strikingly evident, with incisors scoring A1 and A2. The improvement persisted over time. Tooth value also increased compared to baseline. *Conclusions.* This is, to our knowledge, the first report that parathyroidectomy might resolve dental discoloration. This outcome deserves investigation in a meaningful sample size and may eventually prompt the inclusion of dental issues among the consequences of primary hyperparathyroidism.

1. Introduction

Primary hyperparathyroidism (PHPT) is a systemic disease that affects 0.2-1.0% of the general population. Its prevalence is higher in subjects > 65 yrs and in postmenopausal women [1, 2].

The diagnosis of PHPT often is made by occasionally finding elevated serum calcium levels, confirmed by elevated levels of PTH. The treatment of choice for PHPT is parathyroidectomy (PTx) indicated not only in symptomatic patients but also in asymptomatic ones with hypercalcemia, hypercalciuria, and reduced bone density, according to recent guidelines [3, 4]. As a metabolic bone disease, PHPT affects the entire skeleton and may cause abnormalities in the oral cavity, likely by inducing alterations in oral hard tissues or by exacerbating common pathological processes [5].

While most reports about the effects of PTH on dental structures concern experimental models [6, 7], literature regarding oral manifestation of PHPT and/or related biochemical alterations is limited [8, 9]. A very recent systematic review of oral manifestations related to HPT identifies a wide variation in the presentation of the disease concluding that bone pathology, most commonly reported in literature, should not be assumed as the only oral sequelae of HPT [10].

We here report the interesting case of the resolution of tooth pigmentation following PTx in an otherwise asymptomatic woman with PHPT-associated hypercalcemia. This outcome has been reported by patients referred to our clinic

Table 1: Patient's characteristics at baseline and follow-up.

Variable	Normal range	At PHPT diagnosis†	Baseline‡	FU 1 month	FU 6 months	FU 12 months
Age (yrs)		54	59	—	—	60
Biochemistry						
PTH (ng/L)	6.5-36.8	58.2	72.0	48.3	49.9	64.3
Ca total (mmol/L)$	2.10-2.55	2.58	2.76	2.32	2.43	2.37
Ca^{2+} (mmol/L)$$	1.19-1.29	1.36	1.36	1.18	1.15	1.19
u-Ca (mmol/24 h)	2.5-7.5	8.62	8.62	na	na	3.93
p-P (mmol/L)	0.87-1.45	0.91	0.82	na	1.04	0.97
u-P (mmol/24 h)	12.9-42	15.6	19.5	na	na	17.0
25-OH vitamin D (nmol/L)	>75	78	82	na	na	87
Bone mineral density (BMD)						
Lumbar spine L2-L4 *T* score (SD)		-1.6	-1.8	na	na	-1.9
Total femur *T* score (SD)		-1.4	-2.0	na	na	-2.0
Oral assessment						
Teeth (*n*)		27	27	27	27	27
Front upper incisors (vita scale)		A2	C2	C2	A2	A2
Lateral upper incisors (vita scale)		A1	C1	C1	A2-A1	A1
Front lower incisors (vita scale)		A2	C2	C2	A2	A2
Lateral lower incisors (vita scale)		A2	C2	C2	A2	A2
Torus elevation (mm)		na	4	4	4	4

PHPT = primary hyperparathyroidism; FU = follow-up; na = not available/not assessed. †PHPT diagnosis was made 5 yrs prior to surgery. ‡Baseline assessment was performed two months prior to surgery. $Total serum calcium, not adjusted for albumin. $$Ionized calcium, collected and measured according to the current recommendations.

but never addressed before on a formal scientific basis. We believe that it may be overlooked by surgeons and endocrinologists despite its frequent occurrence.

2. Case Report

This is a case report of a nonsmoker Caucasian woman, age 59. Routine biochemical laboratory testing done at menopause in 2010 showed hypercalcemia, 24 hrs hypercalciuria, and elevated PTH. US scan identified a solitary parathyroid adenoma of the upper right gland (12 × 3 mm). The patient was diagnosed with PHPT in 2011. ^{99m}Tc-sestamibi scintigraphy for ectopic sites was negative. PTH, calcemia, ionized calcium, and 24 hrs calciuria were over the upper limit at baseline, two months prior to surgery. Serum and urinary phosphorous, 25-OH vitamin D, serum albumin, eGFR, and all other biochemical parameters were within the normal ranges. Levels were evaluated preoperatively and monitored every month for the first 6 months and thereafter at 12 months (Table 1).

2.1. Medical History. Since age 15, the patient underwent several orthopedic surgeries for traumatic lesions of the ligaments. In all cases, the recovery was complete. Osteopenic at both the lumbar spine and the femur, she underwent i.v. bisphosphonates (zoledronic acid 5 mg) twice, once at 22 months and once at 4 months before PTx, to slow down the HPT-associated bone loss. Home medications included cholecalciferol (7500 UI weekly), antihypertensive therapy, and occasional analgesics.

2.2. Oral Status. The patient had 27 teeth. All four third molars were extracted at age 23 for prophylactic reasons. The second lower left molar was extracted following a trauma at age 24. The patient had no prostheses or implants, and her general oral health was excellent except for gingival recession of the front teeth, more evident in the lower arch. She never smoked nor took any medication known to interfere with dental pigmentation and regularly underwent oral hygiene treatments at 6- to 8-month intervals. She also presented with one right torus mandibularis of 6 mm in length and 4 mm in elevation. The patient had no sialolythiasis. Light microscope analysis of her saliva showed no crystal deposits of any kind. Beginning in 2013, the patient complained of tooth discoloration, particularly evident in the necks of the lower central and lateral incisors. No bleaching was performed.

Tooth shade was evaluated by visual assessment independently by three calibrated examiners (one dentist and two oral hygienists) using a shade guide (Vita Classical A1-D4) [11]. Range covers 16 tooth shades from white to reddish-grey: A1-A4 (reddish-brownish), B1-B4 (reddish-yellowish), C1-C4 (greyish shades), and D2-D4 (reddish-grey). Assessments were repeated during follow-ups (at 1, 6, and 12 months), each performed in the same room, at the same time of the day and under the same artificial central and positional lights. Disagreements were discussed and resolved by a fourth professional, a dentist. Dental pigmentation tended toward green-grey shades in the front teeth and was particularly evident at the neck level of the front incisors where it was C2. Posterior teeth such as molars and premolars did not exhibit the same pronounced pattern, possibly because there was no gingival recession, so the most pigmented area was not visible. Tooth value, a subjective index of the relative brightness or darkness, was negative [12, 13].

2.3. Outcome. For personal reasons, as PHPT was not extremely severe, the patient preferred to delay PTx: it was eventually performed six years after the first finding of hypercalcemia. Histology was positive for chief cell adenoma arranged in solid, trabecular, and pseudoacinar patterns. After surgery, the therapy was integrated for one month with calcitriol 25 μg twice daily and calcium carbonate 1000 mg, in order to prevent secondary HPT following calcium drop. Calcium carbonate was substituted with calcium citrate and finally discontinued due to intolerance. Dietary calcium-containing food allowed a total calcium intake of 500-800 mg daily. One month after PTx, cholecalciferol supplements were resumed according to the preoperative schedule.

The patient's main characteristics before and after endocrine surgery are reported in the table. Biochemical profile was characterized by higher serum calcium and elevated PTH levels. PTH dropped from 130 to 13 ng/L intraoperatively, but increased afterwards, reaching 64.3 ng/L one year after surgery. At a subsequent evaluation at 18 months, PTH declined to 48.2 ng/L (data not shown).

Six months after PTx, the reversal of dental discoloration was strikingly evident with a score of A1 and A2 for the upper and the lower incisors, respectively. This persisted throughout the remaining follow-up period and was recently confirmed at the latest check-up. Tooth value also increased compared to baseline. Dental sensitivity, self-reported by the patient as mild, did not change.

3. Discussion

PTx was accompanied by a dramatic decrease in tooth discoloration and by an improvement in value that paralleled the decrease observed in total and ionized serum calcium levels but was independent of HPT resolution. Indeed, the patient showed a prompt decline of hypercalcemia, while PTH remained over the upper limit, even if at a lower extent compared to the levels recorded before surgery. Such persistence of higher PTH must be considered secondary to the low serum calcium levels. Visible calcium deposition in hypercalcemic states is well described with respect to the eye and also the tooth (in vitamin D intoxication), but changes in teeth color were never reported before [14]. Providing a rationale to this finding is problematic. The tooth being the most calcified structure of the body, a tropism, or selective calcium deposition can be hypothesized with the meaning of storage/scavenger of excess calcium ions at the dentin level, less calcified but more metabolically active than the enamel and therefore more prone to subsequent calcium ion release [15, 16]. This proposition could also explain why the color variation happened so sudden. The actual molecular mechanism needs to be clarified.

Padbury et al. reported a higher frequency of tori in a population affected with PHPT [5], as a consequence of an imbalance between cortical and trabecular bone turnover. The pathogenesis of tori has long been debated and is generally thought to be multifactorial with contributions of genetic as well as environmental factors, such as mandibular shape and occlusal forces [17]. Our patient did not show any reduction in torus size over the follow-up period, nor did substantial changes occur in femoral and lumbar BMD. Note that PTH levels persisted over the upper limit. Also, the times of bone remodeling are quite long so that, in general, tori disappearance may be as slow as their growth.

Today's profile of PHPT manifestations in the oral cavity is more subtle than what was described decades ago [10]. To our knowledge, tooth pigmentation has never been reported as a potential sign. We are aware that tooth-shade assessment would be more objective if carried out with a shade-matching electronic instrument such as the one used in prosthetic restoration. However, in the presented case, the goal was not aesthetic and the measures conducted under controlled and reproducible conditions by healthcare professionals are reliable enough to adequately describe the finding [18], particularly since the shade differences before and after surgery were remarkable.

As we have now entered the "era of outward appearance," both the physical and aesthetic perfections of the body have never been pursued so widely. With all the media and social pressure, much emphasis is also devoted to the harmony and regularity of the mouth and teeth whitening has become a major issue in a person's self-approval [19]. Given these premises, we believe that the oral professionals' role in recognizing unacknowledged PHPT patients may be relevant. In cases of subjects with refractory or recurrent tooth discoloration despite hygiene and whitening sessions, PHPT may be suspected. Checking PTH and calcemia levels would be a simple, cost-effective, and valuable procedure borne of the kind of cooperation among healthcare specialists that should be a basis of public health strategies [20].

4. Conclusions

HPT uncovering could exemplify how different medical branches should interact for the overall benefit of the patient. Consequences of untreated PHPT may be serious and lead to clinically significant complications, with a subsequent economic burden. Nevertheless, a clear marker of the disease is missing and HPT diagnosis is often casual.

The present finding is to our knowledge the first report of dental pigmentation resolution after PTx. We believe it deserves deeper investigation with a larger sample size and may eventually prompt the inclusion of dental issues among the consequences and possible markers of PHPT.

Consent

The patient described in the study has read and signed the informed consent.

Acknowledgments

We are grateful to Mr. Peter Rinearson for his contribution to the English language editing.

References

[1] M. D. Walker and S. J. Silverberg, "Primary hyperparathyroidism," *Nature Reviews Endocrinology*, vol. 14, no. 2, pp. 115–125, 2018.

[2] J. P. Bilezikian, L. Bandeira, A. Khan, and N. E. Cusano, "Hyperparathyroidism," *The Lancet*, vol. 391, no. 10116, pp. 168–178, 2018.

[3] J. T. Adler, R. S. Sippel, and H. Chen, "New trends in parathyroid surgery," *Current Problems in Surgery*, vol. 47, no. 12, pp. 958–1017, 2010.

[4] A. A. Khan, D. A. Hanley, R. Rizzoli et al., "Primary hyperparathyroidism: review and recommendations on evaluation, diagnosis, and management. A Canadian and international consensus," *Osteoporosis International*, vol. 28, no. 1, pp. 1–19, 2017.

[5] A. D. Padbury Jr., T. F. Tözüm, M. Taba Jr. et al., "The impact of primary hyperparathyroidism on the oral cavity," *The Journal of Clinical Endocrinology & Metabolism*, vol. 91, no. 9, pp. 3439–3445, 2006.

[6] Y. Li, Z. Hu, C. Zhou et al., "Intermittent parathyroid hormone (PTH) promotes cementogenesis and alleviates the catabolic effects of mechanical strain in cementoblasts," *BMC Cell Biology*, vol. 18, no. 1, p. 19, 2017.

[7] L. Risom, L. Christoffersen, J. Daugaard-Jensen et al., "Identification of six novel PTH1R mutations in families with a history of primary failure of tooth eruption," *PLoS One*, vol. 8, no. 9, article e74601, 2013.

[8] P. Brabyn, A. Capote, M. Belloti, and I. Zylberberg, "Hyperparathyroidism diagnosed due to brown tumors of the jaw: a case report and literature review," *Journal of Oral and Maxillofacial Surgery*, vol. 75, no. 10, pp. 2162–2169, 2017.

[9] S. Silverman Jr., G. Gordan, T. Grant, H. Steinbach, E. Eisenberg, and R. Manson, "The dental structures in primary hyperparathyroidsm: Studies in forty-two consecutive dentulous patients," *Oral Surgery, Oral Medicine, and Oral Pathology*, vol. 15, no. 4, pp. 426–436, 1962.

[10] B. Palla, E. Burian, R. Fliefel, and S. Otto, "Systematic review of oral manifestations related to hyperparathyroidism," *Clinical Oral Investigations*, vol. 22, no. 1, pp. 1–27, 2018.

[11] R. D. Paravina, "Performance assessment of dental shade guides," *Journal of Dentistry*, vol. 37, Supplement 1, pp. e15–e20, 2009.

[12] D. Tao, J. N. Sun, X. Wang et al., "In vitro and clinical evaluation of optical tooth whitening toothpastes," *Journal of Dentistry*, vol. 67, pp. S25–S28, 2017.

[13] S. Cochrane, "The Munsell color system: a scientific compromise from the world of art," *Studies in History and Philosophy of Science*, vol. 47, pp. 26–41, 2014.

[14] A. Watts and M. Addy, "Tooth discolouration and staining: a review of the literature," *British Dental Journal*, vol. 190, no. 6, pp. 309–316, 2001.

[15] R. S. Lacruz, "Enamel: molecular identity of its transepithelial ion transport system," *Cell Calcium*, vol. 65, pp. 1–7, 2017.

[16] V. E. Arana-Chavez and L. F. Massa, "Odontoblasts: the cells forming and maintaining dentine," *The International Journal of Biochemistry & Cell Biology*, vol. 36, no. 8, pp. 1367–1373, 2004.

[17] A. R. G. Cortes, Z. Jin, M. D. Morrison, E. S. Arita, J. Song, and F. Tamimi, "Mandibular tori are associated with mechanical stress and mandibular shape," *Journal of Oral and Maxillofacial Surgery*, vol. 72, no. 11, pp. 2115–2125, 2014.

[18] D. Kuzmanović and K. M. Lyons, "Tooth shade selection using a colorimetric instrument compared with that using a conventional shade guide," *The New Zealand Dental Journal*, vol. 105, no. 4, pp. 131–134, 2009.

[19] C. J. Schmidt and S. A. Tatum, "Cosmetic dentistry," *Current Opinion in Otolaryngology & Head and Neck Surgery*, vol. 14, no. 4, pp. 254–259, 2006.

[20] M. Warren, "Defining health in the era of value-based care: the six Cs of health and healthcare," *Cureus*, vol. 9, no. 2, article e1046, 2017.

26

Efficacy of the Combination of rhBMP-2 with Bone Marrow Aspirate Concentrate in Mandibular Defect Reconstruction after a Pindborg Tumor Resection

Kamel Alraei,[1] **Jameel Sharqawi**,[2] **Somaya Harcher**,[3] **and Ibrahim Ghita**[4]

[1]*Department of Oral and Maxillofacial Surgery, Al-Noor Specialist Hospital, Makkah, Saudi Arabia*
[2]*Department of Oral and Maxillofacial Surgery, Royal Commission Hospital, Jubail, Saudi Arabia*
[3]*General Dentist, Saudi Arabia*
[4]*Department of Hematology, Al-Noor Specialist Hospital, Makkah, Saudi Arabia*

Correspondence should be addressed to Kamel Alraei; drkamel2@yahoo.com

Academic Editor: Daniel Torres-Lagares

Recombinant human bone morphogenetic protein-2 (rhBMP-2) is an osteoinductive growth factor used in oral and maxillofacial surgery. It offers a feasible alternative for various regenerative procedures, including reconstruction of mandibular defects. In this study, we report a case of a large Pindborg tumor involving the left mandible. The treatment consisted of surgical resection, followed by off-label use of rhBMP-2 in addition to bone marrow aspirate concentrate, together with an allograft in a titanium mesh. The patient was rehabilitated with dental implants, and a good clinical outcome was achieved. We found no evidence of bone resorption or complications in both clinical and radiographic evaluations during the one-year follow-up period. In conclusion, we have demonstrated the efficacy of using rhBMP-2 combined with bone marrow aspirate concentrate, and an allograft with a titanium mesh, for the reconstruction of long mandibular bone defects. Not only is this combination feasible, but it also has the advantages of lower morbidity and cost.

1. Introduction

The reconstruction of mandibular defects poses a significant challenge in oral and maxillofacial surgery, particularly in cases with bone continuity defects [1]. Mandibular defects can be a result of trauma, benign tumors, or malignancies [2]. For successful reconstruction of mandibular defects, the surgeon must establish mandibular continuity, in addition to restoring the height and width of the bone to allow further dental rehabilitation [3].

Autogenous bone grafts are considered the gold standard for surgical repair of most osseous defects [4, 5]; however, there are major drawbacks to this treatment modality, including donor site morbidity and the limited amount of bone that can be harvested [6, 7]. With recent breakthroughs in tissue engineering, many new graft materials and treatment modalities for the reconstruction of mandibular defects have been developed. One of the alternatives to traditional bone grafting is the use of recombinant human bone morphogenetic protein-2 (rhBMP-2), which is a potent osteoinductive growth factor that attracts mesenchymal stem cells, and stimulates them to proliferate and differentiate into osteoblasts [8, 9]. rhBMP-2 can be used alone or in combination with different types of grafts, such as allografts and autografts. Allografts are osteoconductive materials, which maintain space for bone ingrowth, whereas bone marrow aspirate concentrate (BMAC) increases the supply of stem cells and cytokines, thus increasing the osteogenic potential of the graft [10].

In this study, we sought to evaluate the results of using rhBMP-2 combined with BMAC, and an allograft with a titanium mesh, for the reconstruction of segmental bone defects.

2. Case Presentation

A 27-year-old woman presented to the clinic for evaluation of a persistent swelling on the left side of the mandible

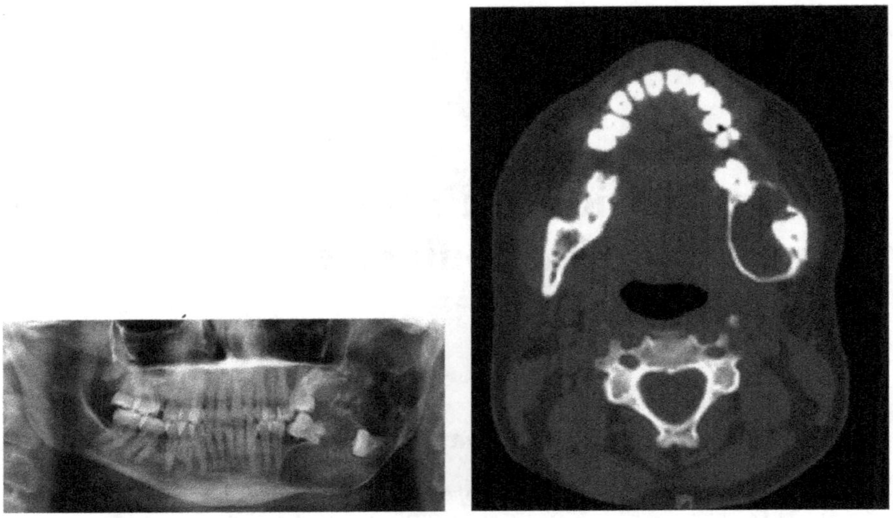

(a) (b)

Figure 1: (a) Orthopantomogram showing an impacted 38 with an associated multilocular radiolucent lesion involving the left posterior mandible, which extends from the second premolar to the left condyle. (b) Axial view of a computed tomographic image of the facial bone showing a hypodense lesion in the left posterior mandible, with expansion and thinning of both the buccal and lingual cortices.

causing facial asymmetry. Radiographic imaging showed a multilocular, radiolucent lesion involving the left posterior mandible, extending into the left condyle (Figure 1). We performed a biopsy which revealed a calcifying, cystic, odontogenic tumor (a Pindborg tumor). As this tumor is aggressive, we decided to proceed with a transcutaneous segmental resection under general anesthesia, followed by immediate reconstruction using a 2.7 mm reconstruction plate (Figure 2). The patient's postoperative course was uneventful. After nine months, the patient returned for the reconstruction of the mandibular defect using rhBMP-2 combined with BMAC, and an allograft with a titanium mesh.

Under general anesthesia, we cannulated the patient's posterior left iliac crest; 60 cc of bone marrow was then aspirated and concentrated using density gradient centrifugation. We placed the patient into maxillomandibular fixation and made a transcutaneous submandibular incision at the scar site of the previous incision. After proper dissection, we exposed the entire defect, together with the reconstruction plate, and recontoured the adjacent bony margins. The titanium mesh was then adapted to reconstruct the mandibular contour, while acting as a protective matrix to contain the graft material. We then secured the mesh in place with a wire. We placed a total of 12 mg of rhBMP-2 (Infuse® Bone Graft from Medtronic Sofamor Danek, Inc.; Tennessee, USA) in four absorbable collagen sponges (1.5 mg/ml). Two sponges were placed inside the mesh, and the two other sponges were cut into small pieces and mixed with 16 mm of allogenic cancellous bone (LifeNet Health; Virginia, USA) in combination with BMAC. The graft material was then packed into the osseous defect. An additional allogenic block (measuring 3 × 1.5 cm) soaked in BMAC was placed in the posterior aspect of the defect, to allow greater dimensional stability (Figure 3). A "watertight" seal closure was performed. The postoperative course was uneventful.

The patient showed radiographic evidence of bone formation three months after the operation; mandibular continuity was regained, as demonstrated both radiographically and clinically (Figure 4(a)). After six months of follow-up, the reconstruction plate was removed as it would have blocked the subsequent placement of implants (Figure 4(b)). Three dental implants were placed under local anesthesia (Figure 4(c)), and prosthetic rehabilitation with implant-supported partial dentures was initiated three months later (Figure 4(d)). After four years of follow-up, a good implant stability and cosmetic outcome was achieved.

3. Discussion

Successful reconstruction of mandibular continuity defects requires the restoration of both vertical and horizontal dimensions of the bone for further functional rehabilitation and implant placement; this step is essential for the creation of an appropriate facial form [11]. In the case of the patient presented herein, we were able to meet these objectives while minimizing morbidity.

Autogenous bone grafts are still considered the gold standard for the reconstruction of osseous defects since they incorporate all the properties necessary for bone regeneration, i.e. osteogenesis, osteoinduction, and osteoconduction. Furthermore, they are histocompatible, meaning that they do not trigger a specific immune response and are not associated with the risk of infection transmission [12, 13]. The most common donor site for obtaining autogenous bone grafts is the iliac crest; the main advantage of this site is the availability of sufficient quantities of bone with the desired quality [12, 14, 15]. Despite all the benefits, the use of autogenous bone grafts is still associated with a high morbidity and a number of potential complications (namely increased overall time of the surgical procedure, risk of hematoma, pelvic instability, sensory disturbances, poor cosmetic appearance,

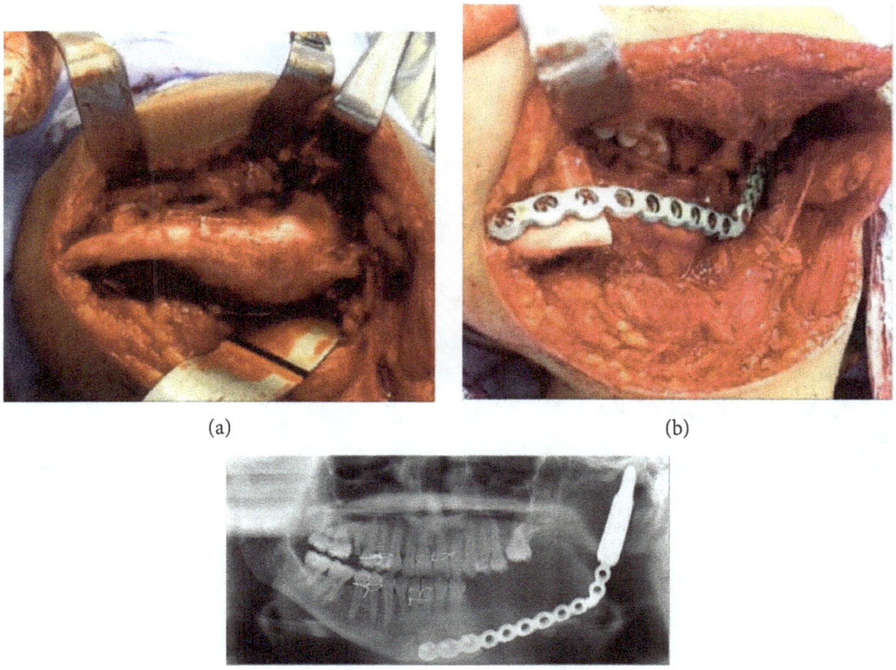

(a) (b) (c)

Figure 2: (a) Photograph showing the tumor and the expansion of both the buccal and lingual cortices. (b) Segmental resection of the left mandible stabilized with a 2.7 mm reconstruction plate. (c) Postoperative orthopantomogram.

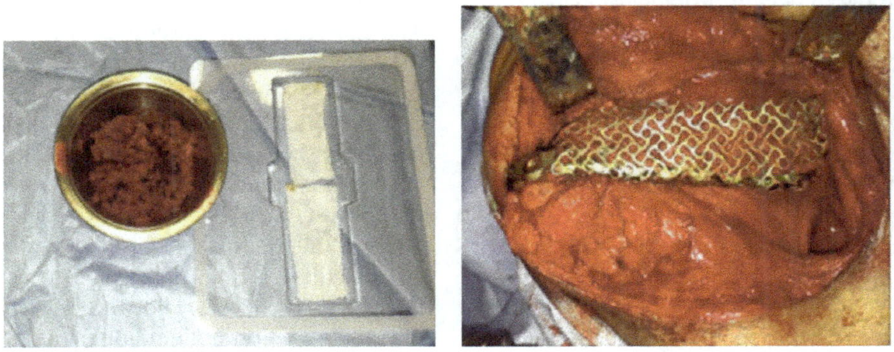

(a) (b)

Figure 3: (a) Absorbable collagen sponges (ACS) impregnated with recombinant human bone morphogenetic protein-2 (rhBMP-2) (right side) and allogenic chips soaked in bone marrow aspirate concentrate (BMAC) with small cut pieces of ACS with rhBMP-2 (left side). (b) Photograph showing the entire defect filled with rhBMP-2 combined with demineralized bone allograft and BMAC.

gait disturbance, infections, herniation of abdominal content, and acute or chronic pain). However, the surgical technique also has an important role in determining postoperative complications [16–18]. The use of autogenous bone grafts in mandibular defects provides a reasonable long-term survival and high success rate (up to 70%); however, the chances of a successful outcome are lower if the defect is longer than 6 cm [19, 20].

Allografts are mainly space-occupying, osteoconductive structures with minimal osteoinductive capability, as they are designed to have minimal antigenicity and risk of infection transmission [21, 22]. Several studies have compared different types of allograft materials in procedures such as ridge augmentation, sinus lift, and bone reconstruction in the maxillofacial region. These studies have concluded that allografts provide an acceptable material for grafting, with the main advantage being the saving of surgical time as no additional bone harvest site is required, as in autogenous bone grafts [23–27].

Members of the transforming growth factor beta superfamily have superior osteoinductive capabilities, with rhBMP-2 and rhBMP-7 being the most extensively studied for the treatment of bone defects. Studies have shown that rhBMP-2 can stimulate osteoblastic differentiation of mesenchymal stem cells, resulting in newly formed bone that has the same composition as that of natural bone [28, 29]. Therefore, rhBMP-2 is one of the most promising growth factors for the regeneration of osseous defects. In addition, it also overcomes most of the problems associated with both autogenous and allogenous bone grafts.

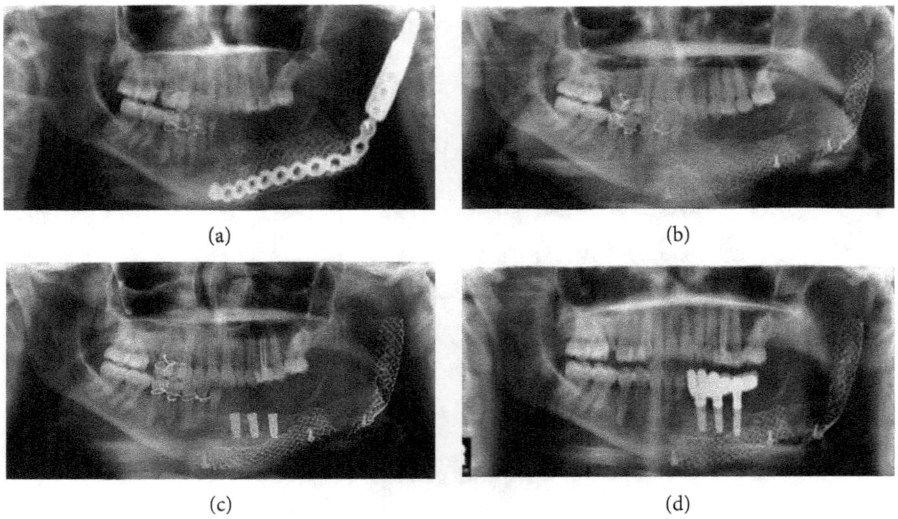

Figure 4: (a) Orthopantomogram (OPG) at the three-month follow-up. (b) OPG after removing the reconstruction plate. Bone regeneration can be observed on the left mandible. (c) OPG showing implant rehabilitation. (d) OPG showing prosthetic rehabilitation with dental implants and an implant-supported partial denture.

Moghadam et al. reported in 2001 the first application of rhBMP-2 in a human mandibular reconstruction. In this study, the authors demonstrated successful bone formation in a 6 cm long mandibular discontinuity defect after segmental resection, with radiographic and histological evidence of new bone formation [30]. Since then, several reports have mentioned the off-label use of rhBMP-2 in mandibular reconstruction [31–34]. For instance, Sheikh et al. reported in 2015 that a predictable reconstruction of continuity bone defects larger than 6 cm could be achieved with the use of rhBMP-2 (12 mg) and BMAC (10 ml), as an alternative to autogenous bone grafting [35].

Studies in animals and humans have shown that when rhBMP-2 is combined with absorbable collagen sponges, it can induce new bone formation even in defects of critical size [34, 36]. Absorbable collagen sponges are ideal carriers for rhBMP-2, as they strongly bind it and provide a continuous release of the protein into the surrounding milieu over a period of three weeks. Nevertheless, absorbable collagen sponges lack structural stability and have a limited ability to prevent soft tissue compression at the surgical site; this further negatively affects vascular growth in bone [35, 37].

Degidi et al. reported in 2003 that titanium mesh has the necessary stiffness for maintaining the space required for bone regeneration, especially in large mandibular or maxillary defects. Furthermore, it can be adapted and contoured into the desired form [38]. Carter et al. have reported in 2008 that one of the possible factors contributing to graft failure in cases of mandibular defect reconstruction was the lack of a space maintainer [39]. An additional benefit of titanium mesh is that it retains the graft material in position with more stability; this was especially useful, as our patient had previously undergone marginal resection [40]. The titanium mesh was easy to handle, molded around the reconstruction plate, and produced successful outcomes with neither wound dehiscence nor infections.

The rationale behind the use of BMAC is that it contains a considerable number of mesenchymal stem cells, which can differentiate into osteoprogenitor cells [41]. Bone marrow aspirate can be easily harvested by aspirating the iliac bone; the procedure is cost-effective and has low morbidity [42]. The aspirate is then concentrated by centrifugation to increase the ratio of mesenchymal stem cells to growth factors [43].

When bone marrow aspirate is combined with graft material, bone regeneration is enhanced; in some cases, it has been shown to be comparable to the results obtained from using an autograft alone. For instance, Taghavi et al. have shown in 2010 that a combination of bone marrow aspirate with allograft is a viable alternative to autogenous bone grafts [44]. Moreover, Hernigou et al. in 2014 studied approximately 1000 patients who were treated with bone grafts for delayed-union or nonunion fractures, and found that the number of adverse events was significantly lower for the bone marrow aspirate group when compared to the autograft group [45]. Furthermore, Carter et al. reported in 2008 that when rhBMP-2 was combined with bone marrow cells, two out of three cases showed successful regeneration of the mandibular defect, while one case failed to form bone due to chronic infection and lack of space maintenance by the graft [39].

The case described in this study shows that it is possible to perform mandibular reconstruction using rhBMP-2 in combination with BMAC mixed with an allograft; it is logical to combine them all with a titanium mesh to bring about bone neoformation. Even if the use of this combination seems to result in a predictable outcome, further studies are needed to determine the ideal combination of grafting materials that would result in maximal clinical and cost-effectiveness.

Consent

We discussed our treatment plan with the patient, including risks and potential complications. We obtained written informed consent from the patient.

Authors' Contributions

Kamel Alraei conceptualized the study and collected the data. Kamel Alraei and Somaya Harcher contributed to data analysis and the writing of the manuscript. Jameel Shrqawi and Ibrahim Ghita contributed to the drafting and review of the manuscript.

References

[1] C. M. Misch, O. T. Jensen, M. A. Pikos, and J. P. Malmquist, "Vertical bone augmentation using recombinant bone morphogenetic protein, mineralized bone allograft, and titanium mesh: a retrospective cone beam computed tomography study," *The International Journal of Oral & Maxillofacial Implants*, vol. 30, no. 1, pp. 202–207, 2015.

[2] A. S. Herford, "rhBMP-2 as an option for reconstructing mandibular continuity defects," *Journal of Oral and Maxillofacial Surgery*, vol. 67, no. 12, pp. 2679–2684, 2009.

[3] J. M. Lane, A. W. Yasko, E. Tomin et al., "Bone marrow and recombinant human bone morphogenetic protein-2 in osseous repair," *Clinical Orthopaedics and Related Research*, vol. 361, pp. 216–227, 1999.

[4] O. T. Jensen, L. B. Shulman, M. S. Block, and V. J. Iacono, "Report of the sinus consensus conference of 1996," *The International Journal of Oral & Maxillofacial Implants*, vol. 13, Supplement, pp. 11–45, 1998.

[5] R. E. Marx, "Clinical application of bone biology to mandibular and maxillary reconstruction," *Clinics in Plastic Surgery*, vol. 21, no. 3, pp. 377–392, 1994.

[6] Z. H. Baqain, M. Anabtawi, A. A. Karaky, and Z. Malkawi, "Morbidity from anterior iliac crest bone harvesting for secondary alveolar bone grafting: an outcome assessment study," *Journal of Oral and Maxillofacial Surgery*, vol. 67, no. 3, pp. 570–575, 2009.

[7] A. Joshi and G. C. Kostakis, "An investigation of post-operative morbidity following iliac crest graft harvesting," *British Dental Journal*, vol. 196, no. 3, pp. 167–171, 2004.

[8] S. D. Cook, S. L. Salkeld, M. R. Brinker, M. W. Wolfe, and D. C. Rueger, "Use of an osteoinductive biomaterial (rhOP-1) in healing large segmental bone defects," *Journal of Orthopaedic Trauma*, vol. 12, no. 6, pp. 407–412, 1998.

[9] M. F. Sciadini and K. D. Johnson, "Evaluation of recombinant human bone morphogenetic protein-2 as a bone-graft substitute in a canine segmental defect model," *Journal of Orthopaedic Research*, vol. 18, no. 2, pp. 289–302, 2000.

[10] H. Dym and J. Pierse, "Advanced techniques in bone grafting procedures," *Dental Clinics of North America*, vol. 55, no. 3, pp. 453–460, 2011.

[11] C. M. Clokie and G. K. Sándor, "Reconstruction of 10 major mandibular defects using bioimplants containing BMP-7," *Journal of the Canadian Dental Association*, vol. 74, no. 1, pp. 67–72, 2008.

[12] T. W. Bauer and G. F. Muschler, "Bone graft materials: an overview of the basic science," *Clinical Orthopaedics and Related Research*, vol. 371, pp. 10–27, 2000.

[13] V. M. Goldberg and S. Akhavan, "Biology of bone grafts," in *Bone Regeneration and Repair*, J. R. Lieberman and G. E. Friedlaender, Eds., Springer, 2005.

[14] G. Schmidmaier, S. Herrmann, J. Green et al., "Quantitative assessment of growth factors in reaming aspirate, iliac crest, and platelet preparation," *Bone*, vol. 39, no. 5, pp. 1156–1163, 2006.

[15] M. E. Elsalanty and D. G. Genecov, "Bone grafts in craniofacial surgery," *Craniomaxillofacial Trauma & Reconstruction*, vol. 2, no. 3-4, pp. 125–134, 2009.

[16] E. D. Arrington, W. J. Smith, H. G. Chambers, A. L. Bucknell, and N. A. Davino, "Complications of iliac crest bone graft harvesting," *Clinical Orthopaedics and Related Research*, vol. 329, pp. 300–309, 1996.

[17] D. W. Boone, "Complications of iliac crest graft and bone grafting alternatives in foot and ankle surgery," *Foot and Ankle Clinics*, vol. 8, no. 1, pp. 1–14, 2003.

[18] A. Barone, M. Ricci, F. Mangano, and U. Covani, "Morbidity associated with iliac crest harvesting in the treatment of maxillary and mandibular atrophies: a 10-year analysis," *Journal of Oral and Maxillofacial Surgery*, vol. 69, no. 9, pp. 2298–2304, 2011.

[19] R. D. Foster, J. P. Anthony, A. Sharma, and M. A. Pogrel, "Vascularized bone flaps versus nonvascularized bone grafts for mandibular reconstruction: an outcome analysis of primary bony union and endosseous implant success," *Head & Neck*, vol. 21, no. 1, pp. 66–71, 1999.

[20] M. A. Pogrel, S. Podlesh, J. P. Anthony, and J. Alexander, "A comparison of vascularized and nonvascularized bone grafts for reconstruction of mandibular continuity defects," *Journal of Oral and Maxillofacial Surgery*, vol. 55, no. 11, pp. 1200–1206, 1997.

[21] J. M. Wozney, "Bone morphogenetic proteins and their gene expression," in *Cellular and Molecular Biology of Bone*, M. Noda, Ed., Elsevier, 1993.

[22] T. Boyce, J. Edwards, and N. Scarborough, "Allograft bone: the influence of processing on safety and performance," *Orthopedic Clinics of North America*, vol. 30, no. 4, pp. 571–581, 1999.

[23] J. D. Kassolis, P. S. Rosen, and M. A. Reynolds, "Alveolar ridge and sinus augmentation utilizing platelet-rich plasma in combination with freeze-dried bone allograft: case series," *Journal of Periodontology*, vol. 71, no. 10, pp. 1654–1661, 2000.

[24] S. S. Noumbissi, J. L. Lozada, P. J. Boyne et al., "Clinical, histologic, and histomorphometric evaluation of mineralized solvent-dehydrated bone allograft (Puros) in human maxillary sinus grafts," *Journal of Oral Implantology*, vol. 31, no. 4, pp. 171–179, 2005.

[25] J. A. Leonetti and R. Koup, "Localized maxillary ridge augmentation with a block allograft for dental implant placement: case reports," *Implant Dentistry*, vol. 12, no. 3, pp. 217–226, 2003.

[26] J. P. A. van den Bergh, C. M. ten Bruggenkate, G. Krekeler, and D. B. Tuinzing, "Maxillary sinusfloor elevation and grafting with human demineralized freeze dried bone," *Clinical Oral Implants Research*, vol. 11, no. 5, pp. 487–493, 2000.

[27] R. D. Roden Jr., "Principles of bone grafting," *Oral and Maxillofacial Surgery Clinics of North America*, vol. 22, no. 3, pp. 295–300, 2010.

[28] T. A. Einhorn and L. C. Gerstenfeld, "Fracture healing: mechanisms and interventions," *Nature Reviews Rheumatology*, vol. 11, no. 1, pp. 45–54, 2015.

[29] A. Valentin-Opran, J. Wozney, C. Csimma, L. Lilly, and G. E. Riedel, "Clinical evaluation of recombinant human bone morphogenetic protein-2," *Clinical Orthopaedics and Related Research*, vol. 395, pp. 110–120, 2002.

[30] H. G. Moghadam, M. R. Urist, G. K. B. Sandor, and C. M. L. Clokie, "Successful mandibular reconstruction using a BMP

bioimplant," *Journal of Craniofacial Surgery*, vol. 12, no. 2, pp. 119–127, 2001.

[31] R. M. Lustosa, L. C. Iwaki, S. Tolentino Ede, M. Chicarelli da Silva, R. de Oliveira Lazarin, and L. Iwaki Filho, "Mandible reconstruction using rhBMP-2: case report and literature review," *Quintessence International*, vol. 45, no. 10, pp. 869–874, 2014.

[32] M. R. Oliveira, L. F. . O. Gorla, M. A. C. Gabrielli, and V. A. Pereira-Filho, "Off-label use of bone morphogenetic protein 2 in the reconstructions of mandibular continuity defects," *Journal of Craniofacial Surgery*, vol. 28, no. 1, pp. 227–230, 2017.

[33] S. C. Desai, A. Sclaroff, and B. Nussenbaum, "Use of recombinant human bone morphogenetic protein 2 for mandible reconstruction," *JAMA Facial Plastic Surgery*, vol. 15, no. 3, pp. 204–209, 2013.

[34] A. S. Herford and M. Cicciù, "Recombinant human bone morphogenetic protein type 2 jaw reconstruction in patients affected by giant cell tumor," *Journal of Craniofacial Surgery*, vol. 21, no. 6, pp. 1970–1975, 2010.

[35] Z. Sheikh, M. Javaid, N. Hamdan, and R. Hashmi, "Bone regeneration using bone morphogenetic proteins and various biomaterial carriers," *Materials*, vol. 8, no. 4, pp. 1778–1816, 2015.

[36] P. J. Boyne, "Animal studies of application of rhBMP-2 in maxillofacial reconstruction," *Bone*, vol. 19, no. 1, Supplement 1, pp. S83–S92, 1996.

[37] P. J. Boyne, L. C. Lilly, R. E. Marx et al., "De novo bone induction by recombinant human bone morphogenetic protein-2 (rhBMP-2) in maxillary sinus floor augmentation," *Journal of Oral and Maxillofacial Surgery*, vol. 63, no. 12, pp. 1693–1707, 2005.

[38] M. Degidi, A. Scarano, and A. Piattelli, "Regeneration of the alveolar crest using titanium micromesh with autologous bone and a resorbable membrane," *Journal of Oral Implantology*, vol. 29, no. 2, pp. 86–90, 2003.

[39] T. G. Carter, P. S. Brar, A. Tolas, and O. R. Beirne, "Off-label use of recombinant human bone morphogenetic protein-2 (rhBMP-2) for reconstruction of mandibular bone defects in humans," *Journal of Oral and Maxillofacial Surgery*, vol. 66, no. 7, pp. 1417–1425, 2008.

[40] R. M. Lustosa, D. . V. Macedo, L. C. V. Iwaki et al., "Continuity resection of the mandible after ameloblastoma - feasibility of oral rehabilitation with rhBMP-2 associated to bovine xenograft followed by implant installation," *Journal of Craniomaxillofacial Surgery*, vol. 43, no. 8, pp. 1553–1560, 2015.

[41] J. E. Block, "The role and effectiveness of bone marrow in osseous regeneration," *Medical Hypotheses*, vol. 65, no. 4, pp. 740–747, 2005.

[42] A. L. Gianakos, L. Sun, J. N. Patel, D. M. Adams, and F. A. Liporace, "Clinical application of concentrated bone marrow aspirate in orthopaedics: a systematic review," *World Journal of Orthopedics*, vol. 8, no. 6, pp. 491–506, 2017.

[43] D. R. Martin, N. R. Cox, T. L. Hathcock, G. P. Niemeyer, and H. J. Baker, "Isolation and characterization of multipotential mesenchymal stem cells from feline bone marrow," *Experimental Hematology*, vol. 30, no. 8, pp. 879–886, 2002.

[44] C. E. Taghavi, K. B. Lee, G. Keorochana, S. T. Tzeng, J. H. Yoo, and J. C. Wang, "Bone morphogenetic protein-2 and bone marrow aspirate with allograft as alternatives to autograft in instrumented revision posterolateral lumbar spinal fusion: a minimum two-year follow-up study," *Spine*, vol. 35, no. 11, pp. 1144–1150, 2010.

[45] P. Hernigou, A. Desroches, S. Queinnec et al., "Morbidity of graft harvesting versus bone marrow aspiration in cell regenerative therapy," *International Orthopaedics*, vol. 38, no. 9, pp. 1855–1860, 2014.

27

Osteochondroma Involving the Ramus of the Mandible: An Unusual Location

Pakki Suresh Kumar,[1] Dola Srinivasa Rao,[2] Swapna Manepalli,[3] Ajit Damera,[1] and Jai Kiran Killada[3]

[1]*Department of Oral Medicine and Radiology, GITAM Dental College and Hospital, Visakhapatnam, Andhra Pradesh, India*
[2]*Department of Periodontics, GITAM Dental College and Hospital, Visakhapatnam, Andhra Pradesh, India*
[3]*Department of Paedodontics and Preventive Dentistry, GITAM Dental College, Visakhapatnam, India*

Correspondence should be addressed to Swapna Manepalli; swapna.manepalli09@gmail.com

Academic Editor: Pravinkumar G. Patil

Osteochondroma (OC) is considered the most common tumor of the axial skeleton, although it is relatively uncommon in the craniofacial region. The present case describes an atypical case of OC in the posterior border of the ramus of the mandible. To the best of our knowledge, only one case has been reported till now in this region. A 35-year-old male patient reported with a complaint of swelling over the left middle one-third of the face and limited mouth opening for six years. Panoramic radiograph (PR) and paranasal sinus (PNS) view showed a well-defined radiopacity located in this region. Computed tomography (CT) and magnetic resonance imaging (MRI) revealed a characteristic mushroom-shaped outgrowth from the inner surface of the ramus of the mandible. The patient was treated with osteotomy, with the cut made at the angle of the mandible. Histopathological examination revealed features suggestive of OC. Subsequently, the patient was able to open his mouth, and there was no evidence of recurrence or postoperative complications in the one-year follow-up.

1. Introduction

Osteochondroma (OC) is a primary benign bone tumor of the long bones commonly involving the axial skeleton such as the metaphysis of the femur and tibia bones [1]. OC of the craniofacial bones is extremely rare because the facial bones exhibit intramembranous ossification, whereas the tumor usually appears in endochondral bones [2]. To the best of our knowledge, the last 30 years revealed a total of 435 patients with OC in the craniofacial region. The most frequently affected site was the mandibular condyle (88.3%), followed by the coronoid process (8.7%) [3]. Only 4 cases have been reported previously involving the mandibular symphysis region [4, 5], and 5 cases were reported involving the mandibular angle region [6], and only 1 case has been reported involving the ramus of the mandible [7]. Herein, we report an extremely rare OC in the mandibular posterior ramus region. Moreover, the present case was unique, because never before has such a large, characteristic mushroom-shaped OC been reported at the mandibular posterior ramus region.

2. Case Report

A 35-year-old male patient reported to the dental clinic with a complaint of swelling over the left middle one-third of the face for six years. History of swelling was provided as gradual in onset, slow-growing, and stable with no regression in size ever. The swelling was not associated with pain, paresthesia, discharge, or difficulty in eating. No significant history of trauma, infection, or medical conditions was reported. Neither similar swelling anywhere in the body was recorded. Facial asymmetry was present with restricted mouth opening on clinical examination, with solitary localized diffuse swelling at the preauricular region, just in front and 1 cm below the level of the left tragus of the ear. The swelling size was approximately 2 cm × 2 cm in diameter with diffuse periphery (Figure 1). The surface appeared to be regular with

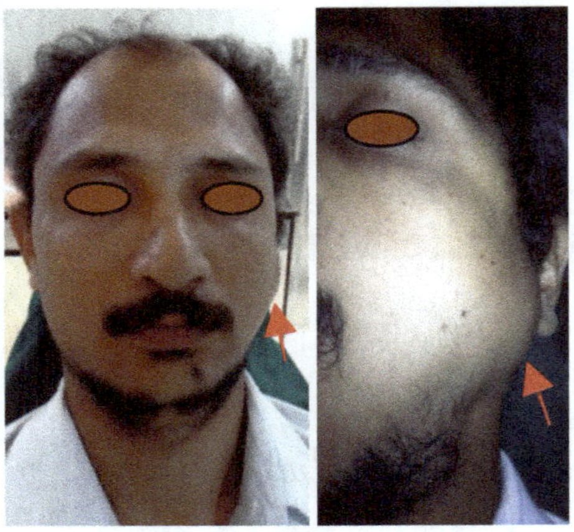

FIGURE 1: Swelling present in the front of the preauricular region on the left side of the face.

similar color and texture as that of the normal adjacent skin. No signs of ulcer, sinus, erythematic, or stretched skin were evident on inspection. Palpation exhibited a well-defined sessile base, fixed to the underlying bone and pinchable overlying skin. It was not tender and bony hard in consistency with no local rise in temperature. Intraoral examination was noncontributory. Based on history and clinical examination, a provisional diagnosis of peripheral osteoma was made with periosteal reactions, exostosis, peripheral osteoblastoma, and osteochondroma as a differential diagnosis.

Panoramic radiograph and paranasal sinus radiograph showed a well-defined radiopacity located at the left posterior ramus of the mandible region (Figures 2 and 3). The axial section of CT showed a well-defined osseous bony outgrowth arising from the posterior edge of the left ramus of the mandible measuring about $3.4 \times 2.9 \times 3.6$ cm (anteroposterior × transverse × craniocaudal planes). The growth showed central medullary with sclerosed cortical bone at the periphery, continuing with the condyle leading to mild elongation and giving a mushroom-shaped appearance on the axial section (Figure 4). MRI scan showed continuity between the medullary cavity of the mandible and the outgrowth. It was isointense on T1 W images and hyperintense on T2 W images with the peripheral hypointense rim on the T1 W and T2 W images. These features were suggestive of the cartilage cap with mineralization. Mass effect was present over the facial nerve, after its existence from the stylomandibular foramen that led to the lateral displacement of the facial nerve (Figure 5). Based on the clinical and radiological features, it was suggested as osteochondroma with lateral displacement of the facial nerve.

Surgical exploration of the growth was performed through the Alkyth-Brameley preauricular and submandibular approach (Figure 6) and osteotomy, with the cut made at the angle of the mandible. After complete surgical excision of the growth, it exhibited a uniformly dense ossified area with few irregular soft tissues at the periphery (Figure 7). The tissue section was decalcified, and H&E staining showed fibrocollagenous tissue overlying cartilaginous islands merging into bone trabeculae separated by fat marrow (Figure 8).

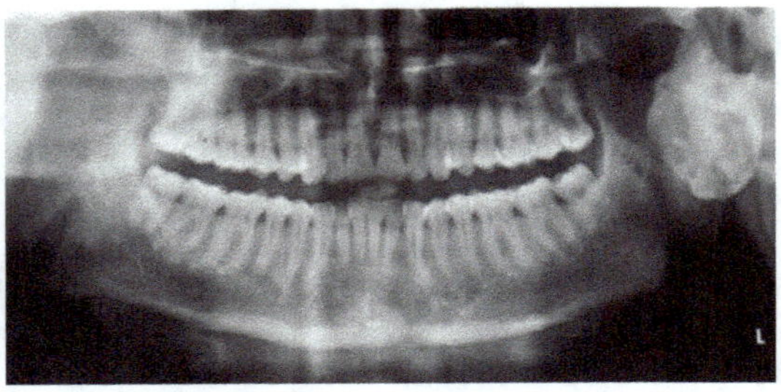

FIGURE 2: Panoramic radiograph view showed a well-defined radiopacity located at the left posterior ramus of the mandible region.

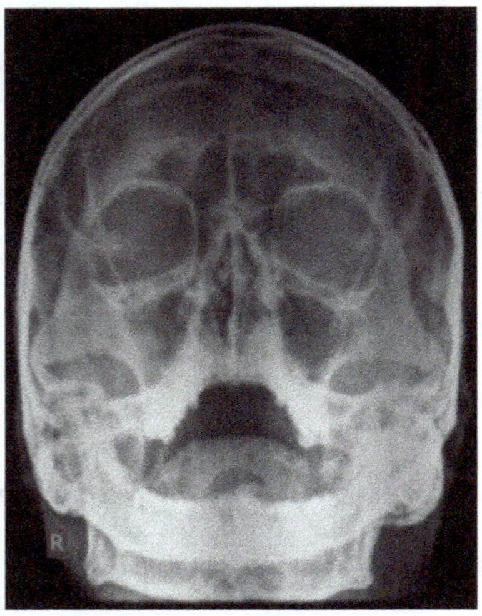

FIGURE 3: Paranasal sinus view showed a well-defined radiopacity located at the left posterior ramus of the mandible region.

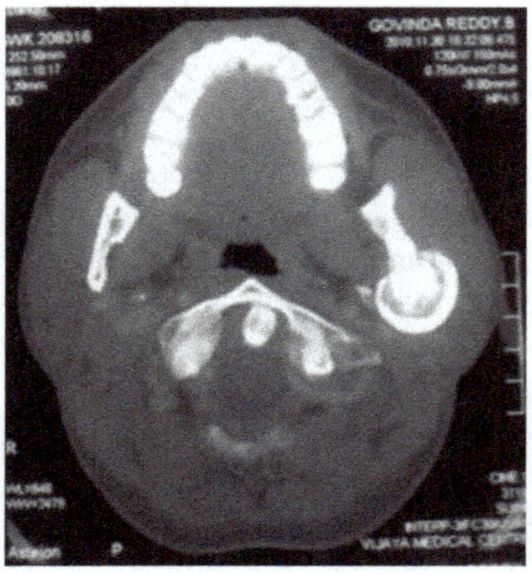

FIGURE 4: Computed tomography axial section showed a well-defined osseous bony outgrowth arising from the posterior edge of the left ramus of the mandible. The lesion showed central medullary with sclerosed cortical bone at the periphery, continuing with the condyle leading to mild elongation and giving a mushroom-shaped appearance on the axial section.

All these features were suggestive of osteochondroma. The patient was kept under observation and was free of recurrence until one year after surgery (Figure 9).

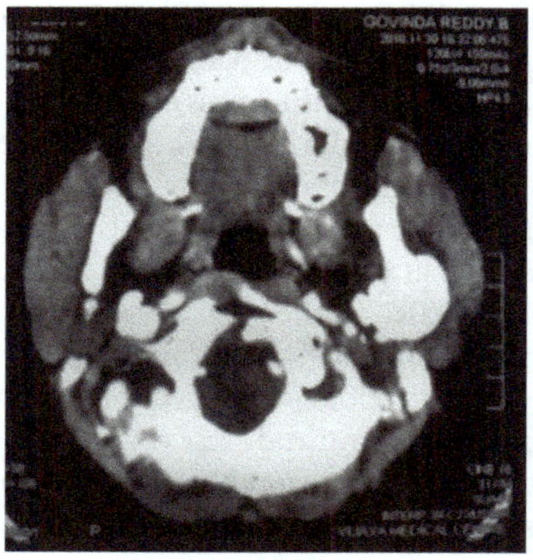

FIGURE 5: Magnetic resonance imaging scan showed continuity between the medullary cavity of the mandible and the outgrowth. It is isointense on T1 W images and hyperintense on T2 W images with the peripheral hypointense rim on the T1 W and T2 W images; these features are suggestive of the cartilage cap with mineralization.

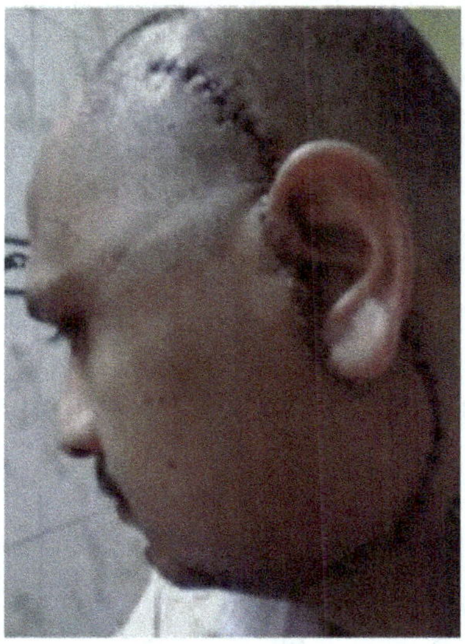

FIGURE 6: Surgical exploration of the growth was performed through the Alkyth-Brameley preauricular and submandibular approach.

3. Discussion

WHO defined OC as cartilage-capped bony projection arising from the external surface of bone containing a marrow cavity that is continuous with that of the underlying bone [8]. Various hypotheses were postulated for the pathogenesis of osteochondroma. Virchow was the first to speak about bony osteochondroma in 1891. Keith suggested that an imaginary defect in the thin cortical bone results in spillage of epiphyseal cells into the metaphysic region, and this commonly occurs in tendon insertion sites. These sites have focal accumulation of embryonic connective tissue with cartilaginous potential. Langenskiold postulated that osteochondroma occurs when limited portions of the undifferentiated cell layer of the growth cartilage are displaced toward the metaphysic peripherally. Lichtenstein and Muller's theory suggested that the periosteum had an inherent potential to form chondroblasts and osteoblasts. Thus, an osteochondroma may arise due to induced or spontaneous metaplasia of the periosteum [7, 9].

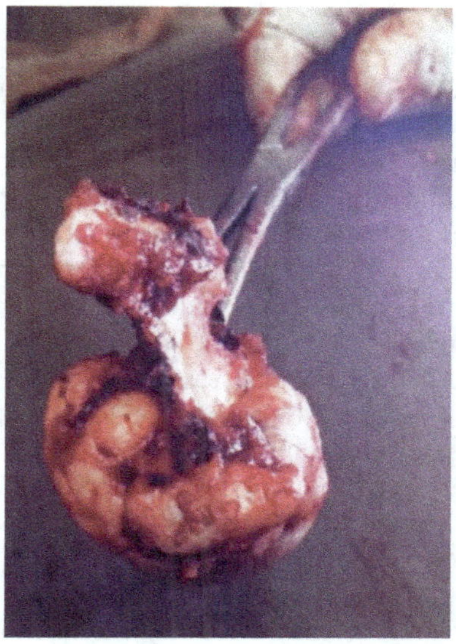

FIGURE 7: On gross examination the lesion exhibited a uniformly dense ossified area with few irregular soft tissues at the periphery.

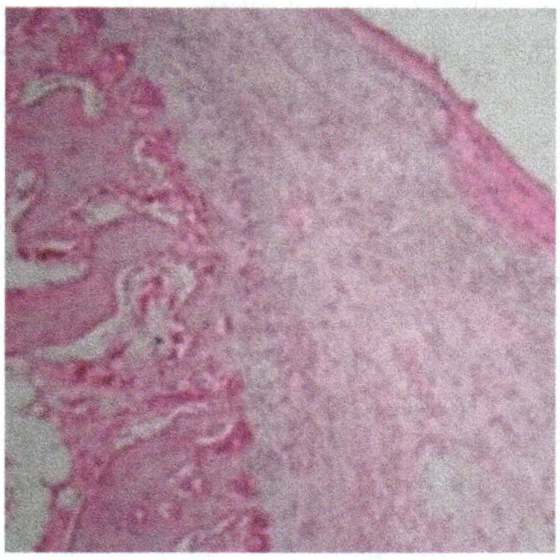

FIGURE 8: H&E staining showed fibrocollagenous tissue overlying cartilaginous islands merging into bone trabeculae.

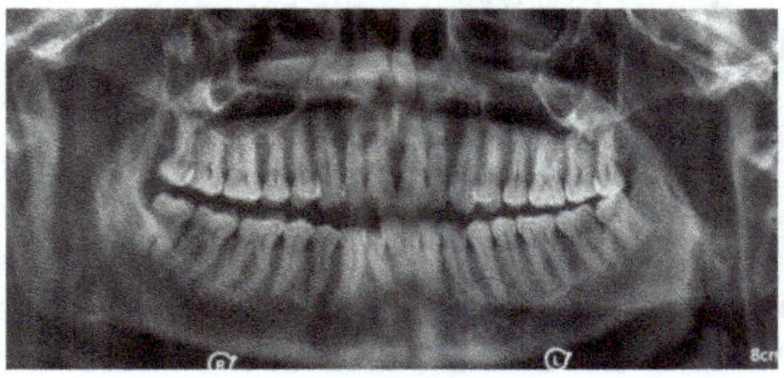

FIGURE 9: Postoperative panoramic radiography showing excision of the lesion and free of recurrence 1 year after surgery.

Osteochondromas are very rare in the maxillofacial region. In 1899, Jacob was the first to explain an OC of the coronoid process; for this reason, this condition has been named "Jacob's disease" [6]. In the craniofacial skeleton, it more commonly occurs around the temporomandibular joint because the region from the mandibular lingula to the anterior process of the malleus is derived from the part of Meckel's cartilage not replaced by mandibular bone, and those remnants of this embryonic tissue may persist in that region [7]. In the mental region, one or two cartilages ossify and form mental ossicles, which become incorporated into the intramembranous bone. Residues of these cartilage precursors in the symphysis appear to form OC of this region. According to cytogenetic analyses EXT1 (8q24,1) and EXT2 (11P11.2-12), loci may be involved in the pathogenesis of hereditary osteochondromas [5, 10].

They have been reported in varied locations of the craniofacial region, where the most common sites are the coronoid process and the condyle [6]. It is a slow-growing, most-of-the-time asymptomatic tumor. Sometimes, the patient may present with facial asymmetry, malocclusion, pain, and hypomobility of the temporomandibular joint. The mouth opening is in the normal range in most of the cases because of the pseudoarticulation around the mass [11].

Panoramic radiography is the primary radiologic examination that is required for diagnosis. An OC appears as a stalk or a flat protuberance emerging from the surface of the bone. On occasion, it ends up as a hook-like formation. Its margins are usually well defined, although the tumor seems to be continuous with the cortex of the bone. A usual finding is that of radiopaque calcified flakes or linear interruptions inside the cartilaginous component of the OC. Panoramic radiography helps in diagnosing the lesion as benign or malignant. Sometimes, an osteochondroma turns into osteosarcoma indicating enlargement of the tumor and the irregularity of its margins. Multiplication of the ossifications, pain, scattered calcifications, and a coexisting radiopaque soft tissue mass may suggest a sarcomatous transformation. In addition, the presence of periosteal reaction with lobulated margins may be present in osteosarcoma [4, 9].

CT and cone beam computed tomography (CBCT) are accurate methods for depicting OC. They can show the bony lesion in detail, as well as show the presence of calcifications and thickness of the cartilaginous cap. But CT and CBCT cannot estimate the metabolic activity, a serious indication of malignancy of any tumor. A scintigraphic method is being used to examine the metabolic activity of the tumor. A poor metabolic activity is only present in benign lesions. Ultrasound radiography helps to examine the cartilaginous cap of the OC as a hypoechoic area above the cortex of the relevant bone [3, 9].

MRI can know the exact morphology of a tumor and any compress over the surrounding structures. MRI is used to verify the continuity of the growth with the cortex of the affected bone. MRI shows a well-defined irregular lesion showing signal intensity similar to that of bone marrow in the center, surrounded by an iso- to hyperintense rim with few hypointense areas predominantly in the posterior aspect suggestive of the cartilage cap. The cartilaginous cap, as it is rich in water, presents a high signal on T2-weighted MRI and a low one on T1-weighted imaging. T2-weighted MRI is preferable because it provides better differentiation of signal intensities, and differentiation in the signaling of a nerve may suggest its suppression or damage. Woertler et al. indicated that the cartilage cap thickness exceeding 2 cm in adults and 3 cm in children should raise the suspicion of malignant transformation. Chondrosarcoma is also characterized by low T1 signal after intravenous contrast infusion (gadolinium), something that is rarely recorded in a benign cartilaginous tumor. So MRI is the gold standard technique for detecting a malignant transformation [6, 9].

Regardless of the etiology, the goal of treatment is complete resection of the lesion and recovery of acceptable mouth opening. After surgical excision, the recurrence rate is found to be 2% in solitary osteochondroma cases all over the body. No signs of recurrence were found in our case until now. Malignant change may occur in about 5% of cases with multiple hereditary lesions, but solitary osteochondromas have a 1% risk of malignant transformation [11].

4. Conclusion

Craniofacial osteochondroma, in the mandibular posterior ramus region, is extremely a rare entity. Panoramic radiography at best can be considered a screening modality in the detection of these lesions. Because of the characteristic radiographic appearance of mandibular osteochondroma, CT and MRI provide a valuable tool to assist in evaluation and treatment planning. The recommended treatment of choice for symptomatic osteochondromas is surgical resection and follow-up because it may transform into osteosarcomas.

Consent

The informed signed consent was obtained from the patient and parent.

Acknowledgments

We cordially thank the patient who consented to using his medical history data for this case report.

References

[1] A. C. Limardo, E. Soza, N. Cumpa, L. Blanco, and R. Padin, "Osteochondroma of the mandibular angle: report case and literature review," *Case Reports International*, vol. 6, pp. 39–42, 2017.

[2] W. Lim, L. K. Weng, and G. B. Tin, "Osteochondroma of the mandibular condyle: report of two surgical approaches," *Annals of Maxillofacial Surgery*, vol. 4, no. 2, pp. 215–219, 2014.

[3] T. Lan, X. Liu, P. S. Liang, and Q. Tao, "Osteochondroma of the coronoid process: a case report and review of the literature," *Oncology Letters*, vol. 18, no. 3, pp. 2270–2277, 2019.

[4] A. Navaneetham, K. A. Rao, H. H. Baweja, and S. Kumaran, "A unique case of multiple osteochondroma: mandibular symphysis and femur," *Annals of Maxillofacial Surgery*, vol. 2, no. 2, pp. 182–184, 2012.

[5] D. N. Kishore, H. R. S. Kumar, K. V. Umashankara, and K. K. Rai, "Osteochondroma of the mandible: a rare case report,"

Case Reports in Pathology, vol. 2013, Article ID 167862, 3 pages, 2013.

[6] R. Abe, I. Miyamoto, H. Sato, D. Saitou, G. Yamaya, and H. Yamada, "An unusually large osteochondroma of the mandibular angle: a case report," *World Journal of Surgical Oncology*, vol. 15, no. 1, p. 201, 2017.

[7] D. Gopinath, V. T. Beena, S. K. Padmakumar, and G. Sugirtharaj, "Osteochondroma of the mandibular ramus: report of a rare case," *Journal of Oral and Maxillofacial Surgery, Medicine, and Pathology*, vol. 26, no. 3, pp. 432–435, 2014.

[8] Q. Zhou, C. Yang, and M. J. Chen, "Osteochondroma of bilateral mandibular condyle: a case report," *International Journal of Clinical and Experimental Medicine*, vol. 8, no. 2, pp. 2989–2992, 2015.

[9] P. Kitsoulis, V. Galani, K. Stefanaki, G. Paraskevas, G. Karatzias, and N. J. Agnantis, "Osteochondromas: review of the clinical, radiological and pathological features," *Invivo*, vol. 22, pp. 633–646, 2008.

[10] S. Mohanty, H. Gupta, J. Dabas, and P. Kumar, "Osteochondroma of maxillofacial region: tumor arising from two different developmental bones," *Journal of Oral and Maxillofacial Pathology*, vol. 20, no. 2, pp. 329–332, 2016.

[11] S. Vaidya, S. Sidana, J. Galinde, and S. Natrajan, "Osteochondroma of the mandibular condyle," *Journal of Contemporary Dentistry*, vol. 2, no. 3, pp. 106–108, 2012.

28

Oral Rehabilitation with Removable Partial Denture of a Patient with Cleidocranial Dysplasia

Ali Jamali Ghomi, Reza Sayyad Soufdoost, Mohammad Saeed Barzegar, and Mohammad Ali Hemmati

Department of Prosthodontics, Faculty of Dentistry, Shahed University, Tehran, Iran

Correspondence should be addressed to Reza Sayyad Soufdoost; rezasoof@yahoo.com

Academic Editor: Mariano A. Polack

This case report describes the oral rehabilitation of a patient with cleidocranial dysplasia who received a removable partial denture along with silicone-based permanent soft liner to improve esthetic and masticatory function. This patient was the candidate of neither implant nor orthodontic treatment due to medical conditions, history of mandible fracture, age, and risk of fracture after mandibular teeth extractions. Cone-beam computed tomography has made it possible to obtain comprehensive information regarding the morphology and positional relationship of impacted supernumerary teeth. Also, proper collaboration between surgeon and prosthodontist helped to achieve significant improvements in patient's self-esteem, masticatory function, and esthetic.

1. Introduction

Cleidocranial dysplasia is a hereditary congenital disorder which results in generalized skeletal dysplasia [1]. The RUNX2 gene mutations that cause cleidocranial dysplasia reduce or eliminate the RUNX2 protein activity in each cell, decreasing the total amount of functional RUNX2 protein. This lack of functional RUNX2 protein can affect the normal development of bones, cartilage, and teeth, resulting in the signs and symptoms of cleidocranial dysplasia [2]. It is characterized by prominent parietal, frontal and occipital bone, underdeveloped paranasal sinus, supernumerary teeth, short shoulder blades (scapulae), an abnormal curvature of the spine (scoliosis), wide-set eyes (hypertelorism), a flat nose, a small upper jaw, and many other abnormalities [1–4].

General dentists can easily diagnose the CCD through a panoramic radiograph taken in addition to other clinical findings [3]. Phenotypic characteristics in the oral cavity include the presence of impacted teeth which could be diagnosed as supernumerary teeth, delayed eruption of permanent teeth, and prolonged retention of primary teeth [4]. Tsuji et al. [5] have reported the average number of supernumerary teeth 7.8 and the average number of unerupted permanent teeth 17.8, in CCD patients aged 15 to 25 years old. In general, supernumerary teeth occur in 6% or more of the normal population [5].

Cone-beam computed tomography (CBCT) has been introduced as the most recent advancement in maxillofacial imaging, enables clinicians to view the morphology of the skull and the dentition in all three dimensions and to design the best treatment plan [6]. The advantages of CBCT over 2D images make it the ideal tool for probing and managing oral and maxillofacial defects [7]. In a patient with CCD, the 3D views by CBCT for evaluation of unerupted, impacted, or supernumerary teeth and their association with vital structures have been essential and inevitable [8].

The treatment plan largely depends on the age [9] and a patient's medical condition [10]. On the other hand, esthetic and masticatory functions are two essential needs, which should be provided by therapists [5]. Dental treatment in the patients with CCD requires an interdisciplinary approach involving orthodontists, maxillofacial surgeons, and prosthodontists [11]. Therapeutic options are varied from the extraction of all teeth followed by the fabrication of denture to implant placement and orthodontic treatment [1]. However, there appears to be a trend in favor of the use of the implant-supported prosthesis instead of conventional removable partial dentures [12].

Over the years, many modifications have been performed in the designing of the complete dentures, but still in compromised cases, residual ridge may be subjected to trauma by the rigid denture base which is in close contact with the soft tissues [13]. Long-term soft denture lining (LTSDL) materials constitute a group of polymer materials using to modifying the trauma associated with wearing complete dentures. They can remain in the oral cavity for at least four weeks. However, their use can extend to several months or even years practically [14]. They reduce the traumatic effect that a denture may have on patients with thin atrophic mucosa, ridge atrophy or resorption, deep anatomical undercuts, bruxism tendencies, or where the oral mucosa exhibits a reduced tolerance to the load applied by a denture, and in congenital and acquired oral defects requiring repair [13, 15]. Soft denture lining materials lead to a more uniform distribution of stress at the mucosa/lining interface, which results in that wearing the complete prosthesis becomes more comfortable for the patient [14]. Currently, two types of soft denture lining material are available: silicone elastomers and soft acrylic compounds. In the clinical situation, the silicone materials are preferred because they remain more stable, while the acrylic materials undergo a more marked loss of cushioning effect over time [14].

2. Case Report

A 60-year-old female came to the diagnosis of the oral disease department of Shahed Dental School for dental treatment with a chief complaint of lack of masticatory capability and poor esthetic for the past 20 years. Her medical history was significant for osteoporosis and congenital heart disease (CHD). Her current medication was the daily use of ASA as an antithrombotic, Digoxin for CHD, Enalapril for her hypertension, and vit D. Also, she had been medicating with Famotidine and Omeprazole for the last two years due to her masticatory hypofunction and digestive problems. Her medical practitioner advised that her dental treatment should be limited to noninvasive dental procedures with minimal trauma. The patient revealed that there was an absence of the lower and upper anterior teeth after exfoliation of deciduous teeth and the history of mandibular fractures 25 years ago in a motor vehicle collision. In extraoral examination, the prominent frontal and parietal, hypertelorism, depressed nasal bridge, mandibular prognathism, and maxillary hypoplasia were observed (Figure 1). Also, the patient was able to move shoulders in front of the chest associated with underdeveloped or absent collarbone (Figure 2).

Intraoral examination revealed a long span bridge in maxilla from tooth #15 to #25 and multiple missing permanent teeth in the anterior and posterior regions of the mandible. A panoramic radiograph and CBCT were captured (Figures 3 and 4).

Radiographic findings revealed multiple impacted permanent teeth in the anterior region of maxilla and anterior and posterior regions of the mandible as well as the fracture of the left angle of the mandible which had been fixed with

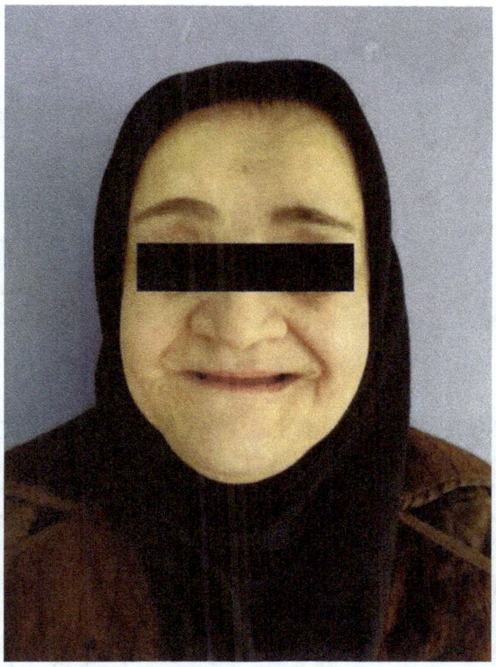

FIGURE 1: Mandibular prognathism with depressed nasal bridge and frontal prominence.

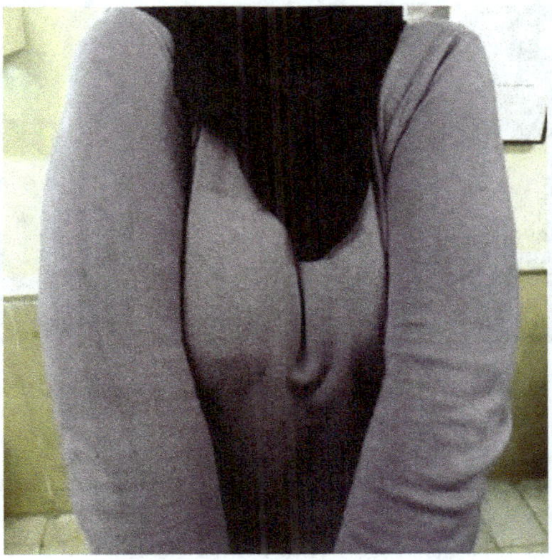

FIGURE 2: Approximation of shoulders in front of the chest.

wire. The patient was diagnosed with cleidocranial dysplasia evidenced by clinical and radiographic findings. After consulting with a maxillofacial surgeon, the extraction of all teeth (erupted and unerupted) and replacement by implants was not suggested due to the medical conditions of the patient including osteoporosis and CHD. The most conservative and minimally invasive treatment recommended by the surgeon. Therefore, removable partial denture (RPD) was planned to restore both arches. The situation was explained to the patient in detail. A treatment plan including RPD after extraction of hopeless teeth was chosen by the patient, which was the same to therapeutic team choice. The long span maxillary bridge was removed and the tooth #15, 13, 23, 24, 25, 36, and 38 were diagnosed hopeless. The extraction of these

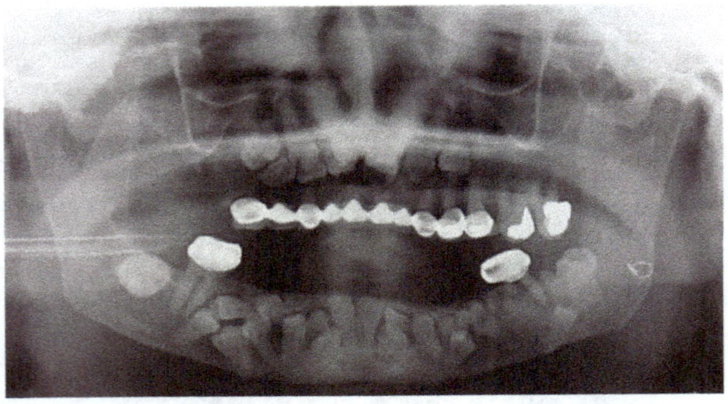

FIGURE 3: Panoramic radiograph before treatment.

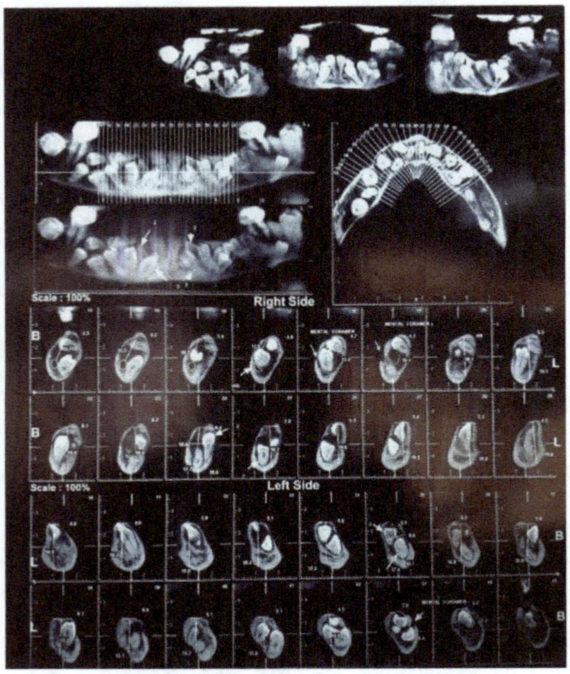

FIGURE 4: CBCT revealed 21 impacted teeth in mandible and 9 in maxilla.

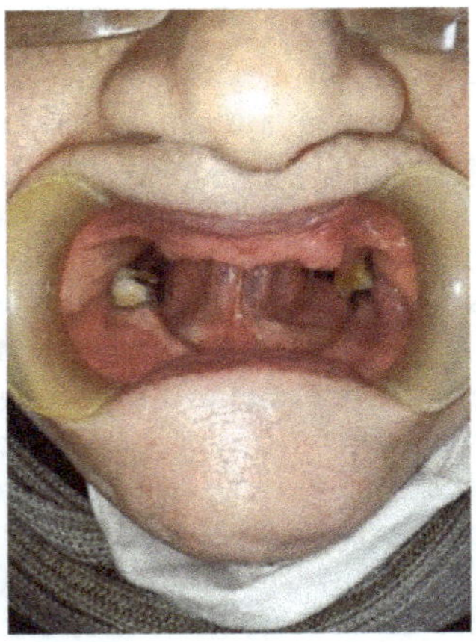

FIGURE 5: Intraoral photograph before prosthodontic treatment.

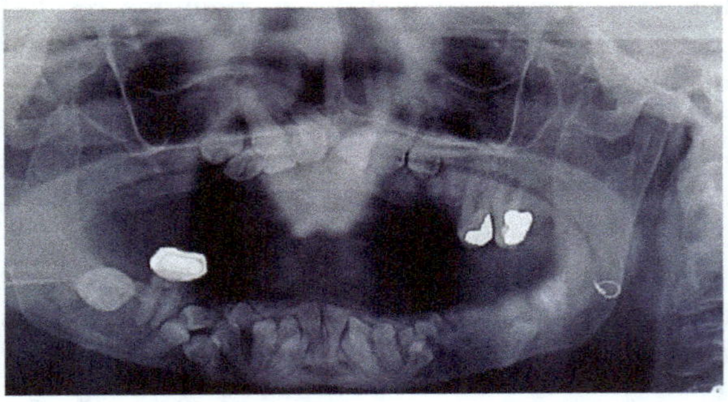

FIGURE 6: Panoramic radiograph 3 months after teeth extraction.

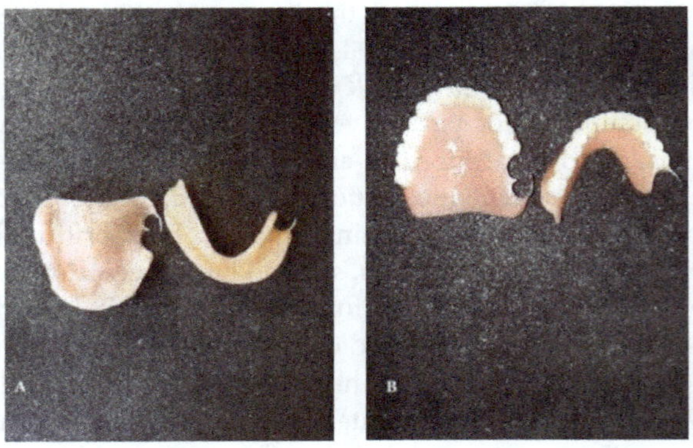

(a) (b)

FIGURE 7: Interior (a) and exterior (b) surfaces of maxillary and mandibular removable partial denture.

teeth was performed under local anesthesia and with minimal trauma. Socket preservation was done with bone graft materials to assist regeneration and healing, and to avoid severe bone loss, particularly in the site of tooth #38. On the other hand, the tooth #26, 27, and 46 were saved due to their stable conditions, increasing the retention and support of the removable partial prosthesis (Figure 5).

After 3 months, a new OPG was captured, which showed no significant mandibular and maxillary bone resorption (Figure 6).

Preliminary impressions were made for both arches using irreversible hydrocolloid impression material (CA37; Cavex Holland BV, Haarlem, Netherlands) in a stock tray. Impressions of both arches were poured to obtain study casts by dental plaster type 2 (Pars Dandan, Iran). Acrylic custom trays were made using auto polymerizing acrylic resin (Bisico-Germany). In the second visit, both custom trays were border molded using green stick compound, the definitive impression was recorded with Panasil initial contact light impression material (Kettenbach, Germany), and final casts were poured in type 3 dental stone (Pars Dandan–Iran). Acrylic resin base and wax rims were fabricated, and maxillomandibular relationships were recorded by facebow. Maxillary and mandibular diagnostic tooth arrangements were prepared to evaluate phonetic and esthetic, teeth position, and to create maxillomandibular relationship. Afterwards, acrylic resin partial dental prostheses were processed from heat-polymerized acrylic resin (Kulzer, Germany) with a heat-cured permanent silicone soft liner (silicone based detax, Germany) and delivered (Figures 7(a) and 7(b) and 8).

Wrought wire retentive arm was designed on tooth #27 and 46 to elevate the retention of partial dentures. In order to minimize the microbial/fungal colonization of liners and

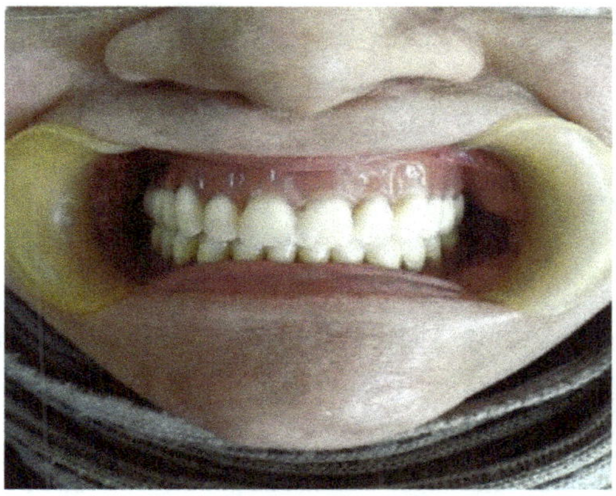

FIGURE 8: Final oral rehabilitation with removable partial denture.

prolong their life, the patient was trained in two sessions on how to maintain the oral and denture hygiene in good condition. Also, the patient was advised to use prostheses except when asleep. An appointment was scheduled after a week for the final adjustment (Figures 9(a) and 9(b)).

The patient was examined clinically and radiographically every 3 months, throughout a year. Her quality of life and mastication function was improved significantly, and the patient was satisfied. The prognosis of the mandibular and maxillary natural molars tooth #26, 27, and 46 were excellent. The maxillary and mandibular partial denture did not need to be relined after a year.

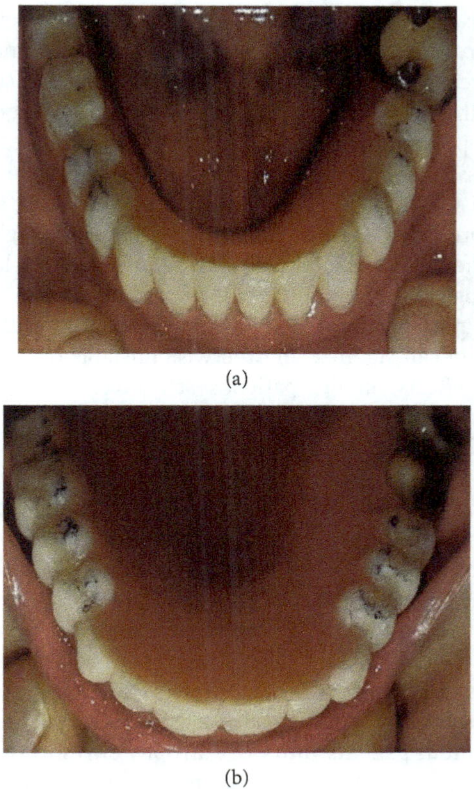

FIGURE 9: Final adjustment of mandibular (a) and maxillary (b) prostheses.

3. Discussion

The treatment of a patient with CCD can be more challenging and complicated, particularly in older adults [16]. To achieve the best treatment plan and satisfaction of patients with CCD, an interdisciplinary dental approach plays an important role [1]. Prosthodontist, orthodontist, and oral surgeon should be involved in creating a comprehensive treatment plan for a patient with CCD [11]. Tailored combination of surgery, orthodontics, and prosthodontics is necessary to provide a functional dentition and reconstruct the smile and facial contour of patients with CCD [1]. The dental treatment in CCD varies and primarily depends on patient's needs, medical conditions, social and economic circumstances, and age of diagnosis, but still the main purpose of treatment is to improve craniofacial and dental function together with aesthetic [5].

Early diagnosis of CCD is very imperative so as to design the best treatment plan and treatment duration [17]. The premature diagnosis leads to a proper orientation for the treatment [16]. There is no consistent protocol for patients with CCD who seek treatment at different ages [1]. In some cases [1, 10, 18], the orthodontic treatment was suggested after the extraction of retained deciduous teeth. In these cases, subsequent orthodontic alignment resulted in a functional and esthetic outcome, and a good facial profile. However, most of these papers just focused on early operation at age 6-12. In our case, orthodontic treatment was not possible with respect to age (60 years), medical conditions, and time of diagnosis. However, if it had been assessed in the earlier age, the orthodontic treatment might have been possible by the extraction of retained deciduous and supernumerary teeth with surgical exposure of impacted permanent teeth and orthodontically guided eruption [17].

In many recent cases, the extractions of impacted teeth followed by implant replacement were suggested as the best treatment plan for patients with CCD [16–18]. In the present case, possible treatment alternatives were discussed with the maxillofacial surgeon with respect to systemic problems, medications, age, and patient's demands. CBCT revealed the numerous impacted teeth in the maxilla (9) and mandible (21), near the inferior border of the mandible, demonstrating the fracture risk of the remaining bone, and damage to the inferior alveolar nerve after extraction. Also, age and osteoporosis were two important factors influencing bone healing after extraction. Petropoulos et al. [19] reported that a genetic defect in patient with CCD may negatively affect the osteoblastic activity around implants and subsequently results in the weaker osseointegration. Considering the above reasons and the history of fracture in angle of the mandible in the left side, treatment planning of full extraction and rehabilitation with implants was ruled out by the surgeon and prosthodontist, despite being a viable alternative.

Some authors suggest that the removal of primary or supernumerary teeth does not promote the eruption of impacted permanent teeth [20, 21]. The lack of cellular cementum is considered to be one of the factors responsible for unerupted teeth in CCD patients [20]. On the other hand, alkaline phosphatase activity has been demonstrated to be consistently reduced in patients with CCD which is another factor associated with delayed eruption in CCD patients [21]. Therefore, it seems that future eruption of the retained teeth in the present case is unlikely. Also, in the present case, maintaining the retained supernumerary teeth could be beneficial for the prevention of more complicated surgeries, severe bone loss, and damage to vital structures [16]. The patient had a history of mandibular fracture, osteoporosis, and systemic problems. These predisposing factors might have raised the risk of mandibular fracture, much bone loss, and psychological trauma in the case of surgery [17].

The preservation of even a single healthy tooth in the oral cavity can stabilize an otherwise unstable denture, have positive effects on the patient's self-esteem, and preserve proprioception and occlusal relationship [16]. Therefore, it was decided to save the tooth number 26, 27, and 46 regarding their stable conditions. In some areas of maxilla and mandible, the mucosa over the embedded teeth was thin, and further resorption expected after wearing the RPD, which might continue to expose the retained teeth. In order to minimize the resorption of residual ridge and mucosa under the rigid base of RPD, silicon-based permanent soft liner was applied. The application of a soft material is intended to increase the comfort of denture wearers and to support prosthetic treatment [22]. The use of LTSDLs is mostly suggested in edentulous patients with ridge atrophy or resorption, bony undercuts, bruxing tendencies, and congenital or acquired oral defects [15]. Also, silicone-based LTSDL materials, which are characterized by more stable hardness, sorption, and solubility than acrylic-based LTSDLs, have been recommended in many studies [14, 15]. As CCD is the rare inherent abnormality, and there is a lack of evidence that what will happen in the future to unerupted teeth, the consistent follow-up is mandatory to monitor patient's conditions [19]. The most challenging aspect in the use of the soft liner was its tendency to support microorganism growth despite the fact that the patient was trained on how to clean and disinfect the denture base in two sessions [14]. In order to solve this problem, and as impacted teeth were not extracted, regular follow-ups were essential to monitor the patient's condition. The patient was examined clinically and radiographically every 3 months for a year.

In the current situation, this case report highlights the importance of this fact that the best treatment is not essentially the complicated one, in contrast, in some cases like our case, noninvasive procedures and realistic expectations are considered as successful treatment, ensuring patient's needs are met. However, long-term follow-ups and more clinical reports are needed to determine the ideal therapeutic approach for CCD patients.

4. Conclusion

Dentists should recognize that the more complicated the proposed treatment plan, the less likely the chance of success. In this case report, functional and esthetic rehabilitation was achieved, using RPD in the maxilla and mandible. The minimally invasive procedure was planned regarding the limitations of using implant replacement and orthodontic treatment.

Consent

Patient consent was obtained from the patients.

References

[1] D. Patel, N. Patel, P. A. Brennan, and J. Kwok, "Multidisciplinary team approach in the oral rehabilitation of patients with cleidocranial dysplasia to achieve a functional aesthetic outcome," *The British Journal of Oral & Maxillofacial Surgery*, vol. 55, no. 9, pp. 932–936, 2017.

[2] M. M. Cohen Jr., "Biology of RUNX2 and cleidocranial dysplasia," *The Journal of Craniofacial Surgery*, vol. 24, no. 1, pp. 130–133, 2013.

[3] N. Suda, M. Hattori, K. Kosaki et al., "Correlation between genotype and supernumerary tooth formation in cleidocranial dysplasia," *Orthodontics & Craniofacial Research*, vol. 13, no. 4, pp. 197–202, 2010.

[4] G. Karagüzel, F. A. Aktürk, E. Okur, H. R. Gümele, Y. Gedik, and A. Okten, "Cleidocranial dysplasia: a case report," *Journal of Clinical Research in Pediatric Endocrinology*, vol. 2, no. 3, pp. 134–136, 2010.

[5] M. Tsuji, H. Suzuki, S. Suzuki, and K. Moriyama, "Three-dimensional evaluation of morphology and position of impacted supernumerary teeth in cases of cleidocranial dysplasia," *Congenital Anomalies*, pp. 1–9, 2019.

[6] T. Matsumura, Y. Ishida, A. Kawabe, and T. Ono, "Quantitative analysis of the relationship between maxillary incisors and the incisive canal by cone-beam computed tomography in an adult Japanese population," *Progress in Orthodontics*, vol. 18, no. 1, p. 24, 2017.

[7] S. Shahidi, B. Zamiri, and P. Bronoosh, "Comparison of panoramic radiography with cone beam CT in predicting the relationship of the mandibular third molar roots to the alveolar canal," *Imaging Science in Dentistry*, vol. 43, no. 2, pp. 105–109, 2013.

[8] S. Singh, S. Sharma, H. Singh, and N. D. Wazir, "Cleidocranial dysplasia: a case report illustrating diagnostic clinical and radiological findings," *Journal of Clinical and Diagnostic Research*, vol. 8, no. 6, pp. 19-20, 2014.

[9] V. Gombra and S. Jayachandran, "Cleidocranial dysplasia: report of 4 cases and review," *Journal of Indian Academy of Oral Medicine and Radiology*, vol. 20, no. 1, pp. 23–27, 2008.

[10] R. Mathur, V. Satish, M. Bhat, and M. Parvez, "Cleidocranial dysplasia: case report of three siblings," *International Journal of Clinical Pediatric Dentistry*, vol. 2, no. 2, pp. 32–39, 2009.

[11] A. J. Ambard, S. Clemens, and D. S. Philips, "Multidisciplinary implant rehabilitation of a patient with cleidocranial dysostosis: a journey from age 13 to 21," *Journal of Prosthodontics*, vol. 28, no. 4, pp. 361–364, 2019.

[12] B. Wöstmann, E. Budtz-Jørgensen, N. Jepson et al., "Indications for removable partial dentures: a literature review," *The International Journal of Prosthodontics*, vol. 18, no. 2, pp. 139–145, 2005.

[13] K. Singh and N. Gupta, "Fabrication and relining of dentures with permanent silicone soft liner: a novel way to increase retention in grossly resorbed ridge and minimize trauma of knife edge and severe undercuts ridges," *Dentistry and Medical Research*, vol. 4, no. 1, pp. 24–28, 2016.

[14] R. Brożek, R. Koczorowski, R. Rogalewicz, A. Voelkel, B. Czarnecka, and J. W. Nicholson, "Effect of denture cleansers

on chemical and mechanical behavior of selected soft lining materials," *Dental Materials*, vol. 27, no. 3, pp. 281–290, 2011.

[15] G. Chladek, J. Żmudzki, and J. Kasperski, "Long-term soft denture lining materials," *Materials*, vol. 7, no. 8, pp. 5816–5842, 2014.

[16] K. Noh, K. R. Kwon, H. Ahn, J. Paek, and A. Pae, "Prosthetic rehabilitation of a cleidocranial dysplasia patient with vertical maxillofacial deficiency: a clinical report," *Journal of Prosthodontics*, vol. 23, no. 1, pp. 64–70, 2014.

[17] F. Atil, A. Culhaoglu, I. D. Kocyigit, Z. Adisen, M. Misirlioglu, and B. Yilmaz, "Oral rehabilitation with implant-supported fixed dental prostheses of a patient with cleidocranial dysplasia," *The Journal of Prosthetic Dentistry*, vol. 119, no. 1, pp. 12–16, 2018.

[18] L. F. da Cunha, I. M. Caetano, F. Dalitz, C. C. Gonzaga, and J. Mondelli, "Cleidocranial dysplasia case report: remodeling of teeth as aesthetic restorative treatment," *Case Reports in Dentistry*, vol. 2014, 5 pages, 2014.

[19] V. C. Petropoulos, T. J. Balshi, S. F. Balshi, and G. J. Wolfinger, "Treatment of a patient with cleidocranial dysplasia using osseointegrated implants: a patient report," *The International Journal of Oral & Maxillofacial Implants*, vol. 19, no. 2, pp. 282–287, 2004.

[20] K. Manjunath, B. Kavitha, T. R. Saraswathi, B. Sivapathasundharam, and R. Manikandhan, "Cementum analysis in cleidocranial dysostosis," *Indian Journal of Dental Research*, vol. 19, no. 3, pp. 253–256, 2008.

[21] S. Unger, E. Mornet, S. Mundlos, S. Blaser, and D. E. Cole, "Severe cleidocranial dysplasia can mimic hypophosphatasia," *European Journal of Pediatrics*, vol. 161, no. 11, pp. 623–626, 2002.

[22] K. Singh, N. Gupta, R. Gupta, and D. Abrahm, "Prosthetic rehabilitation with collapsible hybrid acrylic resin and permanent silicone soft liner complete denture of a patient with scleroderma-induced microstomia," *Journal of Prosthodontics*, vol. 23, no. 5, pp. 412–416, 2014.

29

Treatment of Maxillary Second Premolar with 4 Roots

Z. Allahem[1] and S. AlYami[1,2]

[1]*Department of Restorative Dental Sciences, College of Dentistry, King Saud University, Saudi Arabia*
[2]*Department of Restorative Dental Science, College of Dentistry, Najran University, Saudi Arabia*

Correspondence should be addressed to S. AlYami; shalyame@nu.edu.sa

Academic Editor: Asja Celebic

Aim. To report a case of maxillary second premolar with four roots and four separate foramina and the use of CBCT to help identify the root canal system configuration. *Summary.* A 45-year-old female patient with a no significant medical history was referred for treatment tooth #15. The tooth was diagnosed with symptomatic irreversible pulpitis and symptomatic apical periodontitis. After taking periapical radiographs and expected uncommon morphology, CBCT was taken to help confirm canals configuration and aid in the treatment of the case. Root canals treatment was carried without complication under dental operating microscope using a rotary system and continuous wave obturation.

1. Introduction

The key to successful endodontic treatment lies in understanding the complexity of the root canal system and cleaning all the roots canals [1]. Incomplete instrumentation followed by incorrect obturation is the most common reason for the failure of endodontic treatment [2]. The most common morphology of the maxillary second premolar is a single root (67%), followed by two roots (30%), while the incidence rate of three roots is only 3%. An incidence of 0.3 to 2% has been seen in laboratory studies for maxillary second premolars with three separate roots [3, 4]. A study done in 1974 in the North of America reported that 75% of teeth exhibiting with one canal at the apex with type I, II, and III Vertucci classification in 48%, 22%, and 5%, respectively [3]. A recent study done by CBCT reported that type I, II, III, IV, and V canals configuration in 49.9%, 9.3%, 2.2%, 32.6%, and 4%, respectively [5]. Anatomically, three-rooted maxillary premolars look similar to maxillary molars, and are sometimes called small molars or radiculous [6]. However, to the best of our knowledge, no case report of a maxillary second premolar with four roots has been published. We present here, a case report of a maxillary premolar with four roots: one mesiobuccal, one distobuccal, one mesiopalatal, and one distopalatal. The four roots were identified using cone-beam computed tomography (CBCT). A 45-year-old female patient with a no significant medical history was referred from a prosthodontist for endodontic treatment with the chief complaint of pain in her maxillary right second premolar. There was no swelling, sinus tract, or lymphadenopathy on the extraoral examination. The intraoral examination revealed no sinus tract or swelling.

The tooth responded positively to the cold test (sensitive and lingering) with Endo-Frost (propane-butane mixture; Roeko, Germany) and was positive to percussion. The maxillary second premolar was diagnosed with symptomatic irreversible pulpitis and symptomatic apical periodontitis. Nonsurgical root canal treatment was recommended. Since the periapical radiograph revealed an unusual tooth anatomy and as there are limitations associated with the periapical radiograph, a cone-beam computed tomography (CBCT) was performed to confirm the number of roots and canals in the maxillary right second premolar. The CBCT confirmed the unusual anatomy and revealed four separate roots with four canals (Figures 1 and 2).

Informed consent was obtained from the patient. Local anesthesia was administered (2% lidocaine with 1 : 100,000 epinephrine), and after rubber dam isolation, access preparation was performed. Inspection of the pulp floor under the

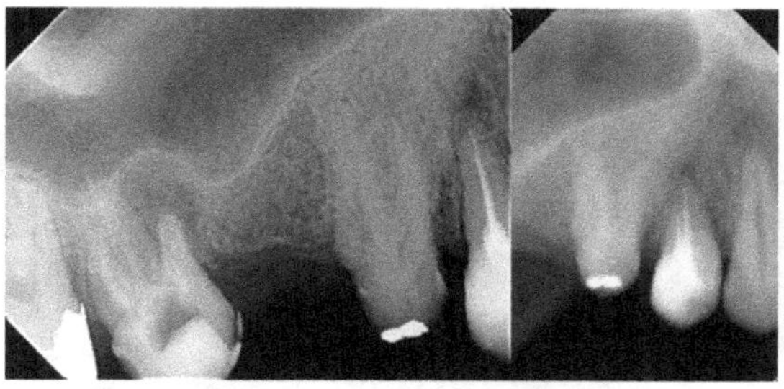

FIGURE 1: Periapical radiograph showing maxillary second premolar with abnormal morphology.

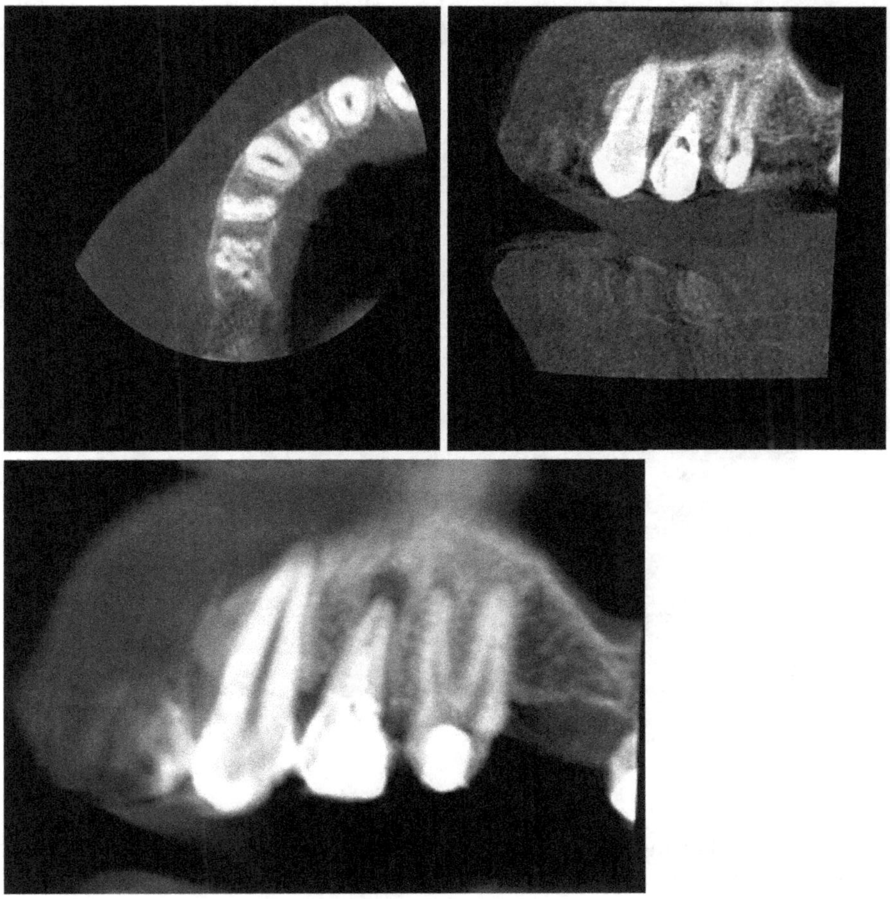

FIGURE 2: CBCT showing maxillary second premolar with 4 roots.

dental operating microscope (Carl Zeiss, Germany) revealed four separate canal orifices (mesiobuccal, distobuccal, mesiopalatal, and distopalatal) (Figure 3). Initial orifice shaping was performed with an SX rotary file (Dentsply Tulsa, Tulsa, OK) starting with a K-file from size 8 and progressing up to size 15 (Dentsply Maillefer, Ballaigues, Switzerland). The root canal length was recorded using an apex locator, RootZX II (J. Morita, Tokyo, Japan), and confirmed with a radiograph. The canals were cleaned and shaped with nickel-titanium rotary instruments (ProTaper Next; Dentsply Tulsa). The canals were enlarged with Protaper X2 to the full working length. All the canals were irrigated with 5.25% sodium hypochlorite after each file, and a final rinse was performed with 17% ethylenediaminetetraacetic acid (EDTA) followed by 5.25% sodium hypochlorite. The canals were dried with sterile paper points (Dentsply Maillefer), and obturation was performed using the continuous wave technique. Four matching gutta-percha cones (Dentsply Maillefer) were gauged and carefully fitted with AH plus sealer (Dentsply Maillefer) under an operating microscope to working length. The downpack that was done with a System B Analytics unit (SybronEndo, Orange Country, CA) was used at a setting of 220°C for each canal. Backfilling was done using Obtura III (Max System, Obtura Spartan, Algonquin, IL, U.S.A). Finally, the access cavity was temporarily filled with Fuji resin-modified glass ionomer filling (ChemFil, Dentsply DeTrey, Germany). The patient was referred back to the prosthodontist for the final restoration (Figure 4). 2

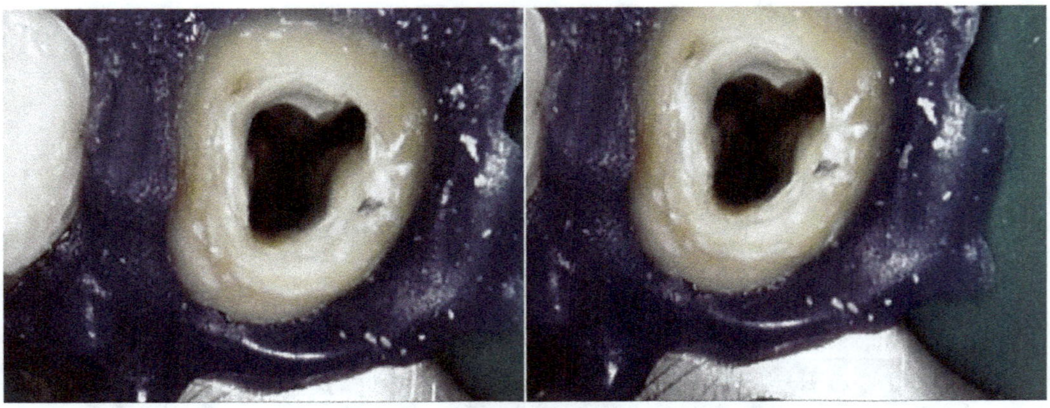

FIGURE 3: Access cavity photograph showing 4 canals orifices.

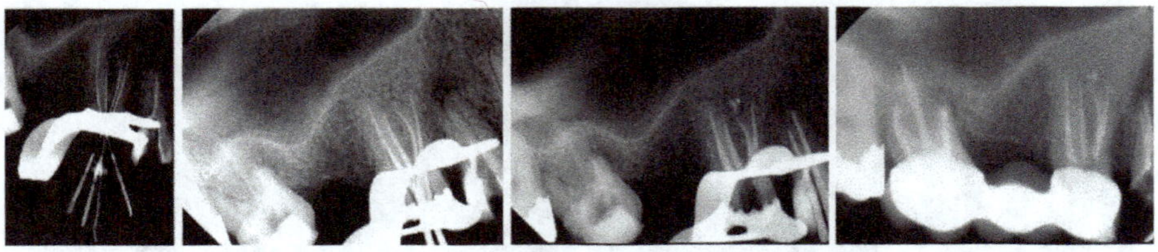

FIGURE 4: Radiographic taken during endodontic treatment, working length measurement, master cone, and final obturation after backfill soften root filling.

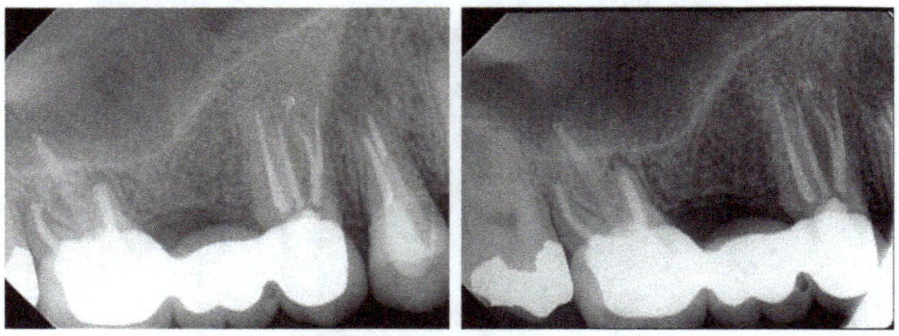

FIGURE 5: Two years follow up showing normal apical tissue.

years follow up clinical examination showing healthy gingiva with probing depth within normal limit, radiographic showing normal apical tissue (Figure 5).

2. Discussion

Adequate root canal therapy requires locating, cleaning, shaping, and obturating all the root canals. Failure of any of these steps can lead to posttreatment disease, pain, and/or complications in the treated tooth [1, 7]. Proper interpretation of conventional periapical radiographs taken in more than one angle is mandatory to detect any morphological variations in the teeth [8]. In addition, using advanced diagnostic radiographic techniques, such as CBCT, is very helpful in detecting such variations if conventional radiographic techniques do not provide adequate information and more details are required [9–12]. CBCT was performed in this case to aid the detection of morphological variations and for management. Furthermore, enhancing visualization by means of an operating dental microscope can aid proper examination of the floor of the pulp chamber, help localize canal orifices, and detect variations that may not be seen easily due to the limited access opening [13–15].

3. Conclusion

The clinical significance is that the second premolar with 4 roots is really a rare case.

References

[1] F. J. Vertucci, "Root canal morphology and its relationship to endodontic procedures," *Endodontic Topics*, vol. 10, no. 1, pp. 3–29, 2005.

[2] J. I. Ingle, "A standardized endodontic technique utilizing newly designed instruments and filling materials," *Oral Surgery, Oral Medicine, Oral Pathology*, vol. 14, no. 1, pp. 83–91, 1961.

[3] F. Vertucci, A. Seelig, and R. Gillis, "Root canal morphology of the human maxillary second premolar," *Oral Surgery, Oral Medicine, Oral Pathology*, vol. 38, no. 3, pp. 456–464, 1974.

[4] J. D. Pecora, M. D. Sousa Neto, P. C. Saquy, and J. B. Woelfel, "In vitro study of root canal anatomy of maxillary second premolars," *Brazilian Dental Journal*, vol. 3, no. 2, pp. 81–85, 1993.

[5] C. O. Lima, L. C. Souza, K. L. Devito, M. Prado, and C. N. Campos, "Evaluation of root canal morphology of maxillary premolars: a cone-beam computed tomography study," *Australian Endodontic Journal*, vol. 45, no. 2, pp. 196–201, 2019.

[6] W. W. Maibaum, "Endodontic treatment of a "ridiculous" maxillary premolar: a case report," *General Dentistry*, vol. 37, no. 4, pp. 340-341, 1989.

[7] U. Sjogren, B. Hagglund, G. Sundqvist, and K. Wing, "Factors affecting the long-term results of endodontic treatment," *Journal of Endodontia*, vol. 16, no. 10, pp. 498–504, 1990.

[8] I. Kaffe, A. Kaufman, M. M. Littner, and A. Lazarson, "Radiographic study of the root canal system of mandibular anterior teeth," *International Endodontic Journal*, vol. 18, no. 4, pp. 253–259, 1985.

[9] S. Patel, "New dimensions in endodontic imaging: part 2. Cone beam computed tomography," *International Endodontic Journal*, vol. 42, no. 6, pp. 463–475, 2009.

[10] C. Durack and S. Patel, "Cone beam computed tomography in endodontics," *Brazilian Dental Journal*, vol. 23, no. 3, pp. 179–191, 2012.

[11] N. Cohenca and H. Shemesh, "Clinical applications of cone beam computed tomography in endodontics: a comprehensive review," *Quintessence International*, vol. 46, no. 6, pp. 465–480, 2015.

[12] T. Venskutonis, G. Plotino, G. Juodzbalys, and L. Mickeviciene, "The importance of cone-beam computed tomography in the management of endodontic problems: a review of the literature," *Journal of Endodontia*, vol. 40, no. 12, pp. 1895–1901, 2014.

[13] A. Castellucci, "Magnification in endodontics: the use of the operating microscope," *Practical Procedures & Aesthetic Dentistry*, vol. 15, no. 5, pp. 377–84; quiz 386, 2003, quiz 86.

[14] G. B. Carr, "Microscopes in endodontics," *Journal of the California Dental Association*, vol. 20, no. 11, pp. 55–61, 1992.

[15] B. G. Khayat, "The use of magnification in endodontic therapy: the operating microscope," *Practical Periodontics and Aesthetic Dentistry*, vol. 10, no. 1, pp. 137–144, 1998.

30

Mandibular Metastasis of Silent Papillary Thyroid Carcinoma: A Rare Case Report with Review of the Literature

Shahzad Gholami,[1] Mahin Bakhshi,[1] Saede Atarbashi-Moghadam,[2] Hassan Mir Mohammad Sadeghi,[3] and Arezoo Rahimzamani[1]

[1]Department of Oral Medicine, School of Dentistry, Shahid Beheshti University of Medical Sciences, Tehran, Iran
[2]Department of Oral and Maxillofacial Pathology, School of Dentistry, Shahid Beheshti University of Medical Sciences, Tehran, Iran
[3]Department of Oral and Maxillofacial Surgery, School of Dentistry, Shahid Beheshti University of Medical Sciences, Tehran, Iran

Correspondence should be addressed to Arezoo Rahimzamani; zamani_arezoo@sbmu.ac.ir

Academic Editor: Ronald S. Brown

Metastasis to the jaws is a rare event; however, it has great importance because it may be the only symptom of an undiagnosed underlying malignancy. Papillary thyroid carcinoma, the commonest histopathologic variant of thyroid cancer, has minimal potential for distant metastasis, and most reported metastatic thyroid carcinomas of the oral cavity have been follicular thyroid carcinoma. The aim of this article is to present a rare case of metastatic papillary thyroid carcinoma, which presented itself as a painless expansion in the anterior region of the mandible in a 56-year-old female, and to review previously published cases of this type of cancer. Reporting rare cases such as this one, together with reviewing previous reports of related rare diseases, will expand the body of knowledge about these uncommon lesions.

1. Introduction

Metastases to the oral cavity comprise about 1% of all the oral malignancies and have been mostly detected in the jaws [1]. Metastasis to the jaw has a marked predilection for the posterior region of the mandible, which is rich in red bone marrow and sinusoidal vascular spaces that may be the cause of tumor deposition [1, 2]. Jaw metastasis is more common among older adults (mean age = 53.4 years) and has a male predilection [1]. Nearly 23% of oral metastases are the first sign of an occult malignant tumor elsewhere in the body [2, 3]. The migration can occur via the bloodstream or the lymphatic pathways. The origin of oral metastasis could be different based on gender [2]. Cancers of the lungs, the liver, and the prostate are the source of most jaw metastases in men, and their origin in women are the breasts, the thyroid gland, and the lungs [1]. Thyroid cancers have accounted for up to 6% of the oral cavity metastases [2, 4], occurring more frequently in follicular variants [5]. Oral metastasis is frequently associated with poor prognosis and quality of life [2], and it usually develops at the late stages of the underlying disease [1]. Thus, oral health care professionals have a crucial role in the diagnosis and management of cancer patients, particularly those with silent primary malignancies [1]. The purpose of the present report is to describe clinical, radiographic, and histopathologic features of mandibular metastasis of a silent papillary thyroid carcinoma in a 56-year-old female. It was also considered pertinent to review previously published reported cases.

2. Case Report

A 56-year-old female was referred to the Department of Oral Medicine, Shahid Beheshti University of Medical Sciences (Tehran, Iran) for evaluation of a rapidly growing painful expansion in the left side of her mandible which by her report had been present for 20 days. The patient reported traumatic luxation of her lower left central and lateral incisors due to a fall and their subsequent extractions by a general dentist. The extraction site had not healed properly and had been

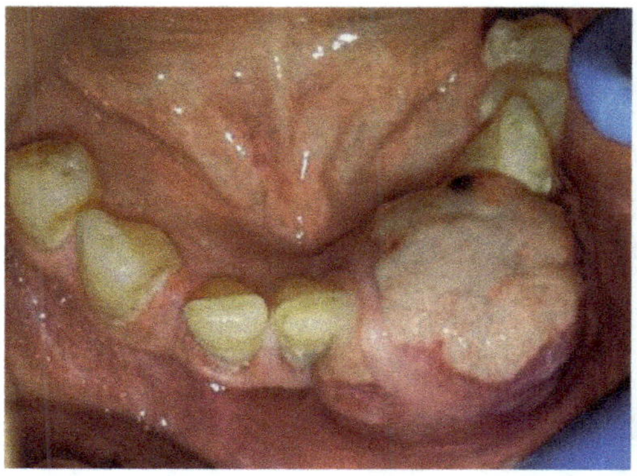

FIGURE 1: An ulcerated mass in the anterior region of the mandible.

expanding. The lesion had been interfering with her eating. Intraoral examination revealed a diffuse swelling in her left anterior mandible measuring 3 × 3 cm and extending from the right central incisor to the left canine. The overlying mucosa was erythematous, ulcerated, and necrotic. The lesion was soft to firm in consistency on palpation (Figure 1).

The patient also suffered from hypertension, diabetes mellitus, and bowel disease.

The panoramic radiograph showed a unilocular radiolucency with ill-defined borders from the right lateral incisor to the left second premolar. Cone beam computed tomography (CBCT) revealed a large destructive lesion with irregular borders associated with a soft tissue mass extending from tooth #26 to the distal of tooth #20, with extensive perforation of the buccal cortical plate. Thinning and erosion of the lingual cortical plate and root resorption of teeth #22, #21, and #20 were also seen (Figures 2 and 3).

There was no cervical lymphadenopathy. According to both clinical and radiographic features, differential diagnoses of aggressive central giant cell granuloma, lymphoma, odontogenic carcinoma, and metastatic neoplasms were considered. The mandibular mass was biopsied, and microscopic sections showed a malignant epithelial neoplasm composed of nests, tubules, and cystic and papillary structures with fibrovascular cores lined by cuboidal and columnar cells. The nuclei showed a ground glass appearance (Figures 4 and 5). Some eosinophilic colloid-like material, hemorrhage, and inflammatory cell infiltration were also seen. The tumor was covered by ulcerated epithelium.

Based on microscopic findings, overall diagnosis of "papillary carcinoma" was rendered. Follow-up immunohistochemical (IHC) staining for TTF1, mammaglobin, CK7, and CK20 was requested for further evaluation and makes difference between metastatic tumors such as papillary thyroid carcinoma (PTC) and papillary breast cancer.

A whole body scan revealed multiple highly metabolically active bony lesions in the chin, the left scapula, the anterolateral arc of the right 7th rib, the right iliac, and the right hip. In addition, both of the thyroid lobes and the isthmus were enlarged and nodular. A calcification was seen in the right nodule of the thyroid lobe, measuring 20 × 10 mm. A compressive effect of the right thyroid nodule on the trachea was obvious. Multiple adenopathies, with a maximum diameter of 14 mm, were evident in different parts of the neck's soft tissue, especially the right side. The tumoral cells were strongly and diffusely positive for TTF1 and CK7 (Figures 6 and 7). No immunoreactivity was seen for CK20.

The microscopic features in combination with the IHC findings were consistent with "metastatic papillary thyroid carcinoma" (PTC). Within 10 days of the patient's first visit, the size of the lesion had nearly doubled, and eating had become difficult for her. In addition, she had been suffering from bleeding of the lesion (Figure 8) and numb-chin syndrome.

The patient was referred to an oncologist for further evaluation and management. According to the decision made by the professional team, a palliative en bloc resection of the lesion was performed. Unfortunately, the patient died one month after the diagnosis.

3. Discussion

Metastasis to the jaws is a rare event, and its early diagnosis is difficult [1]. Factors other than tumor frequency may be involved in oral metastasis, such as biological behavior of cancer, aggressiveness, and predilection for specific oral sites [2, 3]. Metastatic tumors are more commonly found in older adults [1]. The patient in our case was also in her 6th decade of life. Although it has been stated that jaw metastases have a tendency to happen in men, thyroid carcinoma metastasis affects women with a much higher proportion [1]. Metastases to the jaws have a predilection for the mandibular molar/premolar region [1, 4]. However, the anterior region of the mandible was involved in the current case.

Clinical signs and symptoms of jaw metastasis may include pain, swelling, tooth mobility, pathologic fracture, and paresthesia, but it may be asymptomatic [2]. The present case showed a painful swelling with teeth mobility and numb-chin syndrome. Mandibular metastasis with mental nerve involvement may cause numb-chin syndrome [6]. Irani [1] in her systematic review found that anesthesia and paraesthesia were seen in 90% of cases. Thus, it should be considered as a potential sign of metastasis to the mandible from an occult primary tumor [6]. Hirshberg et al. [4] mentioned that about 14% of patients with jaw metastasis had teeth extractions in the metastatic area, with an average time of 2 months between the extraction and the metastatic diagnosis. Our patient also lost her mandibular left central and lateral incisors before the disease was diagnosed. Oral metastasis usually shows simultaneous involvement of multiple body sites, especially the bones [2, 5]. Similarly, widespread skeletal metastasis was observed in this patient.

Most of the previously reported metastatic thyroid carcinomas of the oral cavity had been follicular thyroid carcinoma (FTC), and metastatic PTC was very rare [5, 7, 8]. Hurtle cell, poorly differentiated, and medullary carcinomas have been also reported in the mandible [5]. PTC is the most common microscopic variant of thyroid cancer. Moreover, it has a minimal potential for distant metastasis and tends to spread via lymphatic invasion [2, 5, 6]. It demonstrates an asymptomatic slow-growing thyroid mass, which is sometimes discovered incidentally [5]. Distant metastasis occurs in about 7-23% of patients with thyroid carcinoma [6].

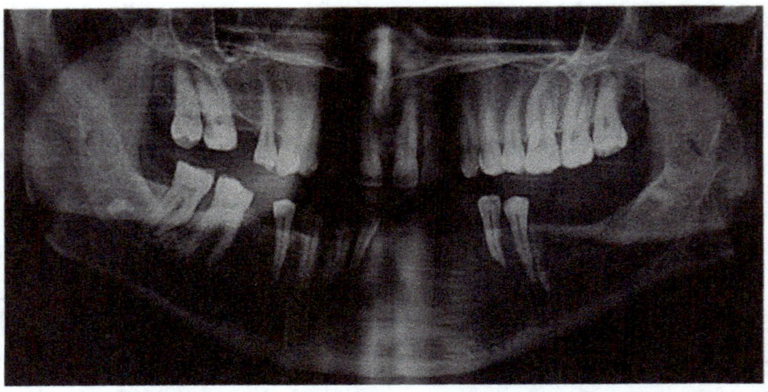

Figure 2: The panoramic radiograph shows an ill-defined unilocular radiolucency extending from the right lateral incisor to the left second premolar, as well as root resorption of teeth 20, 21, and 22.

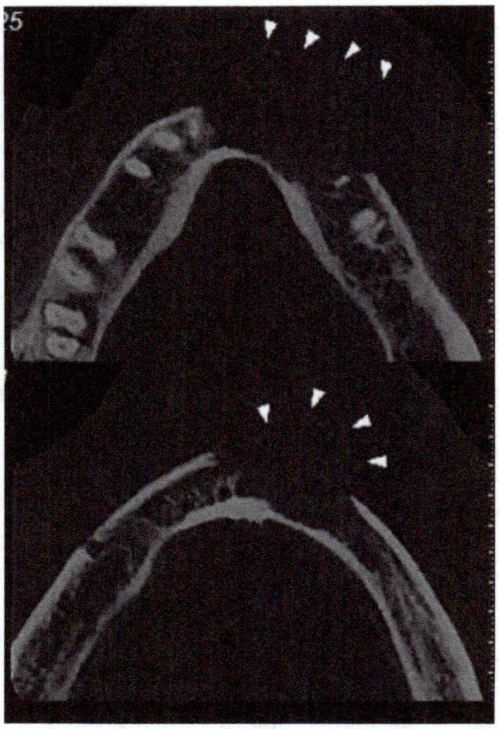

Figure 3: CBCT revealed a large destructive lesion with irregular borders associated with a soft tissue mass causing extensive perforation of the buccal cortical plate.

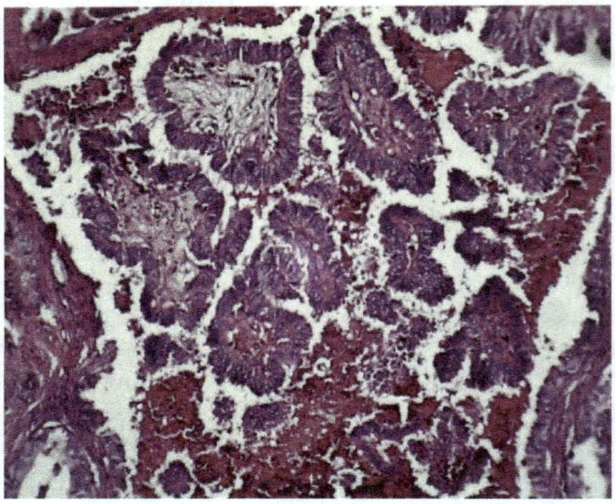

Figure 4: Microscopic sections showed papillary projections with fibrovascular cores lined by cuboidal and columnar cells (H & E ×100).

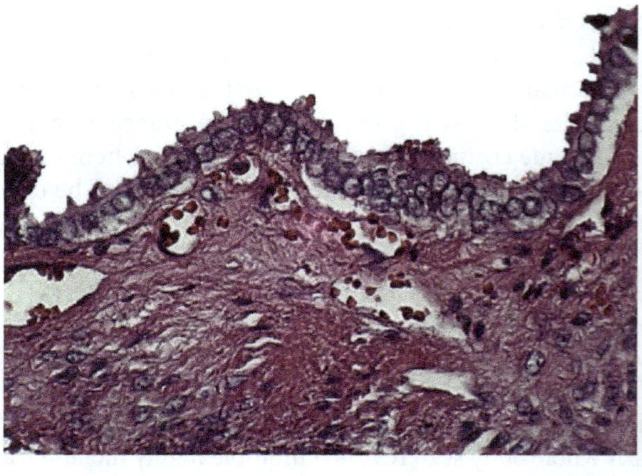

Figure 5: The nuclei showed ground glass appearance (H & E ×400).

Classic osseous regions for thyroid metastasis include the sternum, the vertebrae, and the pelvis [2, 5]. Metastatic PTCs or FTCs usually demonstrate an ill-defined radiolucent lesion in radiographs [5]. A PTC that shows intermediate clinical characteristics between PTC and FTC is considered a follicular variant of PTC (FV-PTC). In microscopy, it demonstrates a follicular pattern with the ground-glass nuclear features of PTC. Bone metastasis in the absence of lymphadenopathy in the setting of PTC may increase the suspicion of FV-PTC [2]. However, in the current case, both the incisional and the excisional biopsy showed a pure PTC pattern. The clinical signs of FTC or FV-PTC may be similar to arteriovenous malformations because they are highly vascular [2, 9]. Our patient also complained about bleeding from the lesion. Thyroid neoplasms are CK7+/CK20-. The panel of antibodies for thyroglobulin, TTF-1, CK7, and CK20 is valuable when the thyroid origin of a metastatic tumor is a possibility [10]. The current case also showed a CK7 +/CK20- and TTF-1+ pattern. Distant metastasis has a

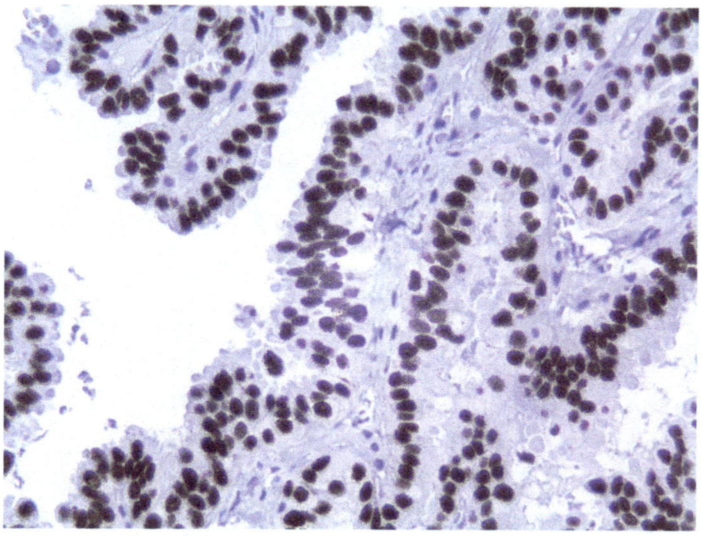

FIGURE 6: The nuclei of neoplastic cells were strongly and diffusely positive for TTF1.

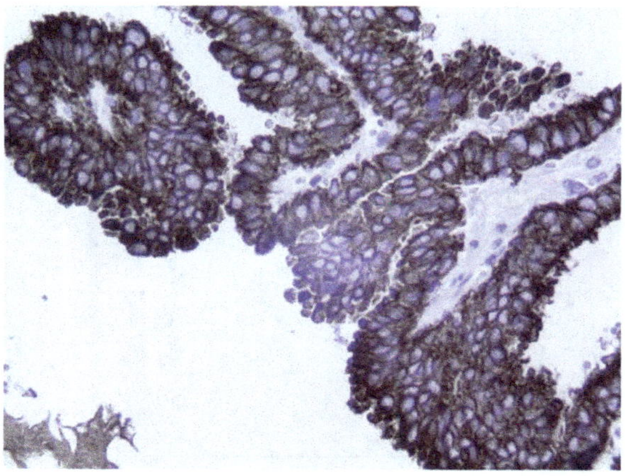

FIGURE 7: The cytoplasm of tumoral cells was strongly and diffusely positive for CK7 (×400).

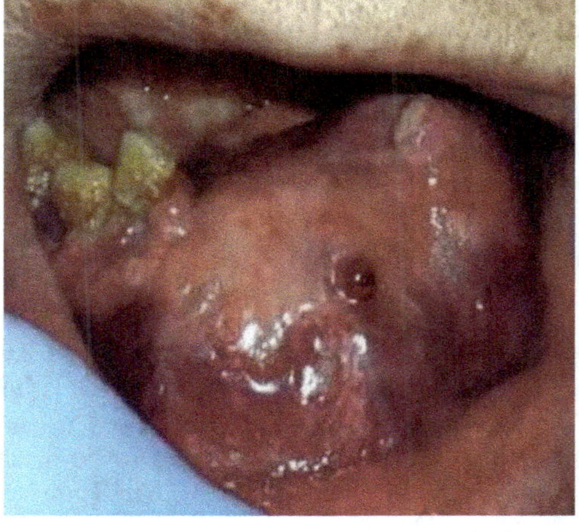

FIGURE 8: Large hemorrhagic mandibular mass 10 days following initial visit.

crucial role in the patients' management, and oral metastasis is a therapeutic challenge for clinicians [10]. It ranges from palliation to several combinations of surgery, radioactive iodine, radiotherapy, and chemotherapy [2]. In our patient, palliative surgery was performed because of the huge mass and its bleeding. The 10-year survival rate for metastatic thyroid carcinomas is 13-21% [6]. Unfortunately, the present case died 1 month after the diagnosis.

Our literature review of metastatic thyroid carcinomas (PTC and FV-PTC variant) to the oral cavity (with sufficient information) resulted in 26 cases from 16 articles including our case. The demographic features are summarized and presented in Table 1 [2, 5, 7–22]. The mean age was 54.4 (ranging from 13 to 69 years). These malignancies occurred most often in the sixth and seventh decades of life, only 3 patients were under the age of 40, and no patient was found in the 8th decade of life. Nikitakis et al. [5] reported that the mean age of the metastatic thyroid carcinoma patients was 60.6 years with a tendency to occur in the 7th decade. Considering the age of occurrence for the primary thyroid carcinoma, which is about 40 to 50 years old, an increase in the mean age of metastasis is related to the amount of time that metastasis needs to develop and be detected [5]. There was a striking female predilection (88.46%) with a ratio of 7 : 66. This high tendency towards females is associated with the high incidence of thyroid carcinoma in women [5]. Among 25 patients with available tumor locations, the mandible was the most common site (80%). Other sites of involvement were the maxilla and the tongue. The tendency for spreading to the mandible may be associated with its greater volume of hematopoietic tissue that delivers easy access to neoplastic cells [18]. They tend to be more common in the jaws in comparison to oral soft tissues (4%). PTC and its FV-PTC variant comprised 53.84% and 46.15%, respectively. Among the 19 cases with available data about the time of metastasis, 42.10% were not aware of their primary cancer. Nikitakis et al. [5] in their review found that

Table 1: Published case reports of metastatic PTC and FV-PTC.

No.	References	Sex/age (years)	Location	Pathologic findings	Metastases found before primary tumor
1	Nishimura et al. [11]	F/51	Man	FV-PTC	Yes
2	Markitziu et al. [12]	F/69	Man and parotid	FV-PTC	Yes
3	Erdag et al. [13]	F/53	Man and infratemporal fossa	FV-PTC	No
4	Colella et al. [14]	F/50	Man	PTC	No
5	Liu et al. [15]	M/66	Man	FV-PTC	No
6	Tamiolakis et al. [16]	F/69	Man	PTC	N/A
7	Antunes and Antunes [7]	F/13	Max	PTC	N/A
8	Nikitakis et al. [5]	M/63	Max	PTC	No
9	Fatahzadeh et al. [2]	F/43	Max	FV-PTC	No
10	Seoane et al. [8]	F/58	Tongue	PTC	Yes
11	Seoane et al. [8]	F/69	Man	PTC	No
12	Muttagi et al. [17]	M/60	Man	FV-PTC	N/A
13	Muttagi et al. [17]	F/63	Man	FV-PTC	N/A
14	Muttagi et al. [17]	F/44	Man	PTC	N/A
15	Muttagi et al. [17]	F/35	Man	PTC	N/A
16	Muttagi et al. [17]	F/51	Man	FV-PTC	N/A
17	Kumar et al. [9]	f/58	Man	FV-PTC	Yes
18	Bhansali et al. [22]	F/60	Max	FV-PTC	Yes
19	Nawale et al. [18]	F/60	Man	PTC	No
20	Nawale et al. [18]	F/42	Oral	PTC	Yes
21	Nawale et al. [18]	F/50	Man	PTC	No
22	Nawale et al. [18]	F/56	Man	PTC	No
23	Anajar et al. [19]	F/52	Man	PTC	Yes
24	Ambelil et al. [20]	F/69	Man	FV-PTC*	No
25	Bingol et al. [21]	F/33	Man	FV-PTC	No
26	Current case	F/56	Man	PTC	Yes

*Man: mandible; Max: maxilla.

oral metastasis had been reported as the first sign of an unknown primary thyroid carcinoma in more than half of the metastatic thyroid carcinoma cases.

4. Conclusion

Although very rare, PTC can metastasize to the oral cavity. Oral metastasis may be the first symptom of a malignancy in other parts of the body. This emphasizes the role of oral professionals in identifying metastatic lesions. CK7/CK20 can be helpful in cases where the primary location of the metastatic tumor is unknown. Metastatic PTC/FV-PTC tends to occur in females, with a very high proportion, most often in the sixth and seventh decades of life. Additionally, there is a striking predilection for mandibular involvement. Reporting rare cases such as this one, together with a review of the pertinent literature will expand the body of knowledge about these uncommon lesions.

Acknowledgments

The authors would like to appreciate Dr. Reza Tabrizi for his help as an oral and maxillofacial surgeon.

References

[1] S. Irani, "Metastasis to the jawbones: a review of 453 cases," *Journal International Society Preventive Community Dentistry*, vol. 7, no. 2, pp. 71–81, 2017.

[2] M. Fatahzadeh, G. Subramanian, and S. R. Singer, "Metstatic papillary thyroid carcinoma to maxilla: a rare case," *Quintessence International*, vol. 46, no. 5, pp. 431–435, 2015.

[3] A. Hirshberg, A. Shnaiderman-Shapiro, I. Kaplan, and R. Berger, "Metastatic tumours to the oral cavity—pathogenesis and analysis of 673 cases," *Oral Oncology*, vol. 44, no. 8, pp. 743–752, 2008.

[4] A. Hirshberg, P. Leibovich, and A. Buchner, "Metastatic tumors to the jawbones: analysis of 390 cases," *Journal of Oral Pathology & Medicine*, vol. 23, no. 8, pp. 337–341, 1994.

[5] N. G. Nikitakis, A. Polymeri, A. Polymeris, and A. Sklavounou, "Metastatic papillary thyroid carcinoma to the maxilla: case report and literature review," *Head and Neck Pathology*, vol. 6, no. 2, pp. 216–223, 2012.

[6] C. Lavanya, "Mandibular metastasis of thyroid carcinoma: a case report," *Journal of Clinical and Diagnostic Research*, vol. 8, no. 7, 2014.

[7] A. A. Antunes and A. P. Antunes, "Gnathic bone metastasis: a retrospective study of 10 cases," *Brazilian Journal of Otorhinolaryngology*, vol. 74, no. 4, pp. 561–565, 2008.

[8] J. Seoane, I. Van der Waal, R. I. F. Van der Waal et al., "Metastatic tumours to the oral cavity: a survival study with a special focus on gingival metastases," *Journal of Clinical Periodontology*, vol. 36, no. 6, pp. 488–492, 2009.

[9] R. V. Kumar, C. Chakravarthy, G. R. Sekhar, S. K. Devireddy, C. Kumaravelu, and A. Kare, "Metastatic thyroid carcinoma presenting as hypervascular lesion of the mandible: a case report and review of literature," *Journal of Oral and Maxillofacial Surgery*, vol. 68, no. 10, pp. 2613–2616, 2010.

[10] P. A. Bejarano, Y. E. Nikiforov, E. S. Swenson, and P. W. Biddinger, "Thyroid transcription factor-1, thyroglobulin, cytokeratin 7, and cytokeratin 20 in thyroid neoplasms," *Applied Immunohistochemistry & Molecular Morphology*, vol. 8, no. 3, pp. 189–194, 2000.

[11] Y. Nishimura, T. Nakajima, H. Yakata, T. Kawasaki, and M. Fukushima, "Metastatic thyroid carcinoma of the mandible," *Journal of Oral and Maxillofacial Surgery*, vol. 40, no. 4, pp. 221–225, 1982.

[12] A. Markitziu, D. Fisher, and Y. Marmary, "Thyroid papillary carcinoma presenting as jaw and parotid gland metastases," *International Journal of Oral and Maxillofacial Surgery*, vol. 15, no. 5, pp. 648–653, 1986.

[13] T. Erdag, C. Bilgen, and K. Ceryan, "Metastatic thyroid carcinoma of the mandibule," *Revue Laryngologie Otologie Rhinologie*, vol. 120, no. 1, pp. 31–34, 1999.

[14] G. Colella, R. Capone, and S. Cappabianca, "Mandibular metastasis from papillary thyroid carcinoma—a case report," *Tumori*, vol. 89, no. 4, pp. 452–454, 2003.

[15] L. Liu, G. Venkataraman, and A. Salhadar, "Follicular variant of papillary thyroid carcinoma with unusual late metastasis to the mandible and the scapula," *Pathology International*, vol. 57, no. 5, pp. 296–298, 2007.

[16] D. Tamiolakis, I. Tsamis, V. Thomaidis, M. Lambropoulou, G. Alexiadis, and I. Venizelos, "Jaw bone metastases: four cases," *Acta Dermatovenerologica Alpina, Panonica, et Adriatica*, vol. 16, no. 1, pp. 21–25, 2007.

[17] S. S. Muttagi, P. Chaturvedi, A. D'Cruz et al., "Metastatic tumors to the jaw bones: retrospective analysis from an Indian tertiary referral center," *Indian Journal of Cancer*, vol. 48, no. 2, pp. 234–239, 2011.

[18] K. K. Nawale, M. Vyas, S. Kane, and A. Patil, "Metastatic tumors in the jaw bones: a retrospective clinicopathological study of 12 cases at tertiary cancer center," *Journal Oral Maxillofacial Pathology*, vol. 20, no. 2, pp. 252–255, 2016.

[19] S. Anajar, J. Hassnaoui, S. Rouadi, R. Abada, M. Roubal, and M. Mahtar, "Mandibular metastasis revealed papillary thyroid carcinoma: rare case," *International Journal of Surgery Case Reports*, vol. 37, pp. 130–133, 2017.

[20] M. Ambelil, S. Sultana, S. Roy, and M. M. Gonzalez, "Anaplastic transformation in mandibular metastases of follicular variant of papillary thyroid carcinoma: a case report and review of the literature," *Annals of Clinical and Laboratory Science*, vol. 46, no. 5, pp. 552–556, 2016.

[21] U. A. Bingol, C. Cinar, and O. Cetinkale, "Mandibular Metastases of Papillary Thyroid Carcinoma Treated by Hemimandibulectomy and Costochondral Rib Graft," *Plastic and Reconstructive Surgery Global Open*, vol. 3, no. 2, article e305, 2015.

[22] A. Bhansali, R. N. Kataria, K. A. Subrahmanyam, B. D. Radotra, and S. K. Mathur, "Maxillary mass as the presenting manifestation of papillary thyroid carcinoma," *Indian Journal of Cancer*, vol. 40, no. 2, pp. 80-81, 2003.

Two Cases of Nonsuicidal Self-Injury Comprising Partial Autoamputation of the Apex of the Tongue

Takashi Moriya,[1] Hitoshi Sato,[1] Kenichi Takeda,[2] Kaori Ikezaki,[2] Ryogo Katada,[2] and Tatsuo Shirota[2]

[1]*Department of Oral and Maxillofacial Surgery, Division of Oral Oncology, Showa University School of Dentistry, Tokyo, Japan*
[2]*Department of Oral and Maxillofacial Surgery, Showa University, School of Dentistry, Tokyo, Japan*

Correspondence should be addressed to Hitoshi Sato; h.sato@dent.showa-u.ac.jp

Academic Editor: Muawia A. Qudeimat

The prevalence of nonsuicidal self-injury (NSSI) in adults is lower than that in adolescents and it is more prevalent in patients with psychiatric disorders. Sleep disturbances such as nightmares are associated with NSSI after accounting for depression; thus, persons with major NSSI sometimes present at medical institutions during the night seeking emergency treatment. Gingival tissues comprise the most frequent target of self-injury of the oral cavity using oral hygiene tools. Most NSSI in the oral cavity is minor because such tools are blunt. Major NSSI such as autoamputation of the tongue is rare. We describe two patients who partially autoamputated the apex of their own tongues using edged tools. Case 1 was a 55-year-old female with depression who had defaulted from psychiatric intervention. She had cut off her tongue using a Japanese kitchen knife and presented with the dry, necrotic amputated portion and blood oozing from the remainder of her tongue. We debrided and sutured the remainder of the tongue without reattaching the amputated portion. Her postoperative course was uneventful, and she was free of adverse events such as functional disability and wound infection. Case 2 was a 69-year-old female with schizophrenia who had defaulted from psychiatric intervention and had cut off her tongue using scissors. The amputated portion of the tongue was lost and the remainder, which was oozing blood, was debrided and sutured. She defaulted on a follow-up appointment. Neither of these patients had suicidal intent. The prevalence of NSSI across all age groups has recently increased, and the risk that self-injury will become normalized has become a concern. Thus, dentists as well as oral and maxillofacial surgeons should be aware of the possibility that patients will present with major NSSI requiring emergency treatment.

1. Introduction

Nonsuicidal self-injury (NSSI) is usually described as the deliberate, direct destruction or alteration of body tissue without conscious suicidal intent [1, 2], and it is a unique risk factor for suicide [3]. Nonsuicidal self-injury occurs among 17.2% of adolescents, 13.4% of young adults, and 5.5% of older adults [4]. It often occurs in patients with psychiatric disorders such as schizophrenia [5–7], autism [8], and depression [9], and the target of NSSI is often the skin, eyes, or genitalia [10]. Much of the described NSSI in the oral cavity has been minor, because the gingival tissues are the most frequent site of injuries and the tools have usually been toothbrushes and brush picks [11–15]. On the other hand, major NSSI is a considerable public health problem because it is also associated with high rates of emergency room utilization [16]. We describe two adult patients who presented at our emergency room during the night with partial autoamputation of the apex of the tongue.

2. Case Reports

2.1. Case 1. A 55-year-old Japanese female presented in November 2011 having autoamputated the apex of her tongue with a Japanese kitchen knife. She had chronic depression but had defaulted from psychiatric intervention and thus was not under prescribed medication for depression. She had endured parasomnia with nightmares for several months. She had cut her tongue after experiencing a terrible nightmare about her son and presented at the emergency room eight hours later at 05:00 hours. Her vital signs were unremarkable, but blood continuously oozed from the remaining part of the tongue (Figure 1(a)). No other lacerations were evident, and the remainder of the tongue had normal mobility (Figure 1(b)). She had also brought the dry and necrotic amputated portion (2.8 × 1.5 cm) (Figure 1(c)). Active bleeding from the lingual arteries was not evident. A bite block was inserted between the posterior molars, and then we debrided (Figure 2(a)) and sutured the remainder of the tongue using an antimicrobial Vicryl® Plus suture coated with polyglactin 910 and triclosan (Ethicon Inc., Somerville, NJ, USA) under local anesthesia with xylocaine 2% and adrenaline (1 : 80,000 dilution) (Figure 2(b)). The amputated portion of the tongue was not reattached. We prescribed loxoprofen sodium hydrate (Loxonin; Daiichi Sankyo Co. Ltd., Tokyo, Japan) 60 mg for pain control and the antibiotic amoxicillin hydrate (Sawacillin; Astellas Pharma Inc., Tokyo, Japan) 3 × 250 mg daily to prevent infection. We provided the patient with postoperative instructions regarding oral hygiene, a soft diet, and smoking cessation and also explained the importance of resuming psychiatric treatment for chronic depression. Her postoperative course was uneventful, and she has remained free of functional disability and wound infection.

2.2. Case 2. A 69-year-old Japanese female presented in January 2011 having autoamputated the apex of her tongue with scissors. She had a 10-year history of schizophrenia but had defaulted from psychiatric intervention and stopped taking prescribed medication. She also had parasomnia with arousal disorders. She arrived at the emergency room three hours after the autoamputation at 03:00 hours. Her vital signs were stable. Although blood oozed from the major portion of the tongue, the lingual arteries were not damaged (Figure 3(a)). No other lacerations were evident, and the mobility of the remaining portion of the tongue was normal (Figure 3(b)). The amputated portion was missing; thus, the remainder of the tongue was debrided and sutured using Vicryl® Plus antimicrobial coated sutures (Ethicon Inc.) under local anesthesia (xylocaine 2% with adrenaline (1 : 80,000 dilution) (Figures 4(a) and 4(b)). The patient was prescribed with loxoprofen sodium hydrate (Loxonin; Daiichi Sankyo Co., Ltd.) for pain control and amoxicillin hydrate (Sawacillin; Astellas Pharma Inc.) to avoid infection. We provided the patient with postoperative instructions including oral hygiene and a soft diet. We also described the importance of resuming psychiatric treatment for schizophrenia and follow-up with us. However, this patient did not keep her first postoperative appointment and was lost to follow-up.

3. Discussion

The prevalence of NSSI has recently increased in both sexes and across age groups in England [17], and the risk that self-mutilation will become normalized has become a concern. Although NSSI is more prevalent among young women and girls in Western countries [17], it is more prevalent among male than female Chinese college students [18]. This prevalence in China is remarkable in rural, but not urban areas [18, 19]. This might be related to coping method with emotional stress that is influenced by culture and gender norms. Since a history of NSSI is a clinical marker for subsequent suicide attempts [3], self-mutilation to cope with emotional stress could have serious long-term public health implications.

Major NSSI are generally associated with severe mental illness [5–9, 20–22] and often result in the permanent loss of organs such as the skin, eyes, genitalia [10], or their functions [21–23]. Davies and Doyle have identified a close association between psychiatric disorders and major NSSI because at least 79.3% of patients with major NSSI also have chronic psychiatric disorders [22]. Some individuals are believed to practice NSSI because of feeling overwhelming guilt, depersonalization, or experiencing hallucinations [1, 24]. Since the degree of NSSI is related to anger, anxiety, or impulsivity [25], nonsuicidal autoamputations are rare [26]. On the other hand, disruptions in sleep are associated with an increased tendency towards emotional dysregulation [27]. Nightmares rather than insomnia symptoms have recently been associated with NSSI after accounting for depression [28]. One of our patients (Case 1) mutilated herself with a knife after a dreadful nightmare about her son, about whom she felt overwhelmed with guilt as he was a juvenile delinquent. However, she had no suicidal intent. The other patient (Case 2) had often experienced hallucinations during arousal from sleep. Thus, sleep arousal disorders and schizophrenic hallucinations might have led her to the autoamputation even though she also had no suicidal intent. Since both these patients had defaulted from psychiatric intervention, relapsing symptoms of their psychiatric disorders might have been involved in their NSSI. Moreover, dentists as well as oral and maxillofacial surgeons should be aware that patients with major NSSI associated with sleep disturbances such as nightmares might present late at night seeking emergency treatment.

Minor NSSI do not lead to major disabilities and are relatively common, whereas major NSSI such as autoamputations can lead to significant disability. Most NSSI of the oral cavity are caused using tools of oral hygiene such as toothbrushes or brush picks, and gingival tissue is a frequent target [11–15]. Thus, most NSSI in the oral cavity such as erosion, ulcers, or periodontal clinical attachment losses are minor. To determine the characteristics of intraoral NSSI using edged tools, we searched the PubMed database in June 2019 using the search terms "self-harm" OR "self-injury" OR "NSSI" OR "self-mutilation" OR "self-inflicted injuries" AND "intra oral" OR "oral cavity" OR "tongue" OR "gum" OR "gingiva" OR "lip" OR "teeth." Data were screened in two steps. The first excluded articles with incomplete text or with missing data. The second step involved filtering by patient age, sex, medical history, tools used for mutilation, and suicidal intent. Table 1 describes five patients with NSSI of the oral cavity that they inflicted using edged tools [20, 21, 29]. As far as we are aware, only three patients who have used edged tools to inflict intraoral NSSI have been described. The mean age of these five patients (including the two described herein) was 46.8 ± 21.0 years, and three were female. Two patients used scissors and three used knives. Three of the major NSSI

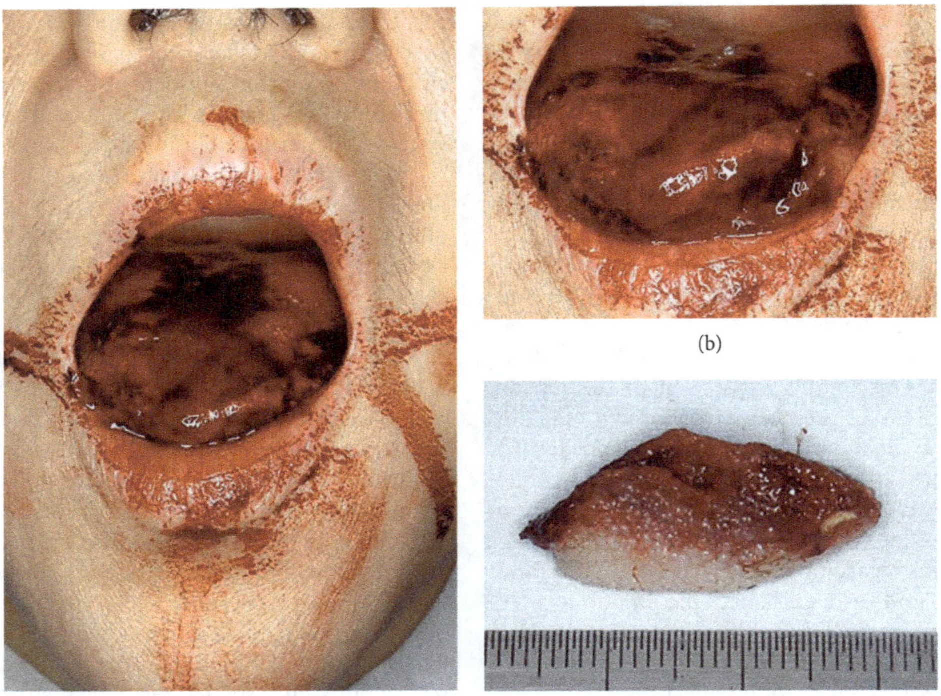

(a) (b) (c)

FIGURE 1: Case 1: preoperative images of the oral cavity. At rest (a), tongue protrusion (b), and amputated portion (c).

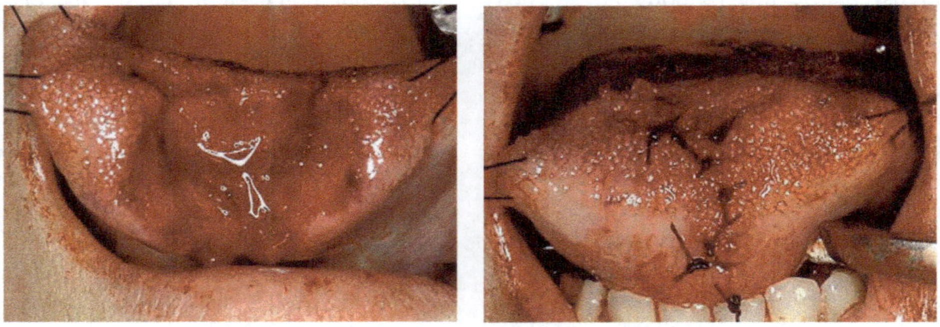

(a) (b)

FIGURE 2: Case 1: operative images of the oral cavity. After debridement (a) and suture (b).

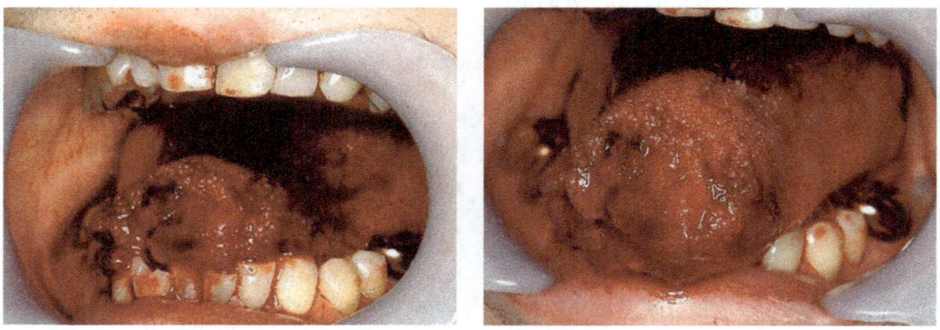

(a) (b)

FIGURE 3: Case 2: preoperative images of the oral cavity. At rest (a) and tongue protrusion (b).

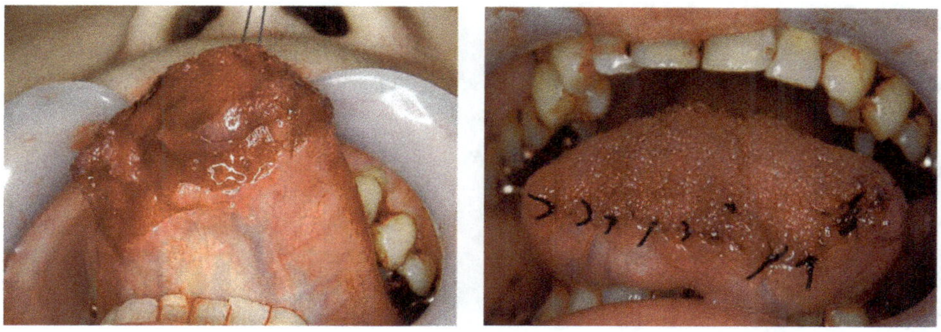

(a) (b)

Figure 4: Case 2: operative images of the oral cavity. After debridement (a) and suture (b).

Table 1: Clinical reports of NSSI of the oral cavity inflicted using edged tools.

No.	Author	Year	Age	Sex	Tools	Lesion	Symptom	Psychological factors
1	Blanton et al.	1977	61	M	Knife	Teeth	Crown fracture	Unknown
2	McGrath et al.	1985	25	F	Knife	Gum	Ulcer	Unknown
3	Hong and Eun	2014	24	M	Scissors	Tongue	Amputation	Schizophrenia
4	Present case	2019	55	F	Knife	Tongue	Amputation	Depression
5	Present case	2019	69	F	Scissors	Tongue	Amputation	Schizophrenia

involved tongue amputations and were associated with schizophrenia or depression.

Treating physicians are faced with challenging decisions when NSSI involves amputation, because some evidence has shown that good rehabilitation and motivated patients are needed to obtain favorable functional outcomes after replantation [20, 21, 30]. Hong and Eun have described successful replantation of an amputated tongue after NSSI in a patient with schizophrenia [21]. That patient was expected to have low compliance and thus remained sedated in an intensive care unit for five days after surgery with a Denhardt mouth gag [21]. Replantation of an amputated tongue portion is challenging, since the tongue is essentially a muscular organ. Another report has described necrosis after replantation of an amputated tongue portion that had remained ischemic for a long time [31]. Our patient (Case 1) brought the dry, necrotic amputated part of the tongue when she presented at the hospital. We did not replant it, because the degree of irreversible damage was likely to be too high. Despite the missing tissue, this patient appeared to be functioning well at one week after surgery. Her articulation and intelligibility were such that relatives could understand her speech over the telephone and she had no difficulty eating any type of food. The other patient (Case 2) did not keep a postoperative follow-up appointment one week after surgery. Therefore, her functional ability and wound condition remain unknown. Patients with psychiatric disorders are expected to have low compliance. Thus, successful outcomes should require intervention with the interdisciplinary cooperation of patients, relatives, healthcare providers, and a medical team that includes dentists as well as oral and maxillofacial surgeons.

Our patient had no continuous arterial bleeding from the tongue and developed no fatal systemic condition after the self-inflicted amputation. However, while people with NSSI do not intend to commit suicide, they might cause more harm than they intended, which could result in severe medical complications or death. Moreover, severe or prolonged self-injury might lead to desperation about lack of control over the causative issue, the self-destructive behavior, and its addictive nature. This might then escalate to true suicide attempts. Therefore, prompt intervention is important for NSSI in the oral cavity to avoid serious bleeding complications, infection, and the possibility of further self-mutilation. On the other hand, the characteristics of intraoral NSSI remain unclear, because it is rare. Tools for assessing NSSI epidemiology in community populations are few and are either limited in the scope of NSSI features assessed [32] or do not include intraoral NSSI. The NSSI Assessment Tool (AT) has been validated and is useful for determining prevalence, form, function, recency, and severity [33]. Future studies should investigate the features of intraoral NSSI using the NSSI-AT. Since the "wound locations" including the lips or tongue are evaluation items in the NSSI-AT, a detailed analysis might reveal relationships between the motivation to inflict intraoral NSSI.

4. Conclusion

We described two nonsuicidal patients who mutilated their tongues using edged tools after sleep disturbances. The prevalence of NSSI has recently increased, and concerns have been raised about the potential normalization of self-mutilation. Although such patients are rare, medical providers including dentists and oral surgeons should be aware of the increasing likelihood that a patient will present with a major NSSI seeking emergency treatment late at night.

Acknowledgments

This case report was supported/partially supported by Takaaki Kamatani and Yuji Kurihara. We are thankful to them who provided expertise procedure to the patients presented by this case report.

References

[1] A. R. Favazza, "The coming of age of self-mutilation," *The Journal of Nervous and Mental Disease*, vol. 186, no. 5, pp. 259–268, 1998.

[2] E. M. Pattison and J. Kahan, "The deliberate self-harm syndrome," *The American Journal of Psychiatry*, vol. 140, no. 7, pp. 867–872, 1983.

[3] P. Wilkinson, R. Kelvin, C. Roberts, B. Dubicka, and I. Goodyer, "Clinical and psychosocial predictors of suicide attempts and nonsuicidal self-injury in the Adolescent Depression Antidepressants and Psychotherapy Trial (ADAPT)," *The American Journal of Psychiatry*, vol. 168, no. 5, pp. 495–501, 2011.

[4] S. V. Swannell, G. E. Martin, A. Page, P. Hasking, and N. J. St John, "Prevalence of nonsuicidal self-injury in nonclinical samples: systematic review, meta-analysis and meta-regression," *Suicide & Life-Threatening Behavior*, vol. 44, no. 3, pp. 273–303, 2014.

[5] M. Rodríguez-Martín, M. Sáez-Rodríguez, J. L. Carrasco et al., "Self-induced paraffinoma in a schizophrenic patient," *Journal of the American Academy of Dermatology*, vol. 56, no. 5, pp. S127–S128, 2007.

[6] R. L. Altom and A. J. DiAngelis, "Multiple autoextractions: oral self-mutilation reviewed," *Oral Surgery, Oral Medicine, and Oral Pathology*, vol. 67, no. 3, pp. 271–274, 1989.

[7] A. J. Paterson, F. Stewart, E. N. Tulloch, and A. M. Hughes, "Self-inflicted mutilation of the dentition in a schizophrenic patient," *British Dental Journal*, vol. 173, no. 9, pp. 314–316, 1992.

[8] C. D. Johnson, M. K. Matt, D. Dennison, R. S. Brown, and S. Koh, "Preventing factitious gingival injury in an autistic patient," *Journal of the American Dental Association*, vol. 127, no. 2, pp. 244–247, 1996.

[9] H. S. Sandhu, V. Sharma, and G. S. Sidhu, "Role of psychiatric disorders in self-inflicted periodontal injury: a case report," *Journal of Periodontology*, vol. 68, no. 11, pp. 1136–1139, 1997.

[10] M. D. Feldman, "The challenge of self-mutilation: a review," *Comprehensive Psychiatry*, vol. 29, no. 3, pp. 252–269, 1988.

[11] B. Blasberg, A. Jordan-Knox, and R. J. Conklin, "Gingival ulceration due to improper toothbrushing," *Journal of the Canadian Dental Association*, vol. 47, no. 7, pp. 462–464, 1981.

[12] G. L. Pattison, "Self-inflicted gingival injuries: literature review and case report," *Journal of Periodontology*, vol. 54, no. 5, pp. 299–304, 1983.

[13] P. Fletcher and D. P. Tarnow, "The interproximal brush and toothbrush abrasion-a case report," *Periodontal Case Reports*, vol. 5, no. 2, pp. 40-41, 1983.

[14] B. A. Pearlman, "A mistaken health belief resulting in gingival injury: a case report," *Journal of Periodontology*, vol. 65, no. 3, pp. 284–286, 1994.

[15] H. Endo, T. D. Rees, W. W. Hallmon, Y. Kono, and T. Kato, "Self-inflicted gingival injuries caused by excessive oral hygiene practices," *Texas Dental Journal*, vol. 123, no. 12, pp. 1098–1104, 2006.

[16] M. Olfson, M. J. Gameroff, S. C. Marcus, T. Greenberg, and D. Shaffer, "Emergency treatment of young people following deliberate self-harm," *Archives of General Psychiatry*, vol. 62, no. 10, pp. 1122–1128, 2005.

[17] S. McManus, D. Gunnell, C. Cooper et al., "Prevalence of non-suicidal self-harm and service contact in England, 2000-14: repeated cross-sectional surveys of the general population," *Lancet Psychiatry*, vol. 6, no. 7, pp. 573–581, 2019.

[18] X. Yang and M. W. Feldman, "A reversed gender pattern? A meta-analysis of gender differences in the prevalence of non-suicidal self-injurious behaviour among Chinese adolescents," *BMC Public Health*, vol. 18, no. 1, p. 66, 2018.

[19] J. Tang, G. Li, B. Chen et al., "Prevalence of and risk factors for non-suicidal self-injury in rural China: results from a nationwide survey in China," *Journal of Affective Disorders*, vol. 226, pp. 188–195, 2018.

[20] K. G. McGrath, R. Pick, E. Leboff-Ries, and R. Patterson, "Factitious desquamative gingivitis simulating a possible immunologic disease," *The Journal of Allergy and Clinical Immunology*, vol. 75, no. 1, pp. 44–46, 1985.

[21] J. M. Hong and S. C. Eun, "Self-mutilation of the tongue in a patient with schizophrenia," *The Journal of Craniofacial Surgery*, vol. 25, no. 2, pp. e116–e118, 2014.

[22] S. J. Davies and M. P. Doyle, "Major self-mutilation leading to complete amputation of the hand during an acute psychotic episode," *Case Studies in Surgery*, vol. 2, pp. 6–9, 2016.

[23] M. Large, N. Babidge, D. Andrews, P. Storey, and O. Nielssen, "Major self-mutilation in the first episode of psychosis," *Schizophrenia Bulletin*, vol. 35, no. 5, pp. 1012–1021, 2009.

[24] J. B. Webb, "Replantation in trauma," *Trauma*, vol. 7, no. 1, pp. 1–9, 2016.

[25] R. D. Goldney and D. Lester, "Ethology and self-injury," *The British Journal of Psychiatry*, vol. 170, no. 2, pp. 192-193, 1997.

[26] D. Simeon, B. Stanley, A. Frances, J. J. Mann, R. Winchel, and M. Stanley, "Self-mutilation in personality disorders: psychological and biological correlates," *The American Journal of Psychiatry*, vol. 149, no. 2, pp. 221–226, 1992.

[27] D. F. Dinges, F. Pack, K. Williams et al., "Cumulative sleepiness, mood disturbance, and psychomotor vigilance performance decrements during a week of sleep restricted to 4-5 hours per night," *Sleep*, vol. 20, no. 4, pp. 267–277, 1997.

[28] C. R. Ennis, N. A. Short, A. J. Moltisanti, C. E. Smith, T. E. Joiner, and J. Taylor, "Nightmares and nonsuicidal self-injury: the mediating role of emotional dysregulation," *Comprehensive Psychiatry*, vol. 76, pp. 104–112, 2017.

[29] P. L. Blanton, W. C. Hurt, and M. D. Largent, "Oral factitious injuries," *Journal of Periodontology*, vol. 48, no. 1, pp. 33–37, 1977.

[30] C. McDonald, "Self-mutilation in adolescents," *The Journal of School Nursing*, vol. 22, no. 4, pp. 193–200, 2006.

[31] C. Davis and J. Armstrong, "Replantation of an amputated tongue," *Plastic and Reconstructive Surgery*, vol. 108, no. 5, pp. 1441-1442, 2001.

[32] K. L. Gratz, "Measurement of deliberate self-harm: preliminary data on the deliberate self-harm inventory," *Journal of Psychopathology and Behavioral Assessment*, vol. 23, no. 4, pp. 253–263, 2001.

[33] J. Whitlock, D. Exner-Cortens, and A. Purington, "Assessment of nonsuicidal self-injury: development and initial validation of the non-suicidal self-injury–assessment tool (NSSI-AT)," *Psychological Assessment*, vol. 26, no. 3, pp. 935–946, 2014.

Permissions

All chapters in this book were first published by Hindawi Publishing Corporation; hereby published with permission under the Creative Commons Attribution License or equivalent. Every chapter published in this book has been scrutinized by our experts. Their significance has been extensively debated. The topics covered herein carry significant findings which will fuel the growth of the discipline. They may even be implemented as practical applications or may be referred to as a beginning point for another development.

The contributors of this book come from diverse backgrounds, making this book a truly international effort. This book will bring forth new frontiers with its revolutionizing research information and detailed analysis of the nascent developments around the world.

We would like to thank all the contributing authors for lending their expertise to make the book truly unique. They have played a crucial role in the development of this book. Without their invaluable contributions this book wouldn't have been possible. They have made vital efforts to compile up to date information on the varied aspects of this subject to make this book a valuable addition to the collection of many professionals and students.

This book was conceptualized with the vision of imparting up-to-date information and advanced data in this field. To ensure the same, a matchless editorial board was set up. Every individual on the board went through rigorous rounds of assessment to prove their worth. After which they invested a large part of their time researching and compiling the most relevant data for our readers.

The editorial board has been involved in producing this book since its inception. They have spent rigorous hours researching and exploring the diverse topics which have resulted in the successful publishing of this book. They have passed on their knowledge of decades through this book. To expedite this challenging task, the publisher supported the team at every step. A small team of assistant editors was also appointed to further simplify the editing procedure and attain best results for the readers.

Apart from the editorial board, the designing team has also invested a significant amount of their time in understanding the subject and creating the most relevant covers. They scrutinized every image to scout for the most suitable representation of the subject and create an appropriate cover for the book.

The publishing team has been an ardent support to the editorial, designing and production team. Their endless efforts to recruit the best for this project, has resulted in the accomplishment of this book. They are a veteran in the field of academics and their pool of knowledge is as vast as their experience in printing. Their expertise and guidance has proved useful at every step. Their uncompromising quality standards have made this book an exceptional effort. Their encouragement from time to time has been an inspiration for everyone.

The publisher and the editorial board hope that this book will prove to be a valuable piece of knowledge for researchers, students, practitioners and scholars across the globe.

List of Contributors

Carlos-Martín Ardila and Efraín Álvarez-Martínez
Titular Professor University of Antioquia, Medellín, Colombia

Yuritza Hernández-Arenas
University of Antioquia, Medellín, Colombia

Kazuhiko Yamamoto, Nobuhiro Yamakawa, Ikumi Yamamoto and Tadaaki Kirita
Department of Oral and Maxillofacial Surgery, Nara Medical University, Japan

Yumiko Matsusue and Tetsuji Kawakami
Department of Oral and Maxillofacial Surgery, Nara Medical University, Japan
Department of Oral and Maxillofacial Surgery, Takita Hospital, Japan

Shinpei Matsuda and Hitoshi Yoshimura
Department of Dentistry and Oral Surgery, Unit of Sensory and Locomotor Medicine, Division of Medicine, Faculty of Medical Science, University of Fukui, Japan

Shamimul Hasan and Shahnaz Mansoori
Department of Oral Medicine and Radiology, Faculty of Dentistry, Jamia Millia Islamia, New Delhi, India

Deepika Bablani Popli and Keya Sircar
Department of Oral Pathology, Faculty of Dentistry, Jamia Millia Islamia, New Delhi, India

Syed Ansar Ahmad
Department of Oral and Maxillofacial Surgery, Faculty of Dentistry, Jamia Millia Islamia, New Delhi, India

Kirti Dua
Faculty of Dentistry, Jamia Millia Islamia, New Delhi, India

Zülfikar Karabıyık
Kütahya Health Science University, Dentistry Faculty, Department of Oral and Maxillofacial Surgery, Turkey

Mustafa Kıranatlı
Kütahya Health Science University, Dentistry Faculty, Department of Oral and Maxillofacial Radiology, Turkey

Manabu Shigeoka
Division of Pathology, Department of Pathology, Kobe University Graduate School of Medicine, Kobe, Japan

Daisuke Takeda and Masaya Akashi
Division of Oral and Maxillofacial Surgery, Department of Surgery Related, Kobe University Graduate School of Medicine, Kobe, Japan

Shogo Hasegawa, Hitoshi Miyachi and Toru Nagao
Department of Maxillofacial Surgery, School of Dentistry, Aichi-Gakuin University, 2-11 Suemori-Dori, Chikusa, Nagoya, Aichi 464-8651, Japan

Jun Sasaki
Department of Maxillofacial Surgery, School of Dentistry, Aichi-Gakuin University, 2-11 Suemori-Dori, Chikusa, Nagoya, Aichi 464-8651, Japan
Department of Maxillofacial Surgery, Okazaki City Hospital, 3-1 Goshoai, Koryujicho, Okazaki, Aichi 444-8553, Japan

Orazio Bennici
Private Practice, Catania 95123, Italy

Alessia Malgioglio, Serena Moschitto, Vincenzo Ronsivalle, Gaetano Isola and Antonino Lo Giudice
Department of Medical-Surgical Specialties, School of Dentistry, University of Catania, Policlinico Universitario "G. Rodolico-San Marco", Via Santa Sofia 78, Catania 95123, Italy

Gianrico Spagnuolo
Department of Neurosciences, Reproductive and Odontostomatological Sciences, University of Naples "Federico II", Naples, Italy

Alberta Greco Lucchina
Regenerative Medicine Research Laboratory, Saint Camillus University of Health Sciences, Rome, Italy

Eugênia Leal de Figueiredo, Carolina Chaves Gama Aires, Bruno José Carvalho Macêdo Neres, Bruna Luna de Araújo and Ricardo José de Holanda Vasconcellos
Department of Oral and Maxillofacial Surgery, School of Dentistry, Universidade de Pernambuco, Camaragibe, PE, Brazil

José Alcides Almeida de Arruda
Department of Oral Surgery and Pathology, School of Dentistry, Universidade Federal de Minas Gerais, Belo Horizonte, MG, Brazil

Amani Mizouri, Oumaima Tayari, AlaEddine Mahfoudhi and Jamila Jaouadi
Complete Removable Prosthodontic Department, Research Laboratory LR12ES11, Faculty of Dental Medicine, University of Monastir, Monastir, Tunisia

Adel Bouguezzi
Oral Surgery Department, Research Laboratory LR12ES11, Faculty of Dental Medicine, University of Monastir, Monastir, Tunisia

Saeed Asgary and Leyla Roghanizadeh
Iranian Center for Endodontic Research, Research Institute of Dental Sciences, Shahid Beheshti University of Medical Sciences, Tehran, Iran

Makiko Okubo-Sato, Kenji Yamagata, Satoshi Fukuzawa, Kazuhiro Terada, Fumihiko Uchida, Naomi Ishibashi-Kanno and Hiroki Bukawa
Department of Oral and Maxillofacial Surgery, Institute of Clinical Medicine, Faculty of Medicine, University of Tsukuba, 1-1-1 Tennodai, Tsukuba, Ibaraki 305-8575, Japan

Ahmed A. Zahrani
Department of Oral and Maxillofacial Surgery, King Saud University and University Dental Hospital, Riyadh, Saudi Arabia

Ahmed Qannam, Ra'ed Al Sadhan and Ibrahim O. Bello
Department of Oral Medicine and Diagnostic Sciences, King Saud University and University Dental Hospital, Riyadh, Saudi Arabia

Leonardo Mancini, Alessia Pisaneschi, Marino Ginoble, Vincenzo Quinzi, Enrico Marchetti and Giuseppe Marzo
Department of Life, Health and Environmental Sciences, University of L'Aquila, 67100 L'Aquila, Italy

Vincenzo Mancini
Private Practice in Via Degli Eroi n.4, 67051 Avezzano, Italy

Artak Heboyan and Anna Vardanyan
Department of Prosthodontics, Faculty of Stomatology, Yerevan State Medical University, Str. Koryun 2, Yerevan 0025, Armenia

Anna Avetisyan
Department of Therapeutic Dentistry, Faculty of Stomatology, Yerevan State Medical University, Str. Koryun 2, Yerevan 0025, Armenia

Hans Erling Skallevold
Christiania Tannlegesenter, Grønland 4, 0188 Oslo, Norway

Dinesh Rokaya
Department of Clinical Dentistry, Walailak University International College of Dentistry, Bangkok 10400, Thailand

Vinay Marla
Department of Oral Pathology, Penang International Dental College, Penang 12000, Malaysia

Erika Antonia dos Anjos Ramos, Luciana Munhoz, Stephanie Kenig Viveiros and Emiko Saito Arita
Department of Stomatology, School of Dentistry, University of São Paulo, 2227 Lineu Prestes Avenue, 05508-000 São Paulo, SP, Brazil

Basílio Almeida Milani
Department of Maxillofacial Surgery, Hospital Municipal do Campo Limpo, 1661 Estrada da Itapecerica, 05835-005 São Paulo, Brazil

Tomás Zecchini Barrese
Department of Pathological Sciences, School of Medicine, Santa Casa de Sao Paulo School of Medical Sciences, 61 Dr. Cesário Motta Junior Street, 01221-020 São Paulo, SP, Brazil

Elif Öztürk Bayazıt
Hacettepe University, Faculty of Dentistry, Department of Restorative Dentistry, 06100 Sıhhiye, Ankara, Turkey

Murat Karabıyık
32 Diş Dünyası Ağız ve Diş Sağlığı Polikliniği, 34940 Tuzla, İstanbul, Turkey

Syed Nabil, Elavarasi Kuppusamy, Rifqah Nordin, Abdul Jabar Nazimi and Roszalina Ramli
Oral and Maxillofacial Surgery, Faculty of Dentistry, The National University of Malaysia, Jalan Raja Muda Abdul Aziz, 50300 Kuala Lumpur, Malaysia

Silas Antonio Juvencio de Freitas Filho, Natália Galvão Garcia and Denise Tostes Oliveira
Department of Surgery, Stomatology, Pathology and Radiology (Area of Pathology), Bauru School of Dentistry, University of São Paulo, Bauru, São Paulo, Brazil

Mário César de Souza
Department of Dentistry, Northern State University of Paraná, Jacarezinho Unit, Paraná, Brazil

Nivedhitha Malli Sureshbabu, Mahalakshmi Nandakumar and Deepak Selvam
Department of Conservative Dentistry and Endodontics, Saveetha Dental College, Saveetha Institute of Medical and Technical Sciences, Saveetha University, 162, Poonamallee High Road, Chennai, 600077 Tamil Nadu, India

Kathiravan Selvarasu
Department of Oral and Maxillofacial Surgery, Saveetha Dental College, Saveetha Institute of Medical and Technical Sciences, Saveetha University, 162, Poonamallee High Road, Chennai, 600077 Tamil Nadu, India

Jayanth Kumar V
Department of Oral Medicine and Radiology, Saveetha Dental College, Saveetha Institute of Medical and Technical Sciences, Saveetha University, 162, Poonamallee High Road, Chennai, 600077 Tamil Nadu, India

Naoko Tsunoda, Kei Onodera, Yu Ohashi, Tadashi Kawai, Ikuya Miyamoto and Hiroyuki Yamada
Division of Oral and Maxillofacial Surgery, Department of Oral and Macillofacial Reconstructive Surgery, School of Dentistry, Iwate Medical University, Morioka 020-8505, Japan

Yasunori Takeda
Division of Clinical Pathology, Department of Oral and Maxillofacial Reconstructive Surgery, School of Dentistry, Iwate Medical University, Morioka 020-8505, Japan

Davide Augusti, Gabriele Augusti, Andrei Ionescu, Eugenio Brambilla and Dino Re
Department of Biomedical, Surgical and Dental Sciences, University of Milan, Italy

Abdulmohsen Alfadley
Department of Restorative and Prosthetic Dental Sciences, College of Dentistry, King Saud bin Abdulaziz University for Health Sciences, Riyadh, Saudi Arabia
King Abdullah International Medical Research Center, Ministry of National Guard Health Affairs, Riyadh, Saudi Arabia

Ahmad Alquraishi
Internship Unit, College of Dentistry, King Saud bin Abdulaziz University for Health Sciences, Ministry of National Guard Health Affairs, Riyadh, Saudi Arabia

Yaser Almazrou
Presidency of State Security, Department of Medical Services, Riyadh, Saudi Arabia

Fahd Aljarbou
Department of Restorative Dental Sciences, Division of Endodontics, College of Dentistry, King Saud University, Riyadh, Saudi Arabia

Hamzah Alkofahi and Mohammad Jarrah
Department of Oral and Maxillofacial Surgery, Jordanian Royal Medical Services, Irbid, Jordan

Alaa Maghaireh and Mamoon Fnaish
Department of Periodontics, Jordanian Royal Medical Services, Irbid, Jordan

Mohammad Bataineh
Department of Endodontics, Jordanian Royal Medical Services, Irbid, Jordan

Nik Abdul Ghani Nik Rozainah and Azih Nurul Farah
Conservative Department, School of Dental Sciences, Health Campus, Universiti Sains Malaysia, 16150 Kubang Kerian, Kelantan, Malaysia

Mohmed Isaqali Karobari
Conservative Unit, School of Dental Sciences, Health Campus, Universiti Sains Malaysia, 16150 Kubang Kerian, Kelantan, Malaysia

Estella Musacchio and Leonardo Sartori
Department of Medicine DIMED-Clinica Medica 1-University of Padova, Via Giustiniani 2, 35128 Padova, Italy

Andrea Piotto
Department of Surgical, Oncological, and Gastroenterological Sciences-Clinica Chirurgica 3-University of Padova, Via Giustiniani 2, 35128 Padova, Italy

Pierluigi Binotto
Private Dental Practice, Via M. Polo 10, 35123 Padova, Italy

Antonio Toniato
Endocrine Surgery Unit, Istituto Oncologico Veneto IOV-IRCCS, Via Gattamelata 64, 35128 Padova, Italy

Kamel Alraei
Department of Oral and Maxillofacial Surgery, Al-Noor Specialist Hospital, Makkah, Saudi Arabia

Jameel Sharqawi
Department of Oral and Maxillofacial Surgery, Royal Commission Hospital, Jubail, Saudi Arabia

Somaya Harcher
General Dentist, Saudi Arabia

Ibrahim Ghita
Department of Hematology, Al-Noor Specialist Hospital, Makkah, Saudi Arabia

Pakki Suresh Kumar and Ajit Damera
Department of Oral Medicine and Radiology, GITAM Dental College and Hospital, Visakhapatnam, Andhra Pradesh, India

Dola Srinivasa Rao
Department of Periodontics, GITAM Dental College and Hospital, Visakhapatnam, Andhra Pradesh, India

Swapna Manepalli and Jai Kiran Killada
Department of Paedodontics and Preventive Dentistry, GITAM Dental College, Visakhapatnam, India

Ali Jamali Ghomi, Reza Sayyad Soufdoost, Mohammad Saeed Barzegar and Mohammad Ali Hemmati
Department of Prosthodontics, Faculty of Dentistry, Shahed University, Tehran, Iran

Z. Allahem
Department of Restorative Dental Sciences, College of Dentistry, King Saud University, Saudi Arabia

S. AlYami
Department of Restorative Dental Sciences, College of Dentistry, King Saud University, Saudi Arabia
Department of Restorative Dental Science, College of Dentistry, Najran University, Saudi Arabia

Shahzad Gholami, Mahin Bakhshi and Arezoo Rahimzamani
Department of Oral Medicine, School of Dentistry, Shahid Beheshti University of Medical Sciences, Tehran, Iran

Saede Atarbashi-Moghadam
Department of Oral and Maxillofacial Pathology, School of Dentistry, Shahid Beheshti University of Medical Sciences, Tehran, Iran

Hassan Mir Mohammad Sadeghi
Department of Oral and Maxillofacial Surgery, School of Dentistry, Shahid Beheshti University of Medical Sciences, Tehran, Iran

Takashi Moriya and Hitoshi Sato
Department of Oral and Maxillofacial Surgery, Division of Oral Oncology, Showa University School of Dentistry, Tokyo, Japan

Kenichi Takeda, Kaori Ikezaki, Ryogo Katada and Tatsuo Shirota
Department of Oral and Maxillofacial Surgery, Showa University, School of Dentistry, Tokyo, Japan

Index